Superclasses in Homeopathy

Rajan Sankaran

Homoeopathic Medical Publishers
Mumbai
www.rajansankaran.com

Homoeopathic Medical Publishers

SUPERCLASSES IN HOMOEOPATHY

First published in India in 2023 by
Homoeopathic Medical Publishers
201, Dinar, 20 Station Road,
Opp. City Plaza, Santacruz (West),
Mumbai - 400054, India
Website: www.onlinehmp.com

First Edition, June 2023

Printed at: Repro India Ltd.

ISBN: 978-81-964098-0-7

Acknowledgment

This book is the result of a team effort.

Dr Meghna Shah and Dr Kshiti Mehta have been pillars of support.
Dr Manish Bhatia and Laurie Dack have given many constructive comments.
Dr Sarah Coutinho is a collaborator in all my recent developments.
Dr Kyle Wulfsohn has been a constant companion in developing these ideas and has also done most of the work in the writing of this book.

Shukrita Sankaran has played a pivotal role in the production of the book.

Mônica and Momchil Stoyanov having carefully understood these concepts created very evocative paintings and the cover page, which add much value to this book.
Dr Abhijit Nanavati has made valuable corrections.

To all these wonderful beings, I express my deepest gratitude.

The Cover design

In the beginning of 2023, we received an invitation to elaborate the graphic design of the book "Superclass in Homeopathy" by Rajan Sankaran. The elaborated concept gave continuity to the work in the production of the paintings, the Superclass Collection.

The initially idealized icons were developed in more detail, one or more icons for each superclass. We chose to select iconic animals that are immediately identifiable by most people (from the first to the sixth superclass, respectively): mollusk, snail, bird, dog, horse, lion.

Even during the production of paintings, we suggest the "window" as a key element to be explored graphically. Each superclass represents a particular view of the world, like a lens through which people view the world. There is a direct correspondence between lens and window, even in such widely used expressions as Shakespeare's "the eyes are the window to the soul". So, we imagined a window and scene for each superclass. The chosen painting would have to be compatible with a room or external view of a building, so not all the paintings produced fit this criterion (example of the painting with the horses running away, "The Last One"). We have included again typical elements for each window like: icon, window geometry, plants, frame. And we put all this together, in a house facade, seen from the outside. What more typical than that, a house with a window and room for each superclass, illustrating the diversity so rich and beautiful in people's life, urban, cultural, emotional life! Thus came the cover of the book "Superclasses in homeopathy". And the same elements are distributed inside the book, in an attempt to illustrate the innovative concept of Sankaran artistically and creatively!

Superclass 1 Window: Is there a better geometric shape to illustrate light than the circle? The window is circular, with thin uprights, closed because the environment is sensitive, the icon of the mollusk above, light curtains, the plant is Pulsatilla. The chosen painting was "Demeter".

Superclass 2 Window: There was no doubt about this choice, as it reflected the story of the first meeting with Sankaran, and the painting itself was once thought of as an illustration of someone looking out the window from behind the shutters. The window is rectangular, but with a circular top and rainbow-shaped divisions. The window is open to the outside, the plant is Cannabis sativa. The painting chosen was "English Naval Blue".

Superclass 3 Window: The window is rectangular and only the top is slightly circular. There is a small grid in front illustrating the tendency of people of this superclass to limit and expand. The icon on the pediment is the bird. The chosen painting was "Copil".

Superclass 4 Window: The architecture of this window is classic, cartesian, orthogonal, fully structured. The window is open and its division into small identical squares. The pediment is triangular and symmetrical, the icon above is the dog. The chosen painting was "Do Not Disturb" which is typical of a hotel room or residence.

Superclass 5 Window: The window is rectangular and has a sturdier, straighter pediment, with the horse icon. There wasn't a painting that fit the concept of the room, so we made a mix. The background of the room is the same as the painting "Euphorbiales", but the inspiration for the scene came from the painting "Must Get Out". We draw another person, instead of jumping over the wall, jumping out of the window, onto the roof of the entrance to the house, making clear the idea that the person needs to run away, escape safely from this room.

Superclass 6 Window: Violence and destruction, the window is being destroyed. The chosen painting was "Asteraceae's" which was completed with fire and shrapnel.

—Monica & Momchil Stoyanov

Contents

Section 2 Two

Section Three

Section Four

Section Five

Section Six

Introduction

This book marks the introduction of the Superclass idea into the homeopathic approach. This latest development is a part of the evolution of the sensation method and is fully grounded in the earlier discoveries and experiences. Thus, the previous concepts should be understood in depth before attempting the integration of these newer ideas.

The Superclass idea is a work in progress and will keep evolving and developing and parts of it may even change with experience. The reason that I am presenting these ideas to the profession at this stage is threefold.

1. Even at this stage I see these ideas are being useful in my practice.
2. Even if the details are not ironed out, these ideas represent a whole new way of looking at homeopathy. They influence our case-taking, our view of remedies etc. They represent a quantum leap in my approach. I felt it important to share this with the profession , especially colleagues who have been following my work for the past several decades.
3. It is an invitation to my valued colleagues to try out these ideas in practice and to send me their feedback, criticism and comments. They could also suggest additions. In this way the idea can become more and more complete. My earlier ideas on plant sensations went through this process. I made a chart classifying different remedies into a specific miasm. Such a chart went out to a group of colleagues especially from WISH (World Institute of Sensation Homeopathy). Based on their clinical experience, they could make additions to this chart and fill many blank spaces. I hope that a similar phenomenon with the Superclass will follow after this book.

How can the Superclass idea help the profession? To answer this, we have to identify what are the problem areas in the profession. In my experience, the problem is not about getting results. Every homeopath will have some cured cases and will be able to show that they can get results. The problem is in getting consistent results, reproducible results, predictable results.

In my over four decades of experience, I have seen that the most consistent results are found when we look at a case from both, the symptom and the system points of view.

Symptoms can be of many types;

- Peculiar symptoms
- Mental symptoms
- General symptoms
- Local symptoms
- Repertorial symptoms (rubrics)
- Keynote symptoms
- Pathological symptoms
- Acute symptoms
- Constitutional symptoms
- Totality of symptoms (a mix of all)

There are also many approaches in case-analysis :

- Drug pictures
- Remedy essences
- Therapeutics
- Mental state
- Miasms
- Constitutional types

With so many approaches and so many types of symptoms there can be confusion. I have found a way in which we can be surer. That is to look at another side of the patient, namely the system point of view.

What is the system?

Thus far the system consisted of two coordinates, namely Kingdom and Miasm. In each case we would need to see that along with the symptoms, the remedy matched the kingdom (and sub-kingdom) and miasm of the patient. With this book I am introducing a third coordinate, namely the Superclass.

With this development, we now have a system with three coordinates. When all three coordinates match, and also the symptoms and the source language of the remedy (if found in the patient), then we can be far more sure of the outcome.

You will see many remedies have not yet been classified into Superclass. It is also possible that one would have to classify remedies more accurately. For example, we have put all reptiles into 6th Superclass. Only experience will be able to justify this. It is possible non-venomous and or constrictor snakes fall into a different Superclass. Similarly, all mammals do not belong to the same Superclass and different mammals can be categorised in various Superclasses.

Molluscs are subdivided into the bivalves, gastropods, and cephalopods and these fall into 1st, 2nd and the 5th Superclass respectively. This kind of refinements are likely to happen as we gather more experience. This book offers a preliminary paradigm. It is the beginning of the idea and is very far from being the final word on the subject. Yet, it is a very exciting development. From my clinical experience I can say that it is likely to have far reaching effects in the way we practice our beloved science.

Contemporary Homeopathic practice

The homoeopathic principle is "like cures like." The fundamental concept is to treat a patient with a remedy that is similar to his illness. What is "like" in this situation? What is it that should match between the patient and the remedy? Homoeopaths have historically relied on symptom similarities. The patient's symptoms and the remedy's symptoms should match.

Additionally, as Hahnemann advised, we should pay particular attention to the patient's unusual symptoms. This led to the development of repertories, the proving of homoeopathic remedies, and the recording of each symptom. The homoeopath looked into the patient's symptoms. The data was compared against a range of remedies to determine which was most similar. Of course, this approach produced a lot of effective remedies. It has been the primary method of practice for the previous two centuries. Failures have also occurred, and these failures motivated us to look at alternative options.

Beyond symptom similarity, the matching can also occur in other aspects. And when that does , the consistency of our results significantly increases.

For the past 25 to 30 years, these other aspects have been the subject of research. The Sensation method is the general name for this. The symptom approach is more grounded in reality. The sensory method operates on a conceptual plane. Our chances of success rise if these two factors match. This Sensation Method's two key components have gained considerable popularity, namely kingdoms and miasms.

The kingdom approach divides the state of a person into the kingdoms of plants, minerals, and animals. A plant type would be a condition whose core experience is sensitivity, adaptation, or reactivity. A mineral type would be someone whose primary experience is of lacking or losing ability. One who has fundamentally experienced victim-aggressor or a survival response would be an animal type. There are sub-kingdoms within each of the kingdoms. Identifying the exact sub-kingdom of the patient improves the precision as well.

The miasm category is a way to categorise a state's pace or degree of desperation. For instance, whether the situations in one's life are generally experienced as acute panic or as something that is fixed or as something that is hopeless, etc, decides what miasm the patient belongs to. Once this is identified, it can be used as another coordinate to match with the remedy thus increasing the degree of assurance in the remedy choice

The classification of the patient's state into a kingdom, subkingdom, or miasm is not to be done superficially. Only until the patient delves deeply into his or her experience or sensation does it happen. This has led to the development of an entire case-taking procedure, guiding the patient based on the data at hand by way of fantasy, illusion and ultimately, sensation. At that level, the kingdom and miasm become clear rather than remaining a mere conjecture.

One can follow the development of this approach in my prior writings, including *The Spirit of Homoeopathy, The Substance of Homoeopathy, The Sensation in Homoeopathy, Structure, Insight into Plants,* and other such publications. *From Similia to Synergy,* is a book summarises such a progression.

In the last two or three years I have been able to discover yet another crucial component of the patients' state. This aspect is the Superclass. For me, the discovery of Superclass and its practical use have completely changed the game. It limits our search for the remedy to one of the six Superclasses. Superclasses are simple to comprehend and use. They relate to a person's fundamental character in some way. It is the fundamental manner in which he reacts to the outside world. Does the person try to maintain stability in various circumstances, fight it out, or shut off? These factors define the Superclass.

The properties of each Superclass have now been very precisely defined. We can observe that each Superclass consists of a particular group of plants, animals, minerals, and nosodes. These groups all exhibit the same dynamic response. It is considerably simpler for us to choose a remedy when we search within that Superclass. Our search is narrowed down.

Final coordinates include characteristic symptoms and source characteristics. The remedy choice is very accurate if these are present in the case.

At this point, we use two factual coordinates and three conceptual coordinates. At the conceptual level, the three coordinates are Superclass, Kingdom, and Miasm. Characteristic symptoms and source characteristics serve as the two coordinates at the factual level. Together, they create a very well-rounded and thorough selection of the remedy, giving far better outcomes than before.

The Superclasses and their importance in homoeopathic prescribing are the main topics of this book. A key component of this is the skilful application of WISE processes and case-taking techniques. In my earlier book, "*From Shadow to Light*", I discuss the application of WISE processes. This is where I want to direct the reader's attention.

In the practice of homoeopathy, the concepts of Superclass and the WISE process are extremely helpful. Nevertheless, they are applicable everywhere. Research has shown that the WISE process has a lot of therapeutic potential on its own. In webinars and retreats, they operate on their own. The concept of Superclasses offers a paradigm through which one can comprehend various human types. This kind of comprehension originates at a far higher level than psychological typology. You will see that the Superclass concept is based on fundamental somatic reactions, hence going deep.

Superclasses are a useful concept that is not just for homoeopathy. It aids in our ability to recognise a person's tendencies. Greater awareness and acceptance result from this contributing to the development of a positive, productive response.

Through the understanding of each Superclass, it becomes apparent that each Superclass is a constellation of qualities. By studying this it becomes clear why artists and entertainers are frequently competitive, why they are hurried, suspicious, and restless. We can see all these expressions as a kind of a package of interlinked qualities. It enables us to understand why dependable, solid, and steady people frequently lack the ability to think creatively. It enlightens us to the fact that every person embodies the characteristics of a particular superclass. A Superclass 3 individual will be nurturing and considerate. They are nourishing and kind, and they are especially perceptive to attachments and connections. They will not be as concerned about success, or power.

It is illuminating to view people through the lens of the Superclasses. Relationships may improve as a result of this. Whether in private, public, or professional settings I have to admit that it has greatly aided me in these areas.

Finding out about the Superclasses has been a great thrill. To see the connections between the various groups that make up a specific Superclass, has been eye-opening. Observing the many categories of animals, minerals, plants, and nosodes that make up one Superclass have a similar dynamic response, this has been very interesting. Also connected to this dynamic in each Superclass are specific neurotransmitters and hormones. Specific mind-altering substances are a part of this dynamic as well. The Superclasses are observable through personality traits, fairy tales, archetypes, movies, and even certain colours.

As a way to share our excitement about discovery, we present our work to the homeopathy field and to all of humanity.

A brief note on the book's structure

There are six sections in the book.

Section 1 Is a discussion of the six fundamental categories of dynamic response and an outline of the six Superclasses. Additionally, each member of these Superclasses has a particular personality type. It would be simple to comprehend and relate to this section as if reading about the Sun-signs. At the end of Section 1 ,we have added brief case extracts for the reader to test one's understanding. Try to be aware of the superclass that the patient is belongs to. The book's conclusion will contain the answers to these cases.

Section 2 of this book describes the six dicotyledon subclasses. This is what ultimately led to the comprehension of Superclasses. The superclass idea is based on or a kind of extension of the discovery of the themes of these six subclasses.

There are five main classes or divisions within the Plant Kingdom namely Gymnosperms, Mosses, Ferns, Monocotyledons, and Dicotyledons

There are six subclasses of the dicotyledons. Magnolidae, Hamamelidae, Caryophyllidae, Dilleniidae, Rosidae, and Asteriidae

Each subclass is further divided into several orders. Each order has several families, and each family has a set of remedies.

When we examine remedies in a certain subclass, we can discover that each subclass shares a common trait. For instance, all of the remedies in the sixth subclass share the theme of aggression, attack, battle, and flight. We will go into great detail about the unique characteristics of each subclass in this section. You will be able to observe how each subclass's remedies exhibit various manifestations of the same attribute. It is this understanding that extended to the understanding of Superclasses.

Section 3 compares each subclass's defining characteristic to categories of remedies from other kingdoms. For instance, there is aggression, fight, and flight in the sixth subclass. One can compare these to remedies from heavy metals like Mercury, Platinum, and Aurum because they have the same essential qualities. These bear comparison to snake remedies. These three groups derived from different kingdoms share a striking amount of dynamism. All of these groupings with a similar dynamic are part of the Superclass. We thus extend the idea of the subclass to the establishment of the Superclass. Later, studying neurotransmitters and hormones, one can observe that specific neurotransmitters and hormones also share the dynamic of specific Superclasses. Putting all this together, we gain a thorough understanding of each Superclass. It then becomes even more applicable in real-world situations. This is the benefit of researching these relevant groups together.

Case studies in Section 4 demonstrate how to use these concepts. The cases demonstrate the case-taking methodology. There is always a synergistic strategy. These examples also show an informational hierarchy. A complete pattern appears when we arrange items in the proper order. It is comparable to how a jigsaw puzzle's components fit together to make the final image.

Section 5: We have thought some readers might learn better visually. We have given visual representations of the Superclasses in this section. These take the style of portraits and emphasise the key characteristics of each superclass. There is also a chart that is helpful for displaying the different remedies for each superclass. It will also serve as an overview of the key ideas.

Section 6: We are aware that putting in place a relatively new system can present a number of challenges. There may be issues, doubts, and several opportunities for mistakes. We designed this section based on the typical issues and inquiries we run into when teaching, which the reader can use to hone his skills and knowledge.

A word of advice:

As you can see, choosing the right remedy requires careful thought and skill in many different areas. It entails synthesising various elements with one another. It appears simple and, when everything comes together, even magical in the hands of a skilled practitioner. This degree of dexterity requires objective observation, which is a skill. With this skill is needed genuine knowledge and information of each aspect such as the source qualities, kingdom, miasm, repertory, keynotes and materia medica.

It necessitates expert case-taking, experience with various methodologies, and knowledge of WISE procedures. It takes a very thorough understanding of the software and resources. Applying the concepts superficially without this foundational knowledge carries risk. There will be limited success. One needs to employ a variety of resources in order to grow in these capacities and learn this knowledge. First, books. You will find a list of books at the end of this book. Second, courses offered both online and offline by organisations like The Other Song Academy (TOS) and H.O.P.E. *The Sankaran Masterclass* falls under this category as well. The Masterclass is structured to lead participants step-by-step from the beginning to the most recent advances. Thirdly, clinical training programmes like the TOS Master's programme. One can observe the skilled practitioner taking a case in real time. There will thereafter be a conversation with the participants. One's skill and knowledge significantly improve after daily practice for six months.

SECTION ONE

An experiment

The best way to learn is to experience. So let us do an experiment to better understand the Superclasses and their corresponding dynamics.

Close your eyes and use your imagination. Imagine yourself resting in bed. It is night-time, and you are by yourself in bed. Imagine the surroundings, the scenario in its entirety, the bed, and yourself. Imagine hearing sounds coming from somewhere else in the house, such as a different room, the kitchen, or anywhere else. These noises wake you up and alert you. It appears as though another person has entered the home. Imagine yourself in the following scenario: There is likely another person present, you have heard noises. It is conceivable that a hostile person has arrived. The noises that you hear cause you to wake up. Imagine yourself in this circumstance as if you were there right now as though it is real. Find out what your instinctive, irrational response would be in this circumstance without using your logical or reasoning mind. It is crucial to refrain from thinking, reasoning, and using logic. Do not ask yourself, "What should I do?" Just concentrate on the natural, instinctive answer you would have. Your logical mind may offer a different opinion but consider the initial reaction. Once you are aware of this, write it down in no more than ten words.

After conducting this experiment on hundreds of patients and participants, it is clear that the majority of them struggle with dread or anxiety. However, this is a typical response to feelings of worry and anxiety. We can see that each person has a unique experience and response, though, when we dig a little deeper, we comprehend the distinctiveness of the responses and the reaction to the dread and anxiety.

Afterward, it is feasible to group these replies into the following major categories:

1. To isolate oneself from the outside, to cover yourself and shut your eyes and ears.
2. To peep out and if there is any sign of danger, quickly shut oneself in.
3. To establish a barrier or boundary that no one should cross (but from which you cannot go out).
4. To obtain safety by requesting assistance from the police or others
5. To feel stuck, and the need to get out of the place, one way or the other.
6. To feel a strong sense of fear that sets off the fight or flight reaction, where one may even take a weapon and become aggressive.

We may observe the six different dynamics of perception and response of the Superclasses from these potential responses. This serves as the proposed classification's fundamental foundation. After doing this exercise, it would be fascinating to check into which group you fall. You ought to be able to detect some resonance between yourself, your life, and the Superclass that your response belongs to after studying the Superclasses.

The six Superclasses stand for the different categories of dynamic reactions. This chapter aims to provide a relatable summary of each of these kinds to the reader. It is not a thorough or in-depth description, more of a first look or introduction. We kept it straightforward and free of references to homoeopathic medicines. To help with the idea, we have added a few instances from popular culture.

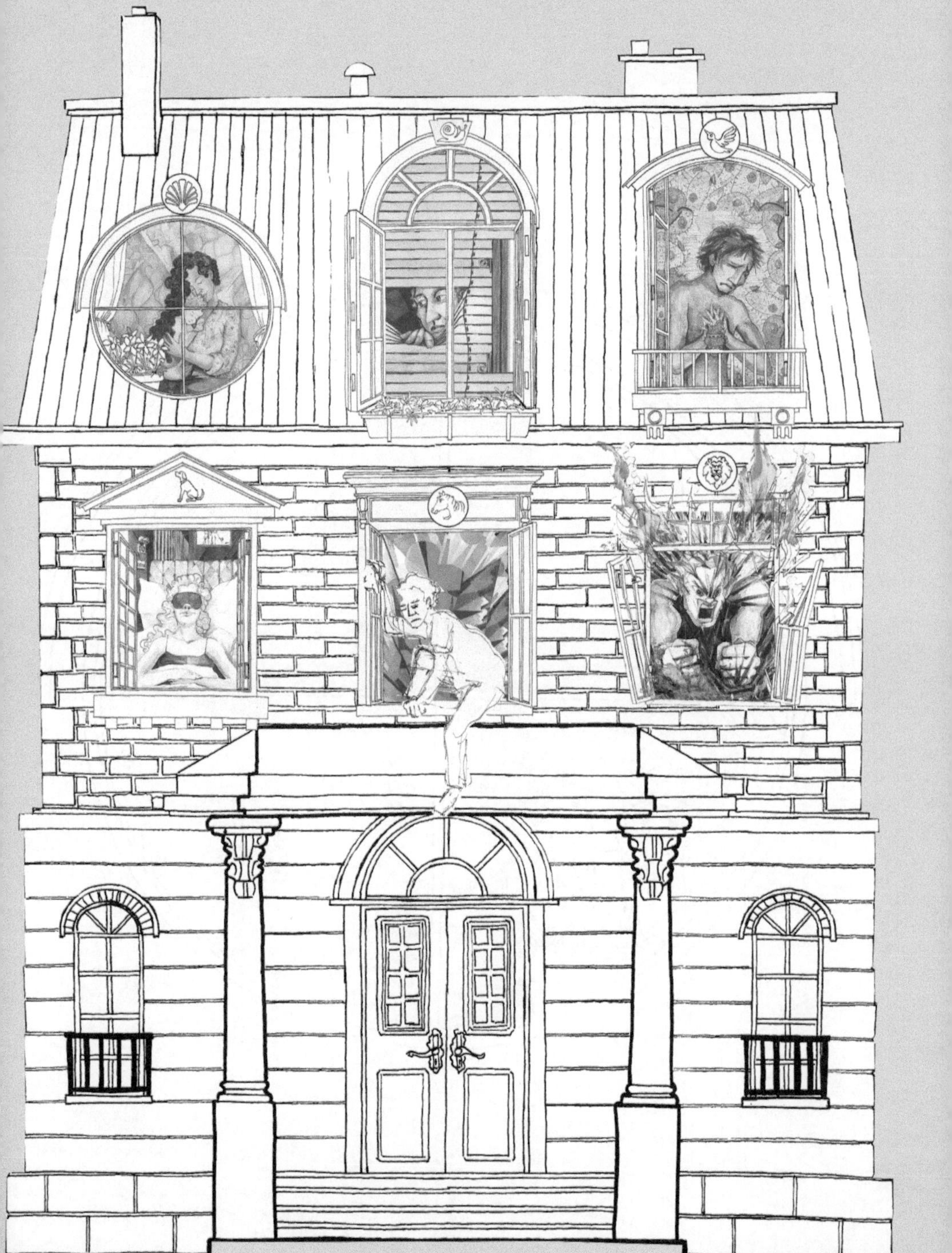

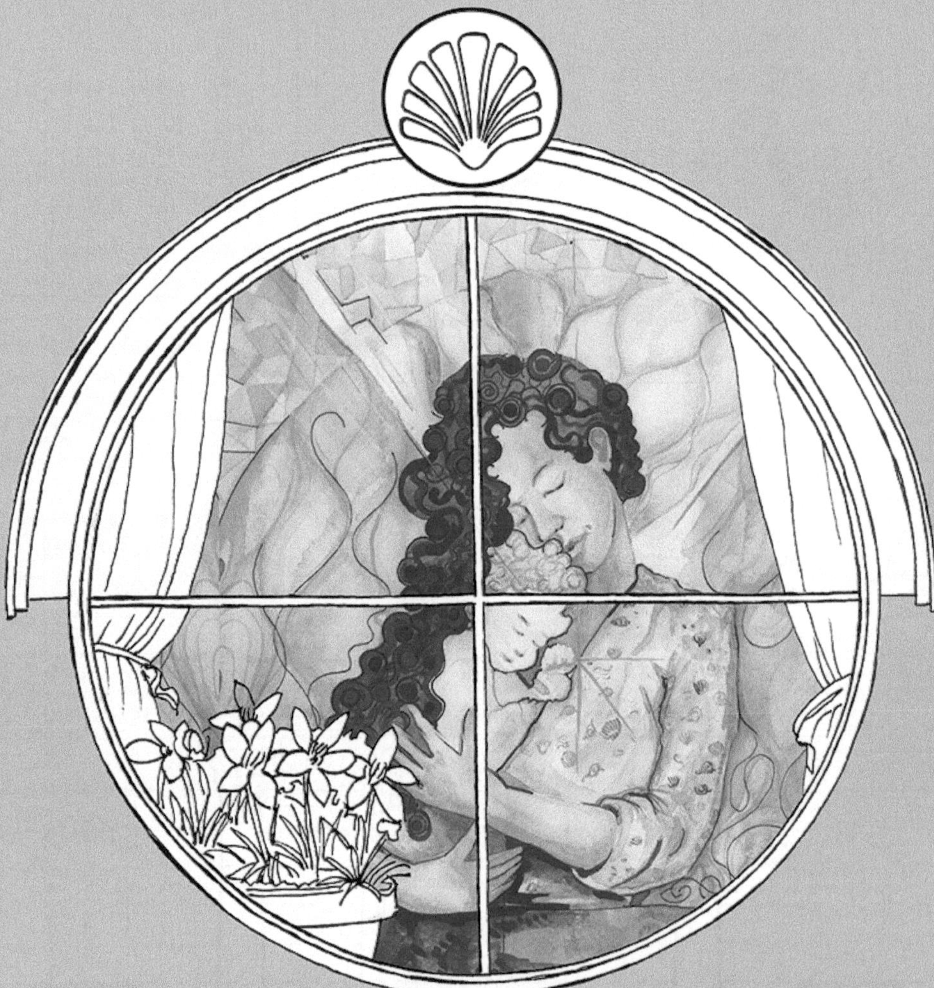

Superclass 1

Oyster Type

Withdrawal and Clinging

The oyster is a creature that fears it is too weak to confront the outside world. As a result, it turns off inside its shell. It hunkers down inside and tightens its shell. The outside world overwhelms and makes this individual feel incredibly vulnerable. As a result, it desires seclusion and seeks out a solid object that she may hold. This kind of protection from the outside world is provided by the shell or even the womb.

In this situation one can feel they are not living fully and that it is incredibly boring and restricting, but they feel that the outside world is too intimidating and so they need to remain within. An additional manifestation of this is a state of anaesthesia or numbness, or a state of not feeling anything. These individuals are also reclusive, introverted people. Usually, non-confrontational and gentle. When they enter the outside world, they often exhibit indecision and confusion. They appear scattered and unfocused. Small things have an impact on them.

Someone who prefers to withdraw themselves from the outside world and stays inside of a cocoon. She feels as though everything around her is too much for her to handle. She enjoys isolating herself from the outside world and retreating into her own universe. She enjoys finding a cosy, safe place where she feels comfortable and is free from any pain or misery. She grasps the secure area or clings to it, stays inside of it.

She does not want to expose herself to the world outside. There is an anaesthetic feeling. It results from an equivalent sense of oversensitivity. Everything has a big impact on her. She retreats within her cocoon as a result. She can amuse herself in the cocoon. They are naturally quite meek, introverted, shy, timid, and modest. They may exhibit less emotion, avoid conflict, and cling to others.

The story of Prince Siddhartha, who was raised by his father in a bubble-like situation, is the life of the Buddha. He lived without any exposure to pain, suffering or misery. He experiences a major shock when he first encounters these. In response to this shock, he withdraws. He muses on how to put an end to or resolve suffering.

After years of deep contemplation, he concludes that craving, aversion, and attachment are the root causes of suffering. Cravings, aversions, and attachments reveal how you interact with the outside world. The Buddha is therefore advocating detachment. It makes sense that the majority of the Buddha statues that we encounter have their eyes closed in a relaxed state of meditation. Naturally, the phrases "so gentle" and "content" come to mind. This is the compensated form.

The uncompensated variant would be extremely sensitive. They cling and are incredibly attached. They are afraid of the outside world. Withdraw quickly and easily. Refuse to show emotion or accept challenges. They are incredibly afraid of losing either this safety or the person who offers it to them. The world gets bigger as you move from the first to the last Superclass. First, the world is incredibly small. They deal with small matters. They are not interested in global issues of a greater scope; they are unimportant for these people. They have basic minds or are trusting and innocent, not cunning or deceitful. They only have a small group of people in their universe. They do, in a way, suffer from agoraphobia. They must protect themselves since they are sensitive to even the smallest things. They will employ phrases like "shield" and "cocoon" or like a "mother's womb," among others. One activity they wish to engage to escape from the world is meditation. In the real world, they become perplexed. They become disoriented or lose their focus. They can be undecided or uncertain. also dependent in a certain way. Coming out into the world is similar to an oyster emerging from its shell or a new-born emerging prematurely from the womb. They may be slow, sluggish, and indolent, barely moving

We might connect the first Superclass with a fairy tale of Sleeping Beauty. According to popular culture, Sleeping Beauty is pierced and sleeps like a new-born. The princess is subject to a curse. By using a sharp item, such as a spindle or a piece of flax, she was pierced and penetrated. She then slips into an enchanted sleep while sequestered in a high tower. This tale has a wide range of interpretations. This typical retelling draws attention to the crucial elements of the original. We see the typical features of the first Superclass. These are sensitivity to piercing and penetrating. The enchanted slumber represented in this story is the dynamic response of withdrawal and isolation from the outside world.

Persons from this Superclass seek out a sense of tranquillity or serenity through drugs, companionship, or meditation, where there will not be any disturbances. Tranquillity is where you are unaffected. At times, they may even appear numb or have thick skin, as if nothing bothers them. They can use entertainment to block out the outside world. They might have their noses buried in their gadgets.

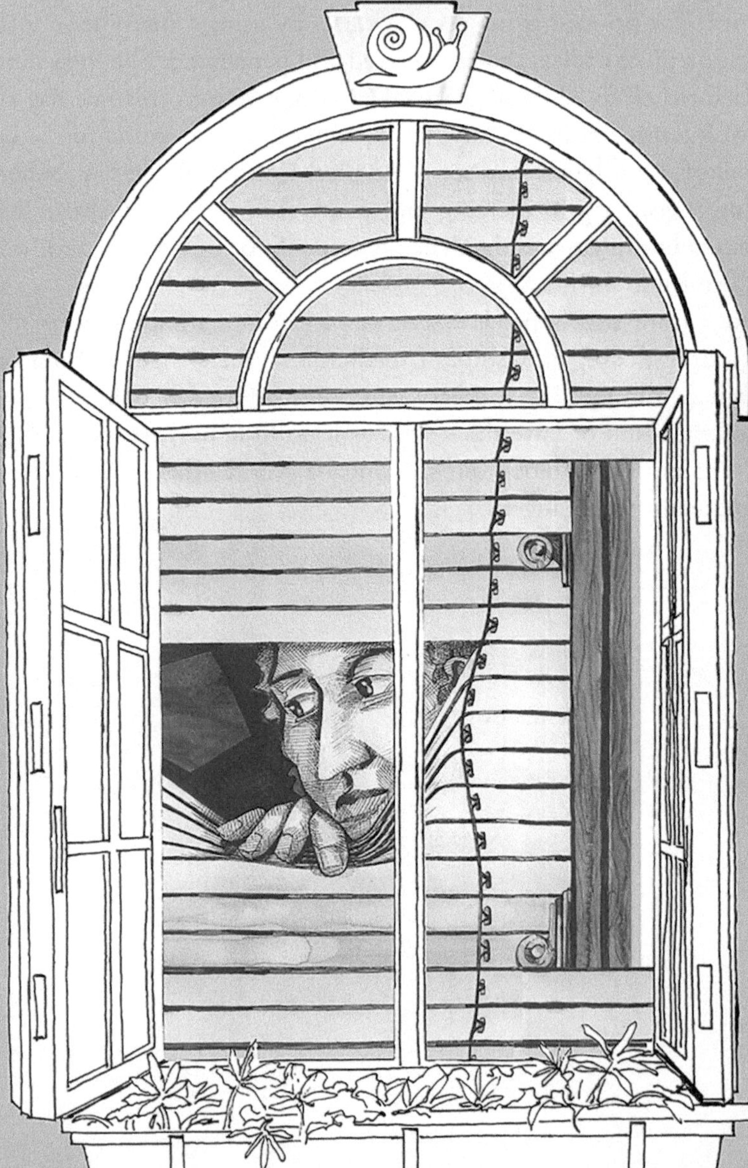

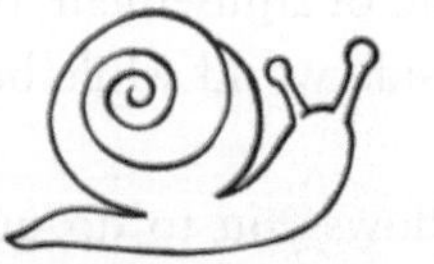

Superclass 2

The Snail type

Opening and Closing

An animal that enters and exits its shell is the snail. It always carries the shell on its back so it can retreat inside in case of danger. It also desires to leave and explore the outside world. A person from this Superclass prefers to be confined in her protected space She is reluctant to speak up. Yet she feels a sense of monotony and a lack of sensory stimulation inside this protected space. a certain level of dullness or gloom. She starts to feel like stepping outside to experience the outside by opening her windows. She just wants to do it when seated in the protected area. She simply adjusts her window's opening and closing to the circumstances outside.

We may refer to her as the dreamer. A person sleeping in her bed is a dreamer. But she travels to other realms and experiences a lot without leaving the security of her bed. She has had experiences as a result of these. As opposed to a person in the first Superclass, who seeks only amusement or entertainment, the person from the second Superclass, while remaining in a somewhat enclosed setting, they want to experience sensory stimulation, excitement and exhilaration. The first Superclass views fun and entertainment as a means of seclusion from the outside world, the second Superclass views it as a means of vicariously experiencing some of it.

For instance, when you are bashful and do not want to look anyone in the eye while seated among complete strangers, you bury your nose as deep as you can, engaging in any kind of amusement, or even addiction which allows you to escape from the outside world while being inside it. This is the first Superclass.

The second Superclass allows you to do quite the opposite. Its purpose is to keep you in the safe zone while also stimulating your senses. They are naturally reluctant to leave their own surroundings and encounter unfamiliar circumstances. They can engage in imaginative flights of fancy while inside their cocoon. They have a lot of creativity. They might design their own personal space, construct their air-castles. They can escape to a world of their senses that is also vibrant, lovely, and exciting, all from within their personal bubble and small universe.

There is a compelling desire to remain inside the secure space that protects them from the dangers of the outside world, to be in an environment free from damage or injury. They begin to perceive this safe haven as being similar to a small, closed area that is dull and devoid of stimulation. While persons from the first Superclass prefer to blend into the background, those from the second dislike doing it. While they are still not ready to leave the safe haven, they want to emerge and become visible in the second superclass. They want to come out and engage their senses. Whether in the shape of a connection, an activity, a colour, or a sound, they want to stand out or start being themselves, yet they are hesitant to do so. They therefore continuously test the waters.

Coming and going, keeping hold of the secure sanctuary while still yearning to travel. The safe refuge has a closed, thick, and dark feeling. The outside, however, feels airy, bright, and open. Both directions are pulling continuously. These individuals possess all the traits of the first Superclass, with the exception of their timidity and shyness. On the other hand, they may be vibrant, alive, artistic, free-spirited, curious and inquiring.

Imagine a little girl who lived in her parental home until she was 25 years old. She senses some level of safety. She begins to have a stimulating interest in interpersonal interactions, intimacy, and even sexuality. She wants to experience something, but she is terrified that she might damage herself. The contrast is as follows: They get excited about the kinds of things they want to do. Regardless of whether they are watching a thriller or smoking a joint, they are all doing it in the protection of their own bubble. It resembles a foetus who has been entirely at ease in the womb in many ways. She needs to exit the womb because it is becoming cramped and small, but she must first determine whether she is prepared. Is she competent? This personality type shifts from time to time. Steps one foot outside very slowly. The second superclass could be compared to a movie character named Walter Mitty, who, despite having a secure career and workplace, yearns to travel.

She still comes across as innocent and straightforward, but there is now a hint of an Alice in Wonderland-style situation where she is appreciating the little things in life. They are having the most amazing adventures while lost in the rabbit hole of their minds, imagining the most amazing situations and incidents they can only accomplish through daydreaming.

Hollywood productions tend to be fantasies. The majority of these fantasies feature heightened perceptions of space, time, colour, and sound. Everything is more expansive, brilliant, and stimulating. One can have a sensory experience while still being in safe confines.

The person from the second Superclass finds great delight in the little things. This person does not need to accomplish a lot or take home a large prize. It is enough to be hearing music while observing the sunset. They too, like those in the first Superclass, have little interest in politics and macro problems.

They may get happy with and show it through small things. However, a mild scolding, harshness, or fear causes them to withdraw and cut off communication. A small event can cause them to smile and chuckle. They do not always stay inside the shell. But if something occurs, they return to the shell. The snail kind is this. The pace is similar same as the first Superclass, but there is some movement.

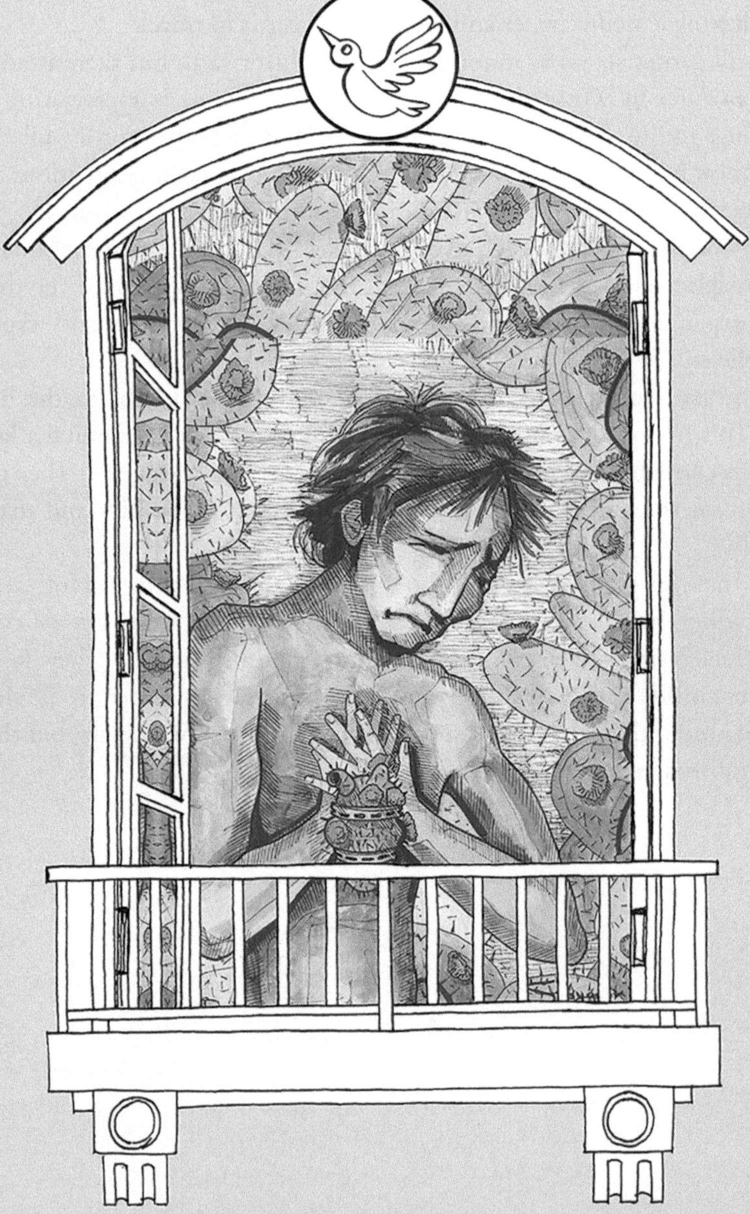

Superclass 3

The Bird type

Limiting and expanding

A creature that looks to fly freely yet remains within bounds is the bird. Remaining within that barrier is crucial for its protection and nutrition. Leaving your comfort zone feels dangerous and daring. The caregiving Superclass is the third one, and she is the people-pleaser by definition. She believes that she should put others before herself. She must lend a hand. She needs to position others before herself. However, a caretaker is also someone who is very concerned with what other people think, expect, and want her to be.

She thinks that the only way she will be taken care of and fed is if she lives up to their expectations or is helpful to them. She thinks that relationships matter. She thinks that the only way to keep a relationship going is to give and put others before yourself. They possess a maternal quality. They are often sympathetic or empathetic towards others. She wants to fulfil their expectations in some way since she cares so much about what they anticipate from her.

She senses a kind of barrier. She can move freely and feel protected inside the boundaries. She believes that crossing this line is dangerous but adventurous. She occasionally struggles to respect this limit. She receives attention and food inside. She belongs, but should she take the chance of stepping out, even if briefly? In that regard, her bounds are defined by her love and care.

They enjoy living within boundaries where they feel safe and protected. These restrictions are either self-imposed or set by societal or familial norms. Conformists are a possibility. They enjoy acting in ways that they believe are required of them. They occasionally enjoy venturing outside the perimeter for brief excursions or to investigate the outer world. They continue to be in need of the sustenance and protection the border offers. If you can picture a philosopher sitting in a comfortable armchair at her house, one who challenges preconceived notions and theories. While they certainly feel constrained and want to grow, they also feel confined and desire freedom.

The cage or the restriction must protect, nourish, and take care of the animal. Relationships can also be like that. You may say that a married individual can see their marriage as a form of confinement. They continue to feel the need for the safety and comfort that jail offers. As a result, they are unable to cross it or escape from it. They occasionally overstep the line and engage in extramarital affairs. While doing so, she maintains her commitment to her marriage's security.

In the third Superclass, value and appreciation are crucial. They question their own sense of worth and value in relation to others. They take actions that can make them feel more valuable in other people's eyes. They feel terrible if something makes them less valuable. They steer clear of certain circumstances as a result.

If they believe they have not done enough for others, they feel guilty e.g. when they feel they have not lived up to others' expectations, particularly when it comes to caring for them. Guilty feelings may accompany the fourth Superclass too, but there is a difference. The guilt in the fourth Superclass has the perception of having committed a crime. They have done something wrong that might cost them money, their position, or their stability.

We generally consider birds to be free. In fact, the bird is usually seen as a symbol of freedom. What I observed is that when unleashed, birds do not fly very far. They stay in the same circumscribed space. The falcon's narrative is the same. The falcon is captured, fed and trained. When released , the falcon does not go beyond a specific circle and is lured back and is not able to leave the boundary.

The bird is in a cage that it has built for itself that is both physical and psychological. Why is there a cage there? Despite the fact that the cage serves as a restriction and boundary, it serves not only as a barrier but also as a place of security and food. It also embodies belonging. Birds of a feather flock together; they are in a community no matter where you see them. This neighbourhood is both a place of belonging and a form of servitude. Your sense of security, nourishment, and even identity come from your group. The majority of the groups we belong to—country, religion, or social group—are in some ways self-made prisons. By staying within these restrictions, you can find protection, nourishment, identity, etc. You can leave it at any time, but doing so puts you at risk.

This presents a dichotomy for a person in the third Superclass. Do I want to stay inside the line and have only a certain amount of freedom, or do I want to wander outside and have an adventure? If I stay indoors, I experience a sense of diminution. Outside, there is a sizable area. It is a development.

The desire to be valuable to others is the other characteristic of the third Superclass. To be of use, to act right, to take care of others. Just like a bird takes care of its own young as well as the young of its entire flock.

These people have a maternal instinct and are carers. Belonging and forming bonds are crucial. They enjoy forming ties, but occasionally those bonds turn into servitude. You will hear about the relationships they care a lot about. When they do not get care, are not given trust, or have their confidence abused, they feel it very keenly. Due to what the connection brings them, they are unable to leave it. At that point, the bond turns into a bondage. They care a lot about what other people think of them. They must fit into a particular stereotype or expectation of other people. They think they can only get love, care, and sustenance if they conform. This is the final superclass where self-sacrifice is involved in giving up. People start to become more self-reliant after the fourth Superclass. Why should I care? They become more "masculine" in a way.

Typical of this Superclass is the fairy-tale of Little Red Riding Hood.

When we look closer at the story, we can see that it is about a young girl who is carrying food for her grandmother (care and nourishment). On the way, she encounters a wolf, who tells her that staying on the path is boring and that by deviating from it, she can have fun and adventure (risk-taking behaviour, straying from the safety of the limit or boundary for adventure). Her mother cautions her before she leaves to stay on the route and avoid deviating into the forest (limitations).

The film "The Titanic" includes similar aspects. A wealthy heiress encounters social limitations in this situation. She must decide between the possibility of crossing the line and losing the support and love of her family. In return, she will have the thrilling experience of falling in love with a young man who is beneath her social status. The movie emphasises these themes of love and limitations frequently. It is helpful in aiding our understanding of the third Superclass's dynamic.

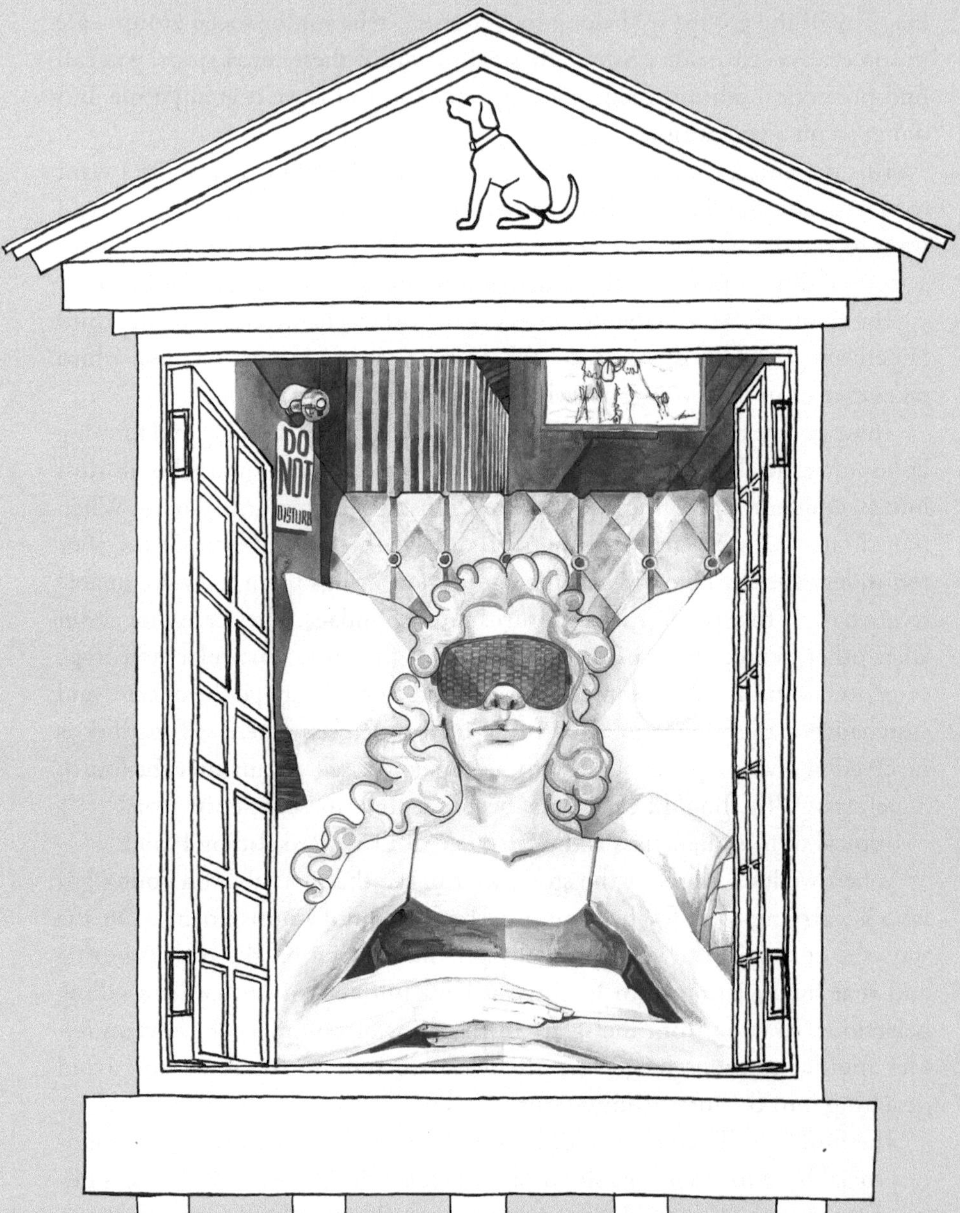
DO NOT DISTURB

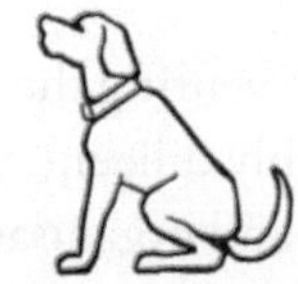

Superclass 4

The Dog type

Stable and settled

The dog is a creature that requires a secure environment, a family, and a clear hierarchy. It desires no change at all and values the stability. The fourth Superclass maintains stability. A steady individual desires consistency and the status-quo in his life. He places a high value on having security in his house, family, career, and health. He takes every action to keep steady. With the exception of the occasional trip, this person's life is more routine. He is someone who will remain in the same position for a long time.

If there is any kind of disruption or change in their lives, they become quite worried. Being steady and safe is the source of all of his concerns. Anything that stands for that must remain intact. Health, family, a job, or money are just a few examples. He is a typical person, a blue-collar worker, and somewhat banal. Any nameless person is known as "John Doe." John Doe does not fit into any certain type of personality. He is the family man who leaves for work and then returns to assess his requirements and by adding to it, whether it be in the shape of a family or a job.

In fact, they attempt to increase the money, housing, social groups, health, etc. These are the blue-collar individuals who have been dependable at their occupations for many years. Any alteration or loss of their equilibrium bothers them. They continue to be devoted and are continuously on the lookout for potentially worrying situations. These are the routine followers. They find comfort and stability in maintaining the status quo. Will I continue to be in good health, etc.?

Another important topic in preventing the impact of catastrophic disasters is insurance. They can also be highly diligent, yet they lack creativity. They are nevertheless capable of efficiency and organisation. They stay out of situations where they might run afoul of the law. In that regard, people frequently follow the law and are afraid to break it.

The dog kind is this. Although there are many ways to view a dog, we are talking about the concept of loyalty. Loyalty would be the key term. When we think of loyalty, we think of sticking to one thing. The term 'stubborn' comes to mind. It refers to sticking with one task, not wanting any sort of change, to be steadfast and steady with one thing, one individual, one residence, and one family.

One may say that the dog sacrifices everything to achieve stability. The owner stands for both food and safety, a type of insurance, a house, a place to stay, and medical aid. A member of the fourth Superclass has a strong desire for stability. Whether the family's financial security, or the stability of his job, home, and family. He wants to make this stability stronger. He steers clear of all instability and change. He typically keeps the same job for years and invests his money in low-risk ventures. Carefully examines his family and his health. He is afraid of anything happening to that steadiness. He is worried about keeping things the same. In order to maintain his stability, he will make an effort to abide by all laws and regulations.

He fears the police, and criminals. Anything that can endanger his health or wealth makes him nervous. He is concerned about natural disasters that might upend the current order. He guards all of these things fiercely. He can defend others since he is sensitive to this type of protection. He could join the military or the police, for instance.

They do not have any notable or unique achievements to their credit, honours, or publications in newspapers.

They are worriers and keep themselves informed of things that can have an impact on their stability such as politics, and natural disasters. They may not only be working in terms of a job or career but also can be homemakers who watch over the family and particularly pay attention when the stability of the family is in danger. They are typically quite organised and well-planned.

They work harder or with more vigour than the first three Superclasses. When things are stable, their anxiety levels might be fairly low. This can change as a result of illness, a family member's passing, a decline in the stock market, etc. They support the organisation. They put forth a lot of effort since the organisation helps keep them stable.

The Three Little Pigs fairy-tale serves as a clear example of the characteristics of the fourth Superclass. In the story, three pigs construct their individual homes using various resources. The construction of the homes for the first two pigs is a little haphazard. The huge, terrible wolf blows them down, effortlessly destroying them. This embodies the 4th Superclass's greatest dread. They will leave behind their stable home. They start to imitate the third pig, who carefully and methodically constructs his home with strong pillars. They make sure it can take any pressure the big bad wolf can throw at it, supplying their security and stability needs.

Another example might be the motion picture *The Pursuit of Happiness*. The main character is a parent who is working alone to support his son. His aspirations are not lofty or ambitious. His main goal throughout the film is to provide him with secure employment that is both dependable and simple. His quest for happiness is really his need for security and stability.

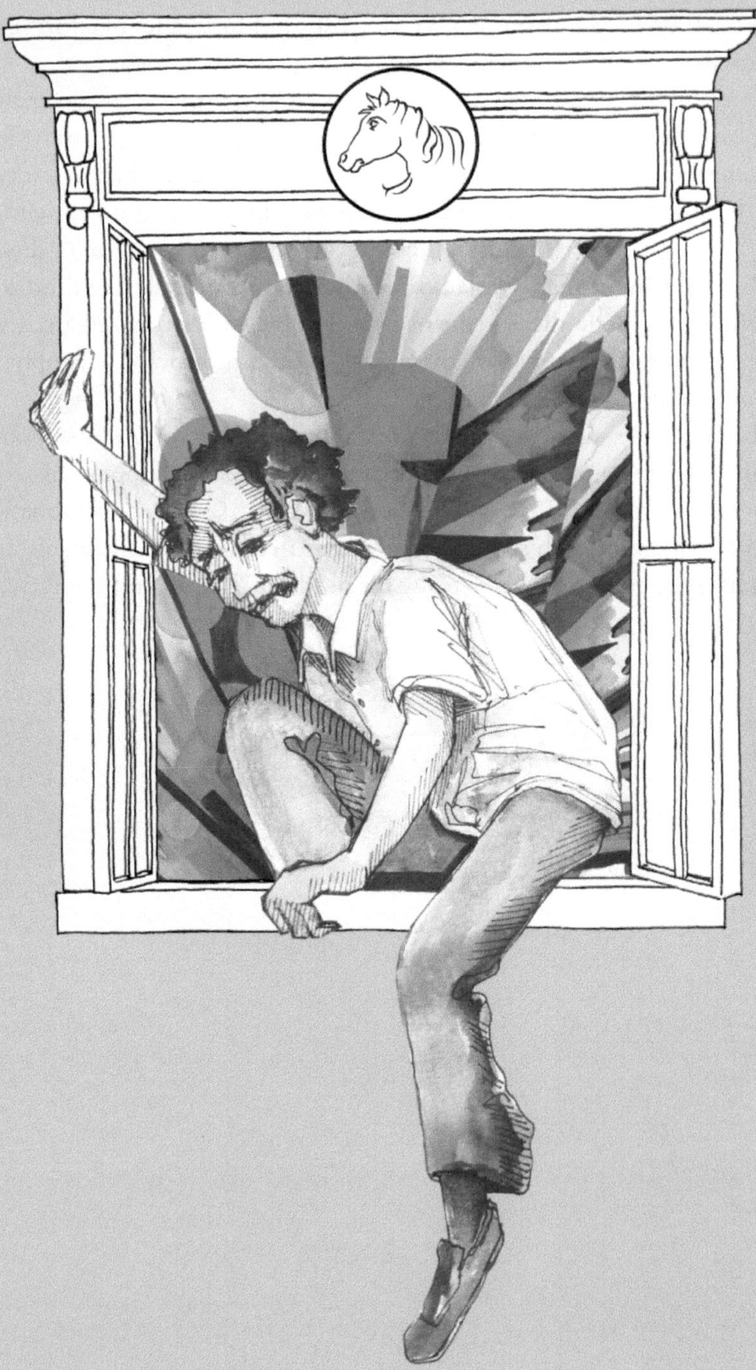

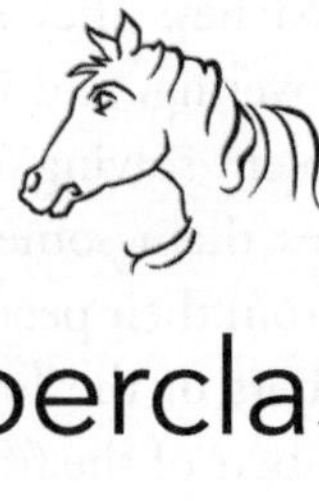

Superclass 5

The Horse type

Restless and must get out

The horse is a creature that despises confinement and longs to escape from it. It desires to move because it is restless. It has a persistent desire to get away from its reins and shackles.

We can say that the person in this Superclass is an explorer. The explorer is unique in that he cannot stay put; he must wander around. He is an achiever, a performer, a man on the move, a jetsetter, and a trendsetter. He cannot be stable in one thing; he requires change constantly. Despite being consistent in his line of work, he continuously wants to switch from one place to another. If requested to remain in the same location, he experiences claustrophobia and suffocation. His basic strategy is to leave or alter the situation. This may apply to relationships as well . They may desire to end the connection because they feel trapped, confined, and tethered by it.

The adventurer/explorer is really brave as well. He is less dependent, more assertive, and even retaliatory. In the midst of difficult situations, he is by himself. The first four Superclasses' need for a safety zone is no longer present. His perception that he has nothing to fall back on makes him more vigilant. He enjoys and revels in his accomplishments. Think of Edmund Hillary who is generally recognized to be the first to set foot on Mount Everest. They push themselves and confront their fears. Being courageous is facing your fear.

They always seek novel approaches. They seek to advance through innovating, changing, evolving, discovering, and inventing. They enjoy the concepts of analysis, planning, problem-solving, and solution-finding. They are performers as well, which makes them somewhat competitive. They enjoy standing out and getting praise from their peers. It is crucial for them to stand out from the crowd. The members of the fourth Superclass are content to maintain a low profile. The members of the fifth Superclass are often egotistical. Being efficient or morally proper is not priority to them. They have to do with being original, imaginative, or with their performance.

This group includes ministers, scientists, novelists, film producers, musicians, architects, engineers, and high-level IT professionals. They move around a lot and are constantly restless. As crisis managers, they are able to navigate challenging circumstances.

This is the horse type. These are the individuals that object to routine, who seek to alter the current situation, aspire to think outside the box. They are the achievers, performers, and risk-takers. They cannot remain still in one spot or with a single thought since; they are so restless. They enjoy risk and adventure. They do not constantly move in and out of the boundaries like the third Superclass does. Professionals, high-level managers, and crisis managers do not wish to enter again once they leave. They must leave it so they can exhale.

The fifth Superclass, in contrast to the fourth which is extremely cautious, can be exceedingly impetuous. These people thrive on being the centre of attention, in contrast to fourth Superclass, who is happy to stay anonymous. The fifth Superclass persons want to be exceptional and out of the ordinary. They thrive on praise and acclaim especially from more experienced individuals or their peers. They are able to put in lengthy hours of work like a horse on steroids.

These people are also keenly aware of their surroundings and vigilant. They are aware of what is going on in their industry. They are aware of the general state of affairs in the world. Often, they see the situation as one that has become desperately too constricting, uncomfortable, suffocating, or dangerous. Additionally, they may become claustrophobic or feel constrained, stuck, or uncomfortable. They become more distrustful, aggressive, and envious as they become further removed from the general population, feeling that they are now even more masculine than the fourth Superclass.

Rapunzel is the character from the fairy tale that can help us grasp the fifth Superclass. Princess Rapunzel has been imprisoned in a high tower without a way out. She is practically isolated. Her every thought and dream revolves around leaving that tower and travelling the globe.

An adventure movie that is high in adrenaline, *"Cliffhanger,"* a film whose title alone inspires imagination, is one that could help us better comprehend the characteristics of the fifth Superclass. Exciting images that thrill and frighten the spectator.

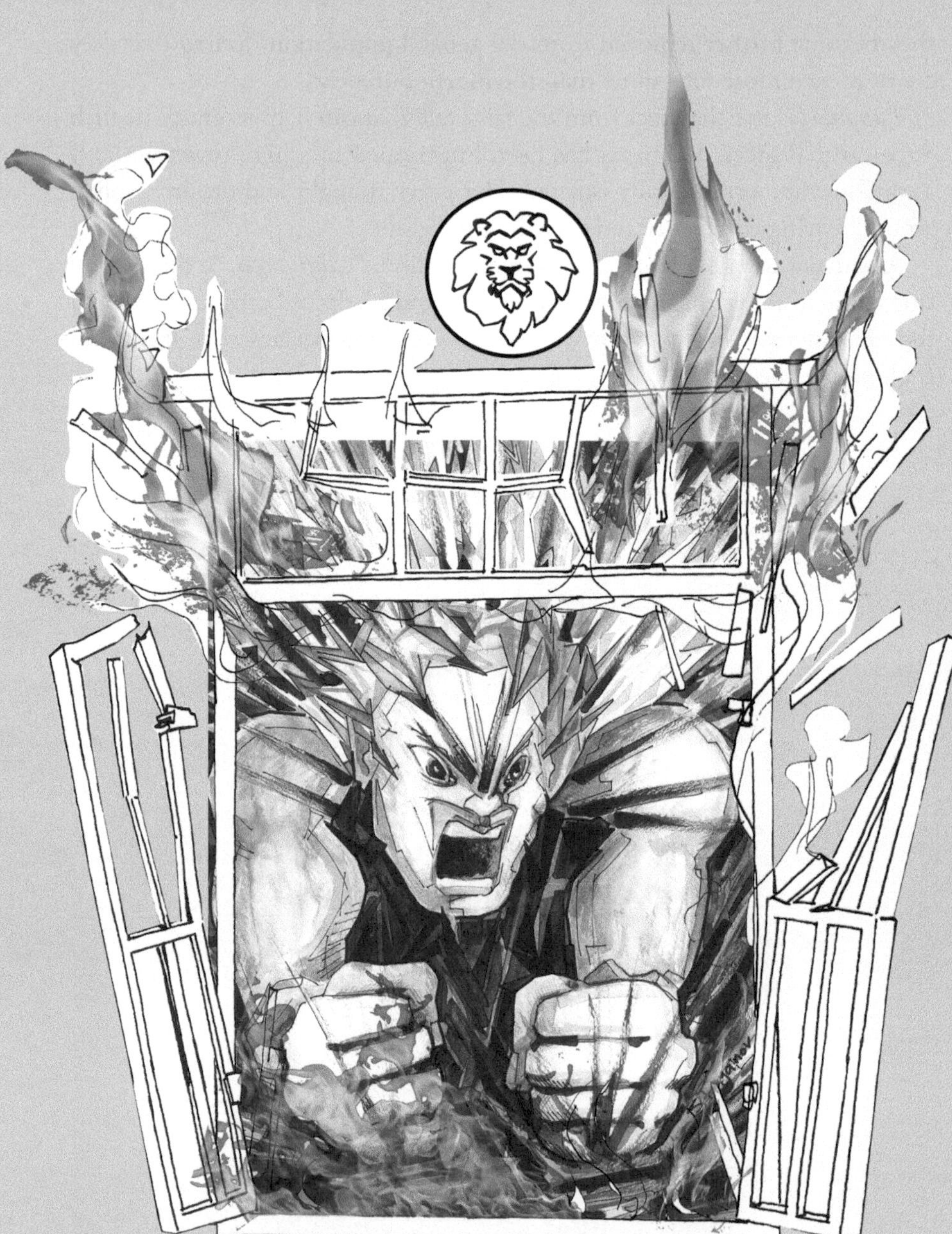

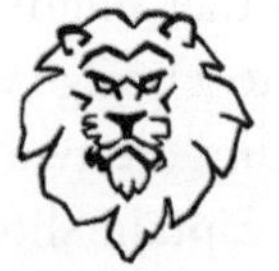

Superclass 6

The Lion type

Destruction and Violence

An animal that can be ferocious, aggressive, and brave is the lion. It reigns supreme in the jungle. It will not give up; the battle will go all the way to the end. It is like a dictator. The dictator is the final superclass; he enjoys exerting power over everyone around him.

Whoever takes the initiative, regardless of success or failure, is the one who leads and directs. The dictator seeks authority and believes that he has been hand-picked to rule the populace in any location he is in. High stakes are involved in this position, and it is even more dangerous than the fifth Superclass. The threat to you is considerably greater, and the sense of solitude is at its highest.

A fall, a death, or destruction are the threats. Failure and loss of confidence are both threats. They put themselves in circumstances that are literally life or death. There will be conflict, violence, and attacks. The possibility of violence exists. They constantly have a rush of adrenaline and are prepared to use anger, violence, and attack. They may be suicidally inclined or exude a strong sense of self-assurance. A person of extremes, their egos can be very high or entirely destroyed.

If they care about other people at all, it is more in the form of controlling and counselling. like a strict father, as opposed to the nurturing motherly trait of the carer in the third Superclass. A certain amount of hardness—you might even call it an uncaring or callous quality—can exist. They are not afraid to make incredibly difficult choices that might even mean losing lives. Sending soldiers into battle or setting fire to a bridge while retreating from a war-front, leaving part of their soldiers behind are two examples. When the ship sinks, the others will leap off, but the captain should go down with it, much like Hitler did at the conclusion of the war. Another common example of all these traits is the mafia boss.

These are the individuals who accept responsibility for their actions, not just for them but also for those nearby. Additionally, it is to them that accountability falls. They are capable of making significant decisions with confidence. They tend to be authoritative and controlling in general. Additionally, they have a tendency to be highly violent and destructive. They approach problems head-on, confront without fear, and adhere to the "an eye for an eye" rule. They exhibit great bravery, tenacity, and violence. Additionally, they are prone to feeling threatened, suspicious, and vengeful. They also experience feelings of loneliness and virtual encirclement by foes. They must deal with the crisis alone, which is also pretty serious. They may hold positions of authority, yet their fall from grace could be just as dramatic. Suicidal tendencies are apparent.

The lion type is this. An expert once told me that the lion fights all the way to the end. Compromise is not an option. The lion reigns supreme in the jungle.The fairy tale *Hansel and Gretel* is a good fit for the sixth Superclass. The story of two kids who wander off in a creepy, dark wilderness They encounter a witch there who makes a threat to cook and eat them. They force the witch into the oven in a kill-or-die scenario. This embodies every aspect of terror and brutality that defines the sixth Superclass.

The well-known mafia film "*The Godfather*" comes to mind when thinking of popular films. The Mafia boss's paternal traits are clear to notice. He has a really strong, manly sense when he looks at his family. He uses horror, violence, and dread as his instruments of control. He exhibits several of the character qualities found in the sixth Superclass. The words "To kill or be killed" are highlighted.

Crisis management

It is important to consider how each of the Superclasses would react in a crisis. Using the Superclass dynamic, we have mapped the six possible replies. The list is as follows:

1. Panic: the situation is overwhelming
2. Inertia: it is a very slow reluctance to face it.
3. Strive: to make an attempt at something
4. Coping: managing to come up with a solution.
5. Mastery: to learn something new, advanced.
6. Leadership: to spread this mastery and make sure that everyone benefits.

We can understand how these reactions would proceed if we use an example. If your house is on fire:

1. The initial reaction is panic. They don't want to face it, they can even faint. It is too overwhelming for them. One may even faint because they do not want to face it. It is too much for them to handle.
2. They enter and exit after taking a second look. It shows a lethargic response, not sure whether they want to face it or not face it.
3. They display a listless reaction, as if they are unsure whether they want to face it or not. They attempt to extinguish the flames. They are acting in this instance, but within specific bounds.
4. They are managing to put out the fire. They would call the fire brigade and cope with the situation.
5. The response would be in developing new ways of firefighting. Here they not only cope with the situation but try to see how to deal with it in the

future. They act not only for themselves but for everyone else. Maybe they design a fire alarm or something innovative. He uses the problem not only to cope but to take it to the next level.

6. And lastly the 6th response would be to introduce a new fire policy. It would be formed and implemented across the entire population. Every building must have enough space in the entrance to allow for emergency assistance. here they are creating a policy for the entire population.

These are stages of response. If you are in the first Superclass you will stop at the first. If you fall in the second Superclass you would progress through the first response but stay at the second. If you are in the 3rd Superclass you will progress through the first two and stop at the 3rd. A person in the 6th, you will pass through all the responses.

Qualities of the Superclass

In order to determine which superclass a person belongs to, we must consider who that person truly is in relation to the characteristics of the Superclasses. We must therefore comprehend some of the fundamental personality traits that characterise the different Superclasses in order to use this. Between the first and sixth Superclasses, we can roughly map out a spectrum of these characteristics. We have noted or emphasised some of the following qualities as seen on the next page.

This chart of traits aims to display a range of two opposite characteristics at opposite ends of the spectrum. Every Superclass occupies a spot on the spectrum. Take the first quality, for instance. It ranges from yielding to stubborn. The most accommodating Superclass would be the first one. The third Superclass would be much less yielding than the second. The person would then appear to be stubborn from the fourth Superclass on. The fifth Superclass would be the most resistant, while the sixth Superclass would be even more resistant. In the same manner, one would consider each quality.

In the first three Superclasses, it is more about others and less about oneself. In the fourth superclass, one really begins to consider their own security. Aggression is the theme in the fifth and sixth. "I will take from you". There is resentment, rivalry, selfishness, and dominance. When we discuss the male hormone testosterone, we talk about money and power. These are the polar opposites of caring. This is the point at which men and women diverge. Females typically are more compassionate and willing to sacrifice their own demands for those of others. She makes an effort to blend in and adapt, living with others' needs in mind. In the second Superclass, this is when the oestrogen component enters the picture. She has a strong sense of dependence on others.

Quality	1	2	3	4	5	6	Quality
Submissive							Stubborn
Laid back							Restless
Mild							Aggressive
introverted							Extroverted
Selfless							Selfish
Naive							Sceptical
Trusting							Suspicious
Dependent							Independent
Flexible							Rigid
Sensitive							Insensitive
Emotional							Practical
Affectionate							Detached
Content							Ambitious
Lazy							Productive
Patient							Impatient
Weak willed							Strong willed
Thoughtful							Impulsive
Peaceful							Destructive
Feminine							Masculine
Humble							Egoistic
Follower							Leader
Slow paced							Hurried
Maternal							Paternal
Weak							Powerful
Romantic							Realistic
Confused							Clear
Fitting in							Rebellious
Soft							Hard
	Violet	Indigo	Blue	Green	Yellow/ Orange	Black/ Red	

They are like creepers in the first Superclass because they are exceedingly clingy. This clinginess gradually lessens as you move through the second and third. However, it is still there. In the fourth, one begins to assemble their own framework. Find a place to live, something comfortable to wear, some money, and some muscle.

As one approaches a case, it is quite helpful to consult this chart to understand where each Superclass falls on the spectrum of each attribute and its polar opposite. It can serve as a form of guide in each case.

Another option is to ask the patient to assess him or herself and indicate on the chart where they believe they fall on the spectrum. We noticed that certain patients provided reliable findings. In other cases, they are dispersed throughout and do not identify any one superclass. One where the majority of the tick marks belong to a single superclass would be a consistent outcome. In general, it is also possible to determine if the majority of the tick marks are located on the chart's right or left side. This indicates the three right Superclasses, or the three left ones.

Also, we often see that if the person belongs to a specific Superclass, he would have marked many qualities in that Superclass and also some in the ones before and after that. In general, we found that that people who are more in touch with themselves at a deeper level tend to be more consistent.

Here are some examples from our experiments in cases of the varying submissions we may receive;

TYPE 1 Where there is a clear grouping around a set of Superclasses

Quality	1	2	3	4	5	6	Quality
Yielding				X			Obstinate
Inert/stationary		X					Restless
Mild		X					Aggressive
Introverted				X			Extroverted
Selfless				X			Selfish
Naive					X		Sceptical
Trusting					X		Suspicious
Clinging		X					Independent
Flexible			X				Rigid
Feminine		X					Masculine
Sensitive			X				Insensitive
Emotional		X					Emotionless
Affectionate		X					Aloof
Content				X			Ambitious
Indolent		X					Industrious
Maternal		X					Paternal
Patient				X			Impatient
Pacifist	X						Violent
Weak willed				X			Strong willed
Thoughtful			X				Impulsive
Peaceful		X					Destructive
Humble					X		Egoistic
Follower				X			Leader
Slow				X			Hurried
Spiritual			X				Materialistic
Weak			X				Powerful
Romantic					X		Pragmatic
	1	9	5	8	4	0	

TYPE 2 Where there is a consistent choice of a specific Superclass

Quality	1	2	3	4	5	6	Quality
Yielding				x			Obstinate
Inert/stationary						x	Restless
Mild					x		Aggressive
Introverted						x	Extroverted
Selfless			x				Selfish
Naive		x					Sceptical
Trusting		x					Suspicious
Clinging				x			Independent
Flexible			x				Rigid
Feminine					x		Masculine
Sensitive				x			Insensitive
Emotional			x				Emotionless
Affectionate		x					Aloof
Content				x			Ambitious
Indolent					x		Industrious
Maternal			x				Paternal
Patient				x			Impatient
Pacifist					x		Violent
Weak Willed					x		Strong willed
Thoughtful						x	Impulsive
Peaceful					x		Destructive
Humble					x		Egoistic
Follower					x		Leader
Slow						x	Hurried
Spiritual					x		Materialistic
Weak					x		Powerful
Romantic		x					Pragmatic
Soft				x			Hard
	0	3	4	5	10	4	

TYPE 3 Where there is a random spread of results, and no clear Superclass emerges

Quality	1	2	3	4	5	6	Quality
Submissive		x					Stubborn
Laid back				x			Restless
Mild		x					Aggressive
introverted					x		Extroverted
Selfless	x						Selfish
Naive					x		Sceptical
Trusting			x				Suspicious
Dependent					x		Independent
Flexible		x					Rigid
Sensitive	x						Insensitive
Emotional							Practical
Affectionate			x				Detached
Content				x			Ambitious
Lazy						x	Productive
Patient		x					Impatient
Weak willed						x	Strong willed
Thoughtful		x					Impulsive
Peaceful	x						Destructive
Feminine			x				Masculine
Humble	x						Egoistic
Follower					x		Leader
Slow paced					x		Hurried
Maternal		x					Paternal
Weak				x			Powerful
Romantic		x					Realistic
Confused					x		Clear
Fitting in							Rebellious
Soft				x			Hard
	4	7	3	4	6	2	

To clarify the idea further, you can see two charts below, one from Superclass 1 to 3 and the other from Superclass 4 to 6. In these two charts you can see the intensity of each quality in a specific Superclass. These charts are not to be given to patients, but can be used by you, the reader, to understand the idea better.

Superclass	1	2	3
Submissive	+++	++	+
Inert/stationary	+++	++	+
Mild	+++	++	+
Introverted	+++	++	+
Selfless	+	++	+++
Naive	+++	++	+
Trusting	+++	++	+
Clinging	+++	++	+
Flexible	+++	++	+
Sensitive	+++	++	+
Emotional	+++	++	+
Affectionate	+	++	+++
Content	+++	++	+
Lazy	+++	++	+
Patient	+++	++	+
Pacifist	+++	++	+
Weak willed	+++	++	+
Peaceful	+++	++	+
Humble	+++	++	+
Follower	+++	++	+
Slow	+++	++	+
Weak	+++	++	+
Romantic	+++	++	+++
Confusion	+++	++	+
Fitting in	+++	++	+
Soft	+++	++	+

4	5	6	Superclass
+	++	+++	Stubborn
+	+++	++	Restless
+	++	+++	Aggressive
+	++	+++	Extroverted
+	++	+++	Selfish
+	++	+++	Sceptical
+	++	+++	Suspicious
+	++	+++	Independent
+	++	+++	Rigid
+	++	+++	Insensitive
+	+	+	Emotional
+	++	+++	Detached
+	++	+++	Ambitious
+	+++	+++	Productive
+	++	+++	Impatient
+	++	+++	Violent
+	++	+++	Strong willed
+	++	+++	Impulsive
+	++	+++	Destructive
+	++	+++	Egoistic
+	++	+++	Leader
+	++	+++	Hurried
+	++	+++	Materialistic
+	++	+++	Powerful
+	++	+++	Pragmatic
+	++	+++	Clear
+	++	+++	Rebellious
+	++	+++	Hard

Sociableness of each Superclass

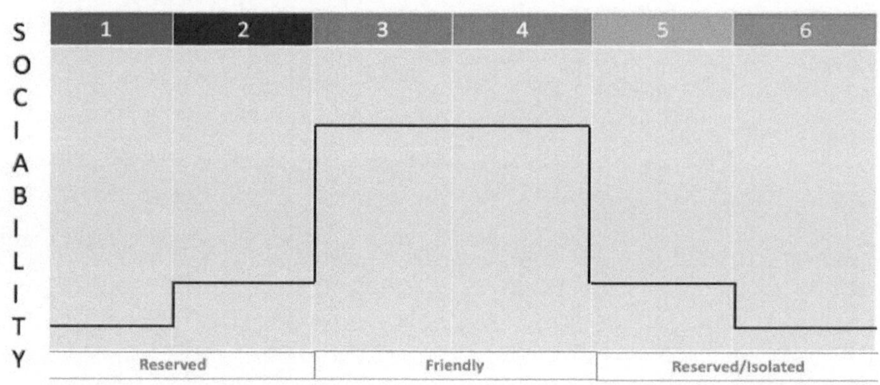

Personality of each superclass:

Superclass 1 and 2 are reserved. Whereas SC 1 is clinging to one or two people, SC 2 is very cautious to come out of the cocoon and mingle.

Superclass 3 and 4 are more social. They need relationships, they need support, they need friends, they need to belong. While Superclass 3 looks for emotional support and company. Superclass 4 tries to build networks which can be supportive in terms of money, health, job etc.

Superclass 5 and 6 are isolated.

Superclass 5 can consider themselves more elite and only interact with a specific group of elite people. Imagine famous musicians, scientists, architects, etc. They will not feel the need to have a large social circle. They may remain in a circle of people of their calibre.

Superclass 6 are the leaders, dictators. People at the top may have many followers but hardly anyone too close to them. Their aggression and temper as well as their high ego keep them away from most. It is lonely at the top and they live alone in their ivory towers.

Examining our knowledge: Brief case studies

Below are a few brief cases that we will offer. Our recommendation is that you read through each one and try to determine what the case's most fundamental dynamic is before categorising it in accordance with your present understanding of the Superclasses. Instead of concentrating on the remedy or kingdom, attempt to connect what you know about the Superclasses, their fundamental dynamics, and their fundamental nature to examples from real-world situations. On page 411, you will find the cases' solutions. Please be aware that these case summaries have been trimmed to concentrate on the key aspects of the case; consequently, the full account is written in the patient's words without any additions from me.

In all cases in this book the abbreviation HG stands for Hand-gesture which is the gesture used by the patient to describe his/her experience.

Case 1

This is the case of a 42-year-old male, the following is some of the key characteristics of his case;

I am very hyperactive. I am emotional by nature. Somebody hitting a stray dog I will not like it. I will feel like kicking that man. I am aggressive. If somebody is hitting some weaker person without any reason, I don't like it. Weaker person would be strength wise, money wise. Powerful person would be just to show his power.

When I need something in work, I expect them to work very fast.

I am very hyperactive. I want results very quickly. e.g., if I have given some work to somebody and it doesn't circle back within that particular time, I feel irritated.

I feel like they are doing a job like a peon. They are performing at low level.

Frustration, anger, irritating. They have not given their due diligence.

At some point of time in life I would even hit the person in front e.g. I used to be on my site and there was a very casual approach from the engineer, and he shifted the burden on somebody else, I gave him a tight slap. Lot of anger and frustration inside. He is doing this because he is the person to be paid. The sufferer is the company and who owns the company. It's not his own company. There is no difference to him. Casual approach. It feels very disturbing. I look after my people very nicely. But when this is not being putting in the work it feels irritable. It also makes you feel whether it was worth it. e.g., sometimes even with dad. Sometimes I feel I do so much for him, love him so much and sometimes in heat of the moment, he says something bad, or does not respond well. It makes you feel doomed.

It is not appreciated in a righteous manner. Rather it comes on the opposite side. I do not have the control over the anger. I might abusive sometimes. Stammering with anger

Perspiration with anger when I scream at top of my voice. My tone goes to a different level.

e.g., Someone has lined my car from behind and there is an argument. If the person keeps quiet, there is no problem. But if the person argues on top of banging my car, then I will first give him a slap and then talk.

e.g., one uber guy was coming from wrong side and was acting smart. I stopped the car and pulled him off the car from the window and just before I would give him slap, he I saw he was under high influence of drinks, so I handed him over to the police.

I get angry when things are not done in proper way

e.g., when I ask my guy to get 2 glasses of water and it takes more time than expected, it makes irritated.

I am very hurried in nature. I would rate myself 8/10 in hurriedness. I am very fast in things and impatient by nature.

Anxiety is work related. There are unpleasant surprises. Things doesn't happen as I had expected. e.g., there is a court case, and the result is only 30% in my favor than coming 70%.

We ask him to relate a stressful incidence for us —

There was a mob attack on me on the site. Company workers had some issues with company so when they saw I had come at the site and I was representing the company, all of them came together on me and there was lot of physical abuse on me by those people. Embarrassed feeling. Without a fault of mine this happened. Rage, revenge to some extent. Tit for tat sometimes. Give an answer at a correct time. I am very ambitious. It was so many things. There was a need for growth in me. Growth for everything. Growth company wise, tenure wise, assets wise.

I did bungee jumping but when I saw it on the show, I couldn't watch it.

But during the bungee jump there was a bit of ego also involved. My son is wrapped around me, so I wanted to show him also.

I have an ego. But more of self-respect. I never allow someone to touch my self-respect

e.g., one friend snaps with you and gets in touch with you at his own sweet time then that comes with a hurt to self-respect.

We ask about his hobbies and interests —

Sky diving, cycling, walking, cricket.
Reading non-fictional or management.

This excerpt sums up the patient's basic nature and the basic dynamic response in the case. We suggest you study this case and try to observe it through the lens of the Superclass and then check in the back of the book to see how you did.

Case 2

This is the case of a 45-year-old male, below is the edited excerpt of his case history focusing on the basic nature and dynamic of the case. Including the WISE processes done with him.

> *I have an interest of keeping fish tanks and an aquarium. They are colorful. I love animals also, but I don't like keeping them as pets because they are small age. They will die someday. Then who will take their place. There is attachment. After them there will be an emptiness. It is like a family member. It is as if some family member has expired. Like my grandmom expired on 8th December 2019. Memories come. She used to do things for me. At present I don't think of anything else, or for anyone else other than my daughter. She cannot talk, she cannot hear. I think a lot about her. How will she do ahead in life?*

What are his fears? —

> *When I stand on sand, I am scared of sea, when pulled inside (HG) pulling sensation inside. As if someone is pulling inside, and I will go down. Like some cyclone is there, like a tornado. As if tornado moves around round and round and all the things go inside it. Inside it gets destroyed. As if from inside someone is pulling (HG with both hands). As if there is something hollow inside. As if there is some hole. What if there is a marshy area. What if I go inside it? I have suffocation problem. "I am stuck in marshy area". I will go inside the hole, so better to go away from here. Breathing will be difficult. I will be restless. No breath, suffocation. I cannot move the hands and legs.*

I need openness. I don't like clothes; I don't even like wearing under garments. Without clothes I am relaxed. There is no bandhan (constriction), not bandhe hue (not tied). I don't like anyone close to me. In train, if there is crowd, I feel suffocated. I can't even sit in one place for 3 hours. I don't even watch movie. Openness, freedom. There is no "bandhan" "bandhe hue" as if tied, lock, stuck. Stuck in one place. If there is something stuck somewhere, then I feel it should immediately get free. I become restless till that time. Something is locked and it is not coming out. Stuck, lock, "fasna" (trapped) I cannot be in this position. I even don't like wearing socks. Again, locked feeling. As if bandhan hai. Tied feeling.

WISE Process Woman 1 – (we show him a picture an ask him to describe the scenario through his imagination)

She is not bothered about anything. She is fearless. There is no tension. She is not even bothered about clothes, happy in herself, doesn't bother about people. She is dancing, she is not looking at anyone. She is not bothered about anyone. "Beparwah" (not bothered). She is carefree. Because this she has worn such clothes and moving like this. At least she will cover her body. Clothes are torn. When there is mental problem then only person moves like this. She is dirty. Not clean. There is no tension. She doesn't care about anything. I will live according to my terms. Experience is of being free. Freedom is there. There is responsibility. Then you are not free. Lot of responsibilities. Again, there is load on mind. Not be in some "bandhan". Beparwah, fearless. No fear. No thoughts about anyone. Fear of falling, of someone killing me. No fear of people. Happy feeling. There is no pressure, no load on mind, weight. As if taking physical load. I feel till when these problems will be till what time. My wife does a lot. My daughter always keeps me on move, active. I don't have time to sit. Even I don't like sitting. I like moving around. Even in rains I will go out. I like travelling more alone, reason is to live on my terms. I don't like to go with someone. I feel fearless, free. I will do everything on my own. Otherwise, other people have their boundaries on me. Boundary equals to "bandhan". Boundary line is round circle. I am in center of the circle. Have to live in boundary. Tied to someone in relation. Not free, azad, fearless. Anything we want to do have to do inside the circle. I want to go out of the circle. Again "bandhan". Being tied down. Someone told you have to be here. I am in that "bandhan". It is responsibility. Outside the circle it is free, you are free, carefree. There were no circles, no boundaries. Everything you have to do in limited. You cannot go out of boundary. This is the limit; you have to be inside this. Again, you are tied. I cannot go out of boundary because of daughter. If she sneezes, I get up immediately. I am extremely anxious about daughter. She cannot speak, talk etc. I want to teach her parlour work, for food and income. Why to depend on someone?

TREE 1 (we show him a picture of a tree and ask him to use his imagination)

I don't like water park, etc. Natural things I like more. This is very beautiful. I love thinking. You can sit and think here. Where I used to be earlier there was a jungle. There is no noise. It is quiet. There are birds chirping. Here there are no birds. Looking at birds you feel free. There is no boundary. No caring for others. Live on your own. You are free. There are no responsibilities. Can fly anywhere. When there is responsibility, they have kids. That boundaries are on them also. "Bandhan" once they have kids. They can't go anywhere; they have to be around the nest only. There are boundaries. Limited area (he shows it with a hand gesture). They can't go away from nest. No one can attack their kids. Attack is to harm. Again circle. He will be in that limited area only. Kids are insecure, anyone can attack them. They might feel boundaries. They are tied down in relation for kids. For kids this is safe, security. They make the security for kids.

SWAN 1 (we show him a picture of 2 swans and 2 ducks)

Family is there. Husband, wife, kids they are roaming. Mother is not looking after kid. Father is shouting on mother please look after the kid. Kid can go around, do something. There can be some accident of kid. Some animal can come and eat. They have to keep them into their boundaries. Kids don't have boundaries, we put it, but they still go. Go out of the boundary it is free. We are free. Crossing the circle. Cross the boundaries. Free. No limit. No responsibilities. Limitless. Once we cross the limit, till where it can go. It can go where it will go. Like a sea. Everything is limitless. You can't measure the limit sea. Like a sky. It is free. No building, no dividers, no boundaries. Dividers like partition. No boundaries.

SWAN 2 (with another picture of swans)

> *Happy family. They are talking something nice. Maybe they are talking about future. Kids are in themselves. They are not concerned what are they talking. They are discussing about kids' future. They are away from the routine work and on vacation. There is new thing, different thing. Outing. In routine work there is same thing going on. Doing same thing again and again. Same things. Dullness, tiredness. It is hectic. Load of mind decreases in outings. They also have to be alert, aware. Surrounding there can be attackers, hunters. My work I used to enjoy. I need to make my mind run fast. Dull mind couldn't work. You have to be alert always. If you are not alert, you are out of market. Every day it was new work.*

Case 3

This is the case of an 82-year-old male whose main complaint was Asthma. He explains what can aggravate his complaints —

> *For example, something is troubling me. I have given some work to the bank, and they haven't done it then I get angry. If I cannot control my temper, then this breathlessness can occur. I feel excited. We in the military are not used to this sort of life. There is a disciplined life in military. Everything is well regulated. All the time you are doing something. When I get very angry, I feel warm in the head. If somebody shouts at me too much and person is not listening to me then I get angry. I feel agitated. Then I try to control myself because I don't want to spoil my health. They try to counteract my instructions. I feel angry. Otherwise, I am a very calm person. I don't get very angry much. I don't keep many worries in my mind. Calm means there is peace of mind, relaxed. Opposite- Anger. I start shouting at the person. I talk loudly. In the process my head and face warm up. E.g.: when I told the person to do job now and person says I will do it my own time. I am not used to this behavior in military. Disciplined behavior. Here it is uncivilized, undisciplined. You have to be civil to another person. Good behavior. Person is talking in calm and relaxed manner. Uncivilized behavior. When you are talking to the person you should not shout. That is uncivilized. You should talk quietly. Everything is to be done in calm and relaxed manner.*

We ask him to tell us more about his nature —

> *I am a type of person, once the superior gave me orders I follow it. The military person is very calm in nature. Our superiors know much more than*

us. Because we need to fight the enemy, so we need to be calm. Number of soldiers sacrifice lives for their seniors. We are trained like that. You have to study and then do exercise and PT. There is not even a single minute free for yourself.

We ask him what the opposite of this is —

Undisciplined, uncivilized – when people don't listen to somebody. You start talking in between and after some time you start raising your voice. You don't reply in nice manner and start abusing the other person.

Some of the dreams he gets —

Somebody has stolen something from my house, and he is running away from me. I am chasing him. Feeling is I must catch him. Why has he done this with me? I must hand him over to the police.

The patient narrates a stressful incident in his life —

When I lost my father, mother, and my elder brother. Most impactful was my brother. We were in boarding school. So, most of our adult life we were always very close to each other. He was like a real elder brother. He was very mature for his age.

When I listened to this, I was sad, but I kept to myself. I cried but not in front of others. When I went to the death bed I didn't shout or howl so much. I was able to control myself. When I was alone at night, I would cry a little bit. People start howling and beating their chest. That sort of behavior some people do. When I was very small, he used to look after me very well. He would protect me. I learnt a lot of things from him. If some other boy would bully me, then my brother would save me and protect me and get me out of that situation. If while running I am bruised, he would immediately take me to nearest clinic. In studies he would help me out. He thought that I was his responsibility and he looked after me very well. He was very calm and could solve any sort of things. Father figure – somebody whom you would look up to. Somebody who is very balance, sane, mature person.

We ask him to talk more about his nature —

I am very punctual. If I don't get up in the morning at a particular time, then I feel guilty. Everything I do at a certain time, lunch, dinner, etc.

Everything is very much in time. I like it that way. In case of appointments, I arrive 10-15mins earlier. I like everything planned earlier. Nothing to worry. I am very clean person. I keep everything very neat and tidy. I keep everything prim and proper. Dish, fork, knife, everything is very neat and proper. House is kept spotlessly clean. There is nothing lying around. For example, if something is fallen on bedsheet, you should change it immediately. It looks dirty otherwise.

The patient tells us about his childhood —

Mostly in the boarding school. It was very good. It was an Irish school. They were well disciplined. We would get up at a certain time. They were so well disciplined. They had a cane and if somebody is being bad or naughty then would hit you. They disciplined us. So, I have been brought up with that discipline. Then I joined the military and again the same story. There was also discipline. So, even now this discipline is my system. Doing everything on time. In our house everything is well organized and well disciplined.

Case 4

This is the case of a 41-year-old male. He came with the complaints of irritable bowel syndrome. The following is the summary of his case including some information from the WISE processes done with him.

There are a lot of stressful reasons in my personal life. I lost my wife last year. She had cancer out of nowhere. It has been rough and traumatic. Now I just want to be sure that I am fit and ready for my son, who is dependent on me. It is quiet draining. I gained a lot of weight since a year due to cholesterol. Sometimes there may be lack of sleep specially after this incidence. My natural mechanism of body is to sleep, but now I have become a light sleeper, I sleep not before 1am now. There is a flip in my personality. I faced same trauma when I lost my parents, I would feel drowsy, sleepy. It was like natural defence. When I heard about my dad's death, I would feel sleepy. Even with my wife's stressful situation I would feel sleepy. I just get very drowsy. I am into deep sleep. My body is trying to tell me that it is uneasiness. Something you can't control, you want to escape, just the way out. To run away, get out of a situation. Blank kind of feeling. It's just like a temporary pause. Like what you feel while sleeping. You are into your own world. It's like meditation, peaceful. No stress. In stress you want to shut off, closed down, go into your shell. No connection from outside world.

Even in hospitals I would just crash, sleep off but since my wife's incident I have not been able to sleep properly. It was very close relationship what we had, and when she got this disease, it was stressful for both of us and seeing her go through all this, was tough in 2017.

Trauma is I am losing lot of things which is very devastating, whatever you are building is going. Its fear. Anything that you love is going away. No control over the situation. Plans suddenly crash. Everything gone for a toss. Now rebuilding without an anchor.

No one to support in that sense when you lose the anchor, the partner. There is lot of responsibility as well. It is very lonely kind of feeling as well. My social interaction is also less as I do work from home. That also adds to loneliness. I am stuck, career wise I feel dead end. Now I need to fix many things, job life, home, son, taking care of myself everything I have to fix at this point of time. Everything seems very unsure, uncertainty about future.

This thing came out of nowhere with my wife. We tried 100 of things, it just kept getting worst. Nothing is steady, fixed. Anchor gives you support, there is something that works. Weight is when things are not working, something can go wrong. What if my job doesn't work? It is also on my own self esteem. I don't have the support, there is fear, what's going to happen? Will I be ok, my child, my career? What will happen to my child's health?

Being alone, how am I going to manage. There is also an uneasiness, helplessness. You have lack of resources, even financially. Support when something helps you when you are in tough situation, something you can count on. Something which helps you taking risk. If that fails something is encouraging, you. Lack of support then you are unsure, you are fearful, you are insecure. There is lot of self-doubt. Insecure is you are not sure how things will work. It is fear – fear of failure, losing something again, unknown. If you know, you can deal with it. Fear of unknown means anything which can happen from anywhere

Now I am fearful for myself, my child. It is in my head. Having her to go through 2nd phase of cancer was very tough. There was lot of back and forth.

20 years back I lost my parents. Same trauma, same fear, same insecurity. It was a sense of shock. You are living in some alternate reality, don't know what can happen. But the difference was sense of responsibility was not that high. Now the child is totally dependent on me. Dependent is that nothing should harm them. Children depend on us for decisions, so it should be right decision, so they don't have to suffer for unnecessary thing. Like those which can affect physically and mentally like drugs, wrong habits smoking and drinking not good for his health and his life. He will not be able to reach the potential that he could. And he might suffer with health issues, like liver problems due to excessive alcohol, or accidents due to alcohol. Excessive smoking can cause problems with lungs. I don't want to think about medical issues right now, that make me anxious. I am scared it can happen with me or my son.

Dreams – wife, my wife and my parents are there, sometimes I wake up during the dream if I am reliving the bad part, I will wake up. I don't want to see her dying, uneasy feeling. It's anxiety, sweaty more on forehead and feel hot means if I have sheet on me, I will kick it away. You feel sad or shaken up. I wake up with a jerk sometimes. Normally also I will not sleep with anything on me. Sometimes I see good dreams also about it.

Fears – health is now one, I always want to do well in my career, financially. Sense of achievement is important for me. Like promotions, or certain job, recognition for something that I did. Having problems like heart, diabetes, hypertension. Thinking about medical upsets me, gives me headache. Parents and wife had many problems so, now I feel what if it happens to me or someone that I love.

Claustrophobia, trapped in small place, HG, I am not able to move, or breathe or not able to see things. You feel suffocated, I don't want to be in closed situation, I don't want to be restricted, not go out. Stuck. You feel trapped. Anxiety my chest, sweaty more on forehead and palms, panicky, helpless, I will cry. Sinking feeling. Faint feeling. Black out. Not in control of your senses. Being alive yet unconscious. You can't see, hear, or feel things.

I am scared of needles or blood. I have also blacked out. Suddenly my body will become cold, I will be sweating on forehead, face, nausea and fading out. Passing out. Body is shutting down. Stopping. Stopping completely. Limp, you don't know what's going on.

When needle is poking you, bringing back some more. In childhood, it was big thorn, which was stuck in my thumb, it was the first time when I had this fainting. And once my dad has the medical procedure and I saw blood and then I passed out, I had sinking feeling, cold metallic taste in mouth. Cold sweat on forehead. I am not good in roller coaster rides. I feel nausea, heart is falling, sinking in stomach and stomach is going around and round and you are feeling like vomiting. Your heartbeat is fast. You feel very scared of it and there is blackout kind of situation. Cold sweat, uneasiness, bad taste in mouth, you feel like lying down on back and hands and legs are by your side. Anxiety and worry have always been there. Taking stress for every situation. Overthinking. What will happen if it goes wrong, how can I deal with it? What if people don't like it if I made a mistake then consequences. What will other people think of me? It will affect the future work that I do.

Childhood —

Quiet, shy kind of kid. I was not naughty or mischievous. I was fearful.

Nature —

Usually, I am a positive kind person, life has given me lot of setbacks. I try to balance and make peace with lot of things. I like to meet people, going out, I enjoy social interaction. I have short attention span if I am doing important work, I get distracted easily, by someone calling me, take a break. I need different stimulus. Doing one thing for long period of time I get bored, I get sleepy, I get headache in the root of nose, temples like something is pressing. Like a force, contracting. It is like a pain. Pushed down. You feel like refreshing, move away. Step away, look away. That makes you feel relaxed. No pain or pressure. You feel energized. I like to try different new things or new experiences. Unless I have specific deadline then I put my concentration into it. Otherwise, I procrastinate a lot.

Sensitive – my family, myself, my ability. If I hear something bad about my family, it will keep on playing in my mind. don't like if there is no air. If it is dry and hot, I don't like that. There is uneasy feeling. Become sweaty and suffocated (hands near chest), feel like there is some kind pressure on chest. Something is pushing you down, making you feel hot around face and chest, you don't feel like moving, restricts. Less energy, lethargy. Opposite is high energy, wanting to be active.

WOMAN 1 —

There is great suffering she is having. Something is approaching her which she doesn't want. She wants to go away. Hide somewhere. She can't take too much suffering. It is too much for her. She wants to go away. She closes her eyes. This is better. There is peace. It is as if there is no connection to what is happening outside. The senses are cut off. No feelings. Absolutely no feeling. You are into your own world. it is calm. Quiet. Nothing is there. It is blank.

Where there are no sufferings. You don't want to see so much suffering, so you shut yourself off.

WOMAN 2 —

She is tired, thirst. Quenching thirst. Wants cold water. She is standing in the desert. Everyone has gone away. She is alone, by herself. She feels lost. She is not knowing where to go, what to do? She is scared. It feels lost. Don't know way out and stuck in the middle. In this one spot, don't know where to go, no directions or clarity how to get out. In the middle of nowhere. Don't know what to do, where to go. Not clear which is right path. Lost. Don't know right path. Don't know what to do, can't think. Thoughts are shut of completely. Stuck in the middle and you don't know. Stuck means no thoughts. Like pause, stop, blank. There is nothing. No thought. Complete blankness. Fade out. Zoned out.

Case 5

This is the case of a young man who came with chronic hepatitis. He complained of an acute, intermittent pain in the region of the liver. This is the summary of his case which he begins by talking of his career as a painter.

Mostly I paint for nightclubs and discotheques, and a lot for art collectors. Actually, I've been painting ever since I can remember. My father was an artist, but he didn't pursue it. My grandfather had a school in my hometown, and my father had to take care of that. But I made a career of it. I like to paint wildlife. I love animals. They make this world look good. I really like them. I have strong love and liking for animals and for nature, for trees especially. My brother tried to cut down a tree, and it gave me a very bad shock. I like children also. I like very dramatic subjects. I am not a landscape man, they do not inspire me. If it is vibrant, like the huge bark of a tree trunk and dramatic blue water, that inspires me.

We ask him what dreams he gets —

Too many dreams, hundreds every night. I have very restless nights, my mind keeps working. I'm very restless in my sleep, and am still tired on waking, not fresh, as if I am working all night. I have dreams with friends, my fiancée, animals, robbers coming, and trying to escape, paintings; thunderstorms excite me. I rarely get romantic dreams. I dream of my family being unwell or on the deathbed. That was a shock to me so I remember that one. I only paint an hour at a stretch, before I get restless and impatient, and have to stop. I lose concentration. I am sorry, I forgot the question.

(I noticed how his speech wandered from one subject to another, all over the place)

I always feel insecure or doubtful about everything I do. People may not approve of it. It may not go through. I am scared about the future, about the stability of business, whether I should be in Bombay or abroad. Everything is a question with me. I do not want to leave my family, but I am not very happy in Bombay. I do not like peace and quiet. I don't like the silence of peaceful areas, it makes me very uncomfortable. I hate to be alone, that scares me, I like people around. I am cold all the time. I cannot remain on one thing for a long time, I have to switch. I cannot sleep alone in a flat. I feel as though the emptiness, loneliness will come and eat me up. I feel weird; I want to run away from this place.

Why should I be inspired by something that does not actually exist? Why should I be so attached; this planet does not really exist. I will have to leave such a beautiful place. Why should I be happy to see a blue sky? The sky is only a chemical reaction, it does not exist. Why do I feel art is so beautiful? Everything means nothing. Death means nothing, I cease to exist. Everything is nothing. My father used to be happy with the work I did. But I used to have those thoughts also. It makes no difference whatsoever. What is the use? I get these thoughts when I am alone. Why be in love? We should never be attached to anything. If you stay detached, you will never feel good or bad about anything. I sleep alone in my studio, and if I hear weird noises, my sleep is lost and I have to turn on all the lights. I think weird thoughts and can see spirits coming. I cannot be in the dark and alone. Walking alone at night, I feel as if a spirit is following me. Emptiness scares me, darkness scares me.

I do not like grey, brown, and deep colours. I like blues and violets and yellows.

Death is a very depressing thing. Nothing exists; it is all a chemical reaction. It will all vanish. I don't mind dying basically. This whole planet will not exist in a few million or trillion years. Everything we see is all going to go off one day. Nothing is for me. I am seeing the sky, the planets, good-looking things, getting inspired and attached, and nothing exists. I am too attached to everything. I feel sad to leave the shoes I have worn for two years, they have been with me so long. I am attached to my family and fiancée, and her family and my friends, the smell of my house, trees around me, the atmosphere around me. This attachment only makes me sad, that I will have to leave this planet. It is not even proven that the soul exists. On the other side, I feel a doubt that probably I won't be written off, that the soul probably does exist. The thing I really do not want is to be lying in bed and dying. I would rather not exist; I would rather commit suicide.

He mentions that he likes flying and paragliding so we ask about this —

You can see things from above. It feels so light. Flying makes life so very beautiful. I wanted wings, so I could fly. You can have an aerial view of everything, and can see things as an onlooker, better perspective.

Case 6

Case of a 40 year-old male with knee pains and chest pains. The following is an extract of the case to highlight his basic nature and dynamic in the case.

I do a lot of exercise. So, when I can't do the exercise because of the pain, I get depressed. If I don't exercise I will gain weight. I go for martial arts classes also. If I don't do that, I feel my time will run out, I will not learn it properly. Even if I get hurt little bit, the pain is excessive. Like say I have to do something by December and if I can't do it then I will not catch up and lag behind.

So, if there is pain, I am tired. The amount of headache I get with the amount of work I do is not proportionate. I do a lot of exercise because I am into cinema also. I have just finished two films and they will be releasing in the end of August. I feel like I have to finish all this so I have to go for black belt in December. So, if I am not regular in classes because of ill health, I can't go for this black belt and again I will be delayed for one year. I feel very anxious, very tensed. If I will be left behind, I will lag behind in the competition. I feel others will go past me faster. So, in proper time if I don't finish faster, I will not be able to do it. Other people are also learning with me, so I feel that they will get their black belt faster and I will be left behind. Then I will feel depressed because I have not kept up with this thing, with my expectation. Like mentally I have a goal, in this time I must do this. Like I expect talks are going on with the producers, so I am supposed to do these films. Now if I don't finish this and because of ill health and pain I am not doing proper work, then time is running out and then I may not get in or I may be late, you feel insecure. Then of course I will be depressed and I actually always wanted to be in the cinema.

But my family background is not from cinema. My father is a doctor. He wanted me to take up medicine. From childhood I always wanted to be into acting. In my native town I did some theatre. So, I came down here and took up a job and I am just trying to get into it. From young days I liked to work with art and liked creativity, theatre, acting. So, it's my love for acting, so decided that I will do it. I used to go for rehearsals, meet with everybody and did it well. When you do well in something, you get acclaimed and cheered up by people. Just to feel, I feel nice. Something with creativity just gives me pleasure and then there is money and fame also into it. So, everything put together, I liked acting. I used to also write short stories and then screenplays.

I have a very bad quality, I have very less patience. Like if I want something, I want it very fast. Like even my college days, when there used to be an emergency, I would tell the sisters to give this medicine; I want them to be given instantly. Then I get irritated if it's little late. I feel the patient might die and why are they not sincere? These things count a lot of for me. Sincerity, sense of time. I am always punctual about my time and even if I am late I feel very guilty because I don't like somebody waiting for me.

Sometimes nowadays I feel a lot of fatigue.
I get little irritable faster.

We asked him what it is like if he doesn't meet his expectations —

It is like being in a jungle and there is no path and you have to just make the path and move. Make your own path. There is nothing like somebody will tell you go follow this path, so you can reach this. There is no guidance. You just make your path, cut the trees, make your own path and move and you make the path in the wrong way, you move in the wrong way. I feel much tensed of course. But it's not that I give up and then wait for some spiritual guidance or something like that. It's not that. I don't just go. To fight back. I mean, in spite of the obstacles, just put all your strength and move forward. Like make the path. So, I feel good about it.

Obstacles means, like I don't know people. Obstacle is something which is causing a barrier to your movement. Barrier is something on your way which is not allowing you to move forward, something which is stopping you.

SECTION TWO

Subclasses and the evoluion of the Superclass

Initially in practice I observed that cases prescribed on general and mental symptoms did better. This sparked the development of the Sensation method. These cases had better and deeper results compared with cases prescribed on local symptoms alone. This began the investigation into the idea of disease as a delusion (see *The Spirit of Homeopathy*). And with this thinking further elements developed including the kingdoms and the miasms. These ideas proved to be helpful in clinical practice. When applied, the results spoke for themselves.

The idea of the three kingdoms gave an immense insight into the case taking and analysis. This is the understanding that we all perceive reality through a specific viewpoint. For example, in the animal kingdom we will see the perception of reality of survival. The features of one vs the other or victim and aggressor themes. In the mineral kingdom we can see that the perception of reality is of structure. Either its loss or capability. And in the plant kingdom reality perception is of sensitivity and reactivity.

Further experimentation and much research has taken place after this. A commonality between certain remedies in each kingdom came to light. This commonality lay deeper to the mind state or its perceptions. This developed quickest in the plant kingdom, ultimately becoming the idea of sensation. Here we could see that within the same family there was a common thread between the remedies.

For example, if we take the remedy Bryonia we can study some of the rubrics such as;

- head; PAIN, headache; motion; agg.; slightest
- extremities; PAIN; knees; motion; agg.
- chest; PAIN; motion; agg.

From these rubrics we can see that Bryonia is a remedy which is worse from least motion. This way of looking at the remedy like this comes from Boenninghausen. He termed this grand generalisation, implying that what is true for the part must be true for the whole.

And when we take this idea a bit further, we look at a rubric like;

- Generalities; Motion; eyes, of; agg.

Again, we will find Bryonia in this rubric. We will also notice another remedy of interest in this rubric, namely Colocynthis. And then when we look at another rubric:

- Mind; Disturbed, disturbance; averse to being

In this rubric too we will find Bryonia as well as Colocynthis. Bryonia and Colocynthis belong to the same order, the Violales. So, this connection becomes very interesting for us.

What happens when we apply Boenninghausens grand generalisation to the order? We must infer that all the remedies within the order will have aversion to being disturbed. They will be worse from motion and will be better from rest and better by retaining the same position.

Using this understanding of Boenninghausen we were able to extract the common themes. These themes of the remedies belonging to the Violales can be seen below.

Family	Sensation	Passive Reaction	Active Reaction	Compensation
Violales	At physical level: Cutting Stabbing Lancinating Sharp Stitching Pinching At mental level: Vexation Chagrin Disturbed Main feeling is: does not want to be disturbed.	Prostration Morose Averse to being disturbed Wants total rest Avoidance of people	Irritability when questioned Violence Malicious Rage Restless	Quietness Calmness Stillness

At this point we have understood the sensation of about 30 different plant families. I have written about these in my book *Insight into plants*.

So, at this point the knowledge which we had was
symptoms of the remedies
generals of the remedies
generals of the family
knowledge of the kingdom.

This information can be displayed as a pyramid.

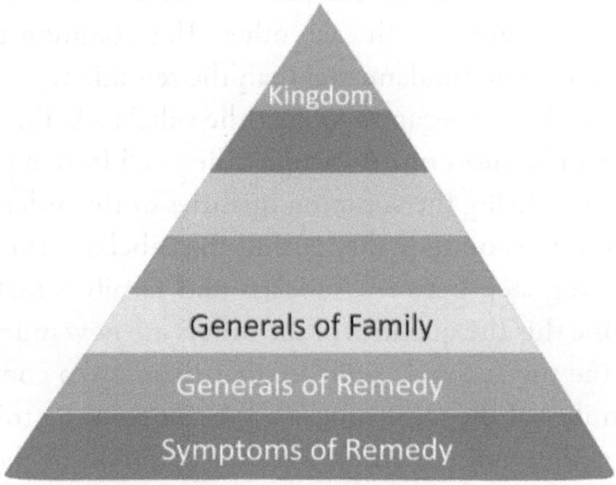

But as we can see from this pyramid there are three steps missing. These are the Generals of the order, Generals of the subclass and Generals of the class, as seen below.

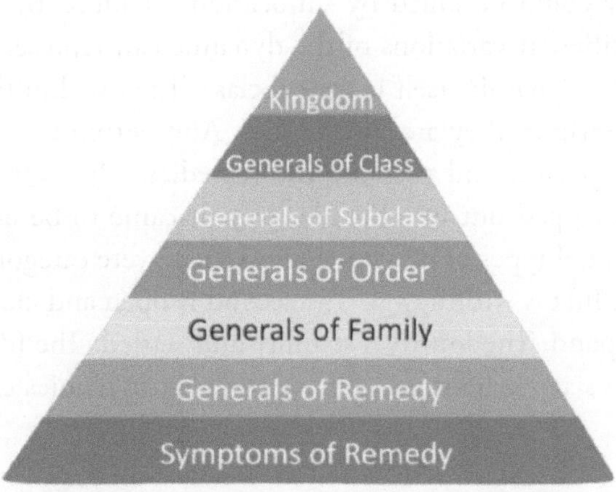

What is the common thread between the families within the same subclass? This was our next question. We had to find the connecting thread between families in the same subclass in the same way we looked for the connecting thread between remedies in the same family. Much work and research has gone into this and it should also be mentioned that inspiration has been drawn from the great work done on this topic by homeopaths such as Michal Yakir, Jan Scholten, Mahesh Gandhi and others.

However, there was a different approach in understanding the subclasses. Whereas they have approached the work from a psychological and or evolutionary standpoint, I have developed this work along the framework of the understanding of the sensation. Families within the same subclass should have something in common with each other. This common thread must be something which is more fundamental than the sensation.

Some may ask why we began to look at the subclass before looking at the orders. Since we only know one or two families well from a given order this was difficult. Generalising the common qualities of the order was not possible. Yet, we found the commonality within the subclass. This made it easier to find the missing step between subclass and family which is the order. After having done this the qualities of the orders are now much clearer to us.

In studying the subclasses, I could see that there was a common dynamic between the families of the same subclass. We can consider this as a dynamic between a perception and a reaction which is common to the subclass. It is broader than the sensation and under which different sensations can be found. For example, if there is a crisis and someone is being killed. The impulse could be to escape or fight back, this is the dynamic. There can be many different variations of this dynamic. So, in this example the person could be killed by injury. They could be killed by suffocation, or killed by an unexpected attack. These different variations of the dynamic can represent the orders of the subclass. The dynamic itself is the subclass. Then within the orders there are specific sensations, they are the families. And within these families there are specific symptoms, and they are the remedies. This was how the plant kingdom was mapped out in a broader way. It came to be understood that there are 6 essential types of dynamics. And these were categorised into the 6 Subclasses. The first is withdrawal. The second is open and close. The third is to limit and expand. The fourth is stability and settled. The fifth is stuck and get out and the sixth is fight and flight. These six dynamics came to be well understood.

Subclass 1

Magnolidae

To understand the common dynamic of this subclass, we need to have a look at some of the remedies we know which are in it. We have Nux-moschata, Camphora, Helleborus, Pulsatilla, Opium among others. What can we see as the common dynamic of these remedies? We can see they all have a kind of numbness, anaesthesia, confusion, withdrawal into their own world. These are the main qualities of the dynamic of this subclass.

Magnolidae	
Typical remedy	Opium
Common features	Trifles aggravate Sensitive Slightest pain & emotions Excited Agitated Strange aggravated Unfamiliar aggravates Addictions Into one's own world Shut off Withdrawal

(*Continues*)

(*Continues*)

	Go into a shell Confusion Anaesthesia
Sensation	Raw Exposed In his own world
Perception	Assault on senses
Dreams/fears	Suffering Pain Insult
Sensitivity	Pain Suffering Animals Slights
Response	Withdraw Numb Anaesthetic
Energy pattern	Inward
Pleasure	Bliss Peace Eyes closed Addiction
Music	Blissful Peaceful
Example	Meditation
Situation	Monk
Pathology	Autism
Modalities	Trifles
Other features	Penetrating Confused
Symbol	Buddha
Words	Numb Slightest causes Anaesthesia Shell Own world Withdraw Confused Touchy

All the orders (and remedies) of a Subclass will have all the qualities of that Subclass. But each one will have one aspect more prominently demonstrated. As we go through the Orders you will see the evolution of the sensation of the subclass.

Magnolidae
Magnoliales (confusion) • **Annonaceae:** Asim, Guat • **Magnoliacaea:** Magn-gr • **Myristicaceae:** Myris, Nux-m
Nymphaeales (Extreme sensitivity for others, dependence, connection with the divine) • **Nelumbonaceae:** Nelu • **Nymphaeaceae:** Nuph
Illiciales • **Schisandraceae:** Anis
Piperales (Monotony, desire for excitement, entertainment) • **Piperaceae:** Cub, Mati, Pip-n, Pip-m • **Sauraceae:** Anemps, Saur
Laurales • **Lauraceae:** Benzo, Camph, Cinnam • **Monimiaceae:** Bold
Aristolochiales • **Aristolochiaceae:** Aristo-cl, Asar
Ranunculales (As if no skin, mix of emotions, change.) • **Berberidacaeae:** Berb, Caul, Podo • **Ranunculaceae:** Acon, Act-sp, Cimic, Hell, Puls, Ran-b, Staph • **Menispermacaeae:** Cocc, Menis, Pareir
Papaverales (Extreme sensitivity to pain and suffering, Anaesthesia) • **Papaveraceae:** Arge, Chel, Cod, Morph, Op, Sang

Magnoliales: (example: Nux moschata): No cover.

- Feels he is in a strange unfamiliar world.
- There is a sudden change
- Confusion
- Faintness
- Numbness
- Sleepiness
- Absent minded

Nymphaeales: (example: Nuphar) extreme sensitivity

- Extreme sensitivity to pain and suffering in the world, especially of animals.
- They turn to spiritual things (Lotus)
- They connect to the spirit or God

Piperales: (example: Piper methysticum): diversion

- Much sensitivity to pain and suffering
- Want to divert mind to material things
- Entertainment, occupation
- Food. Taste, shopping, excitement

Laurales: (example: Camphor): early cover

- Withdraw into their world and shut the outside world out.
- Create their own world which is safe, and outside is dangerous and bewildering.

Aristolochiales: (example: Asarum): Don't want invasion

- They don't want anything from outside to come into their space.
- Aristolochia; everything is dirty, they need to wash hands frequently.
- Asarum: extremely sensitive to penetrating noise.

Ranunculales (example: Pulsatilla): Touchy

- Sensitive and reactive to slight emotions, insults, mortification.
- Reacts with anger, trembling, weeping, etc.
- Adaptable (puls), yielding.
- Changeable (berb)

Papaverales: (example: Opium): Anaesthesia

- Extreme pain
- Suffering
- Thick-skinned. Anaesthetic, Numb
- Fearless.

When studying a remedy, we can see some similarities with remedies from a different Superclass. That is when it becomes important to differentiate between them. Let us take up the example of Camphora —

- A lot of anxiety and fear like Stramonium (6th Subclass)
- Clinging, grasping.

- Desire company at night.
- Panic, danger.
- mind; DELUSIONS, imaginations; world; she has her own little, in which things are clear, outside is uncertain
- mind; DELUSIONS, imaginations; world; world, he is moving in a new
- mind; DELUSIONS, imaginations; danger, of

What is the main difference between Camphora and Stramonium —

- In Stramonium: the reaction is violence, Fight or Flight.
- In Camphora: the reaction is to withdraw into his own world which is safe. (Like an oyster)

Excerpt from Camphora case in Sankaran's insight into plants —

Sankaran's P... Type to search

"I have an overwhelming sadness about my missed childhood and youth. When I was young I tried to commit suicide 5 or six times; life was too overwhelming for me. It feels as if there are two of me - one is the "outside" me, strong and confident, the other one just wants to hide in my little closed shell."

Some other features of Camphor

- Suddenness (Acute Miasm)
- Senses acute or senses blunted (Increased smell or loss)
- Painlessness of complaints usually painful
- Fainting, collapse… Sudden collapse

From Phatak —

It is a remedy for sudden collapse, from over-powering influences acting on nervous centers. Patient becomes ICY COLD; YET HE IS AVERSE TO COVERS or wants them off; and then on alternately with internal burning heat and anxiousness. Sudden; weakness; fainting spells growing worse. Dry collapse, with little vomiting and purging; in cholera.

Subclass 2

Hamamelidae

We can get an insight into the dynamic of the second Subclass through its most well-known remedy : Cannabis indica. We see that Cannabis indica has two polarities. On the one hand there is the excitement, the sensory stimulation, where everything appears bigger, more colourful, more beautiful. It is as if the pores of the skin and senses open up to receive more, as if they are hungry for stimulus. On the other hand, Cannabis indica also has dullness and a weighed down feeling "as if leading a vegetable existence". These two polarities represent the two poles of the second subclass.

We can see that open and shut is a very important theme in the 2nd Subclass. They shut themselves in, in times of challenge. They cannot remain like this for a long time. They have to open because they feel they are living a vegetative existence. They are safe inside but then everything feels monotonous, dull, grey and boring. The outside is interesting but scary.

Hamamelidae	
Typical remedy	Cannabis sativa
Common features	Open & shut Window Heavy & Light Flying Floating Laughing Dancing Fancies Imprisoned Allergies
Sensation	Grey Colorless Boring, or less contact with outside
Perception	Lack of sensory stimulation
Dreams & Fears	Flying
response	Close & open
Energy pattern	Opening & closing
Pleasure	High Floating Laughing
Music	Uplifting Divine
Example	Window
Situation	Bored wife of a rich man
Modalities	>open <in the house
Symbol	Hippie
Words	In & out Windows Colours Heavy & light
Animal	Mollusca: Gastropoda
Mineral	Carbon
Plant	Fern
Miasm	Typhoid Malaria

The main sensations/dynamic in the Hamamelidae;

- Open and closed
- Heavy and light
- Transported to another world outside of himself
- In and out. Window
- Free

This sensation of the Hamamelidae can be better understood through the following;

- Oppression and pressure
- Allergies, pricking, itching, stitching, tickling
- Conflict between higher existence and worldly existence
- Confusion
- Delusion and fancies
- Addictions
- Contact with and withdrawn in the same person
- Laughing
- Protection
- Moving

The conflict between higher existence and worldly existence is important in this Subclass. It can be seen as follows;

Enclosed:

- Mind; Delusions, imaginations, hallucinations, illusions; wall, walls; surrounded by high, is
- Mind; Delusions, imaginations, hallucinations, illusions; vegetable; existence, thinks he is leading a

"Surrounded by walls" gives the idea of being enclosed in space. This could cause a sensory deprivation. The feeling is similar to a vegetative existence.

- Mind; Delusions, imaginations, hallucinations, illusions; body, body parts; able to go out of, and walk around, looking down upon
- Mind; Delusions, imaginations, hallucinations, illusions; soul; body was too small for, or that it was separated from

There is the feeling of being enclosed and compressed in his own body. The body is heavy and restricting freedom, hence the soul escapes from the body and can be free.

- Mind; Delusions, imaginations, hallucinations, illusions; existence; form without, in vast space, illusion of

The form encloses him and the formless frees him.

Light & Heavy:

Lightness is a feeling of the spirit or in the realm of spirituality.

Heaviness is a feeling of worldly existence.

More Rubrics —

- Mind; Delusions, imaginations, hallucinations, illusions; light, penetrates through body
- Mind; Delusions, imaginations, hallucinations, illusions; light, incorporeal, immaterial, he is
- Mind; Delusions, imaginations, hallucinations, illusions; lighter than air
- Mind; Lightness, feeling of
- Mind; Delusions, imaginations, hallucinations, illusions; flying; she or he is
- Mind; Delusions, imaginations, hallucinations, illusions; floating; air, in

Heavy & Dragged down —

- Mind; Delusions, imaginations, hallucinations, illusions; marble statue, felt as if he were – Here we can see the idea of being heavy
- General; Sensations; largeness; single parts feel larger and thicker (Knerr) – this suggests a feeling of heaviness, of becoming more material, and more dragged down.

Absorbed:

There is a kind of shutting off from the world, when you go into a meditative state or one's own inner reality. In the first subclass remedies like Opium are related to Buddha. He never opens his eyes, permanently shut off from the world. In the 2nd subclass there is periodical withdrawal into a meditative state.

- Mind; Meditation – Cann-i, Cann-s, ham
- Mind; Meditation; desire for – ham
- Mind; Absent-mindedness – bros-g, Cann-I, Cann-s, fic-I, fic-mac, ham, jug-c, querc-r,
- Mind; Absorbed, buried in thought – bros-g, cann-I, cann-s, ham
- Mind; Fancies; absorbed in – cann-I

Absent minded and absorbed means the mind is not there, it is somewhere else.

Open & Shut:

- Head; Open; sensation – cann-I, cann-s
- Head; Open; sensation, opening and shutting – Cann-I, Cann-s
- Mind; Air; open; amel – Cann-I
- Mind; Absorbed, buried in thought; eyes, with closed – Cann-I
- Mind; Thoughts, sublime – Cann-I
- Mind; Unconsciousness, coma; closing eyes on – cann-I, cann-s
- Mind; Unconsciousness, coma; transient – cann-I
- Mind; Unconsciousness, coma; frequent spells, absences; loses himself every few moments – cann-I

Oppression:

Oppression is a compressed feeling, everything is enclosed. I want to open or release is the other side.

Some words used for the sensation of compression could be —

Load, tunnel, iron mask, anchor, soda-water bottle, controlled, rigid, limited time and space. There is the feeling of compression and of things closing in.

- Mind; Delusions, imaginations, hallucinations, illusions; cylinder, seemed to be a
- Mind; Delusions, imaginations, hallucinations, illusions; coating around him, has a white
- Mind; Delusions, imaginations, hallucinations, illusions; soda water, thinks he is a bottle of
- Mind; Anguish; oppression and tightness, with
- Mind; Anguish; oppression and tightness, with, air, amel, in open
- Mind; Anxiety; oppression, with
- Mind; Delusions, imaginations, hallucinations, illusions; room; walls; gliding together, seem

Allergies:

An allergy is basically a hypersensitivity to foreign agents. There are various nut remedies – Hazelnut, Walnut, Beech nut, White nut, Chestnut, Sweet Chestnut. Nuts are some of the most common allergens. There is a sensation of pricking, stitching, tingling and urticaria in remedies of the 2nd Subclass.

- Generalities; Allergy; poliallergic – jug-r
- Skin; Eruptions; urticaria; food, after – urt-u
- Skin; Eruptions; urticaria; liver disturbance, with – myrica
- Skin; Eruptions; urticaria; nodular, wheals, hives – cann-s, jug-c, urt-u

Confusion:

- Mind; Confusion of mind; knows not; where one is; nor whenever objects came around her – cann-s
- Mind; Confusion of mind; location, about – bros-g, cann-I, cann-s
- Mind; Confusion of mind; loses his way in well-known streets – bros-g, cann-I
- Mind; Fancies; confused – ham

The confusion: where am I? what is around me?, can be compared with Nux moschata from the 1st Subclass. And in the rubric 'loses his way in well-known streets' we also have Cann-i and Bros-g. Each Subclass has some of the quality of the subclass before it and the one after it. The major differences in the subclass are not the words used but in the reaction. The reaction in the 2nd subclass is to open or shut and not to withdraw as in the first Subclass.

Delusions & Fancies:

Delusions are connected to something higher, floating, free, spiritual, sublime.

We can see the desire for dancing and singing . The type of dance – one in which he is absorbed – in which there is freedom, and floating – more meditative and sublime, like Sufi dancing.

Delusion and fancies are a closing out of the outer reality. There is an opening of an inner reality by which they experience freedom and lightness.

Theorising – gigantic – they build air castles and move into them. Everything exaggerated, bigger, more beautiful, more colourful as if the sense organs had opened up.

Unfit for work and for the world - I am not ready to face the outside world. The opposite of this are fantasies that he is superhuman.

- Mind; Conversation; desires; hear sublime, to
- Mind; Delusions, imaginations, hallucinations, illusions; music; fancies he hears; sweetest and sublimest melody

- Mind; Thoughts, sublime, with eyes closed
- Mind; Dancing; desire for
- Mind; Delusions, imaginations, hallucinations, illusions; music; fancies he hears
- Mind; Delusions, imaginations, hallucinations, illusions; angels
- Mind; Dreams; god, goddess, of
- Mind; Delusions, imaginations, hallucinations, illusions; heaven; is in
- Mind; Theorizing; gigantic
- Mind; Delusions, imaginations, hallucinations, illusions; Christ
- Mind; Delusions, imaginations, hallucinations, illusions; flowers; gigantic
- Mind; Delusions, imaginations, hallucinations, illusions; better than others, that he is
- Mind; Delusions, imaginations, hallucinations, illusions; unfit; work, for
- Mind; Delusions, imaginations, hallucinations, illusions; unfit; world, for
- Mind; Fancies; vivid, lively
- Mind; Fancies; exaltation of

Addiction:

An escape from a boring, mundane, vegetative reality which is safe but boring. Makes them feel, free, light, beautiful, ecstatic. It could be spirituality, music, drugs like cannabis, travelling, seeing beautiful places, meditation, dancing, singing.

In the 2nd Subclass a little bit of movement is involved, unlike the 1st Subclass which is complete withdrawal

- Mind; Drug addiction, morphinism
- Mind; Sensitive, oversensitive; drugs, after recreational
- Mind; Delusions, imaginations, hallucinations, illusions; opium, felt as if he had taken
- Generalities; Tobacco; desire for tobacco
- Generalities; Tobacco; desire for tobacco; smoking, desire for
- Mind; Excitement, excitable; wine; after
- Mind; Wine, after
- Mind; Cheerful, gay, happy; intoxicated, as if
- Mind; Excitement, excitable; intoxicated, as if
- Mind; Vivacious; intoxication, as from
- Mind; Stupefaction, intoxicated as if

Contact with and withdrawn in the same person:

They need contact with the world but there are times when they need to withdraw as well. So, there are phases when they are in contact and communicating. Other times when they are shut off and in their own world of fantasy.

Laughing:

Laughter also means what is not funny seems funny. Also, what is not colourful seems colourful. What is not melodious seems melodious. This is how he is able to get his sensory stimulation.

- Mind; Laughing; every word said, at
- Mind; Laughing; uncontrollable
- Mind; Laughing; silly, foolish
- Mind; Laughing; involuntarily
- Mind; Laughing; immoderately
- Mind; Laughing; causeless
- Mind; Laughing; trifles, at
- Mind; Laughing; serious matters, over

Protection:

> The idea of cannabis is like a safe prison – safe, but isolated and unstimulating.
> Inside – seeing the same grey walls
> Outside – exciting, colourful but risky, so the need for protection arises.
> e.g. the situation of a woman in a colourless marriage

From Dr Sankaran's proving of Cann I from the book *The Substance of Homeopathy*:

Prover no. 15 puts it very clearly in the end where she says it is a common theme in the west when a teenager is exposed (too soon) to all of the danger of the world and he misses the security and safety of his/her home, so the child seeks warmth, security, and a community and often tries to achieve this through drugs.

Movement:

The feeling of compression may account for the need to move. The patient does not want to be confined to one place. This is reminiscent of travellers who move about, enclosed in their mobile homes but are able to look out of the windows.

Here are the main orders in the 2nd Subclass and some of the remedies

Hamamelidae
Urticales — • **Ulmaceae:** Ulm • **Moraceae:** Bros-g, Fic • **Cannabaceae:** Cann-I, Cann-s • **Urticaceae:** Urt-u • **Cecropiaceae:** Cecr
Hamamelidales — • **Hamamelidaceae:** Ham • **Platanaceae:** Platan
Juglandales — • **Juglandaceae:** Jug-c, Jug-n, Jug-r
Myricales — • **Myricaceae:** Myric
Fagales — • **Betulaceae:** Aln, Betul • **Fagaceae:** Cast-v, Fagu, Querc

Subclass 3

Caryophyllidae

When we consider the 3rd Subclass, we need to look at the most prominent remedy, namely Cactus grandiflorus. The main sensation of this remedy is that of CONSTRICTION. In the chest you have the symptom: "FEELS CLUTCHED AND RELEASED ALTERNATELY BY AN IRON BAND, or feels it expand and contract". This idea of expansion and contraction or limiting and expanding becomes the main dynamic of this subclass.

Caryophyllidae	
Typical remedy	Cactus Grandiflorus
Common features	Shrink & expand Grow smaller Clutched & Released Need to be useful Limit oneself Pressure No space Contract Compress

(*Continues*)

(*Continues*)

Caryophyllidae	
Sensation	Limited Cut off Expanded Bigger
Response	Shrink
Energy pattern	Shrinking Expanding
Pleasure	Expansion Merging
Music	Expanding Merging
Example	Sponge
Words	Clutched Released Constricted Limited Bigger Smaller Expanded
Animal	Birds
Mineral	3rd row

1. Cut off by shrinking

There is aversion to company and cutting off the world by *shrinking*. When shrinking he goes *within,* and the *world is out.* The feeling of being *useless* and *meaningless* accompanies this. The reaction of the 3rd subclass could be defined as *shrinking* and *growing smaller* with *indifference* to surroundings, pain, and death.

Rubrics —

- Generalities; smaller, shrinking sensation – **CACT**
- Generalities; Constriction; caged, as if, with wires twisted tighter and tighter – **CACT**
- Generalities; Contractions, strictures, stenoses – **CACT,** fago, phyt, rheum

- Mind; Delusions, imaginations, smaller – anh, **Cact,** cere-b
- Mind; Delusions, imaginations, smaller, he is – **Cact,** cere-b
- Mind; Curl up, desire to – phyt
- Mind; Delusions, imaginations; smaller; things; grow – cact
- Mind; Sadness; lies curled up into a ball – phyt
- Mind; Delusions, imaginations; meaningless, everything is – phyt
- Mind; Delusions, imaginations; life; meaningless, is – phyt
- Mind; Delusions, imaginations; useless, is – phyt
- Mind; Meaningless, feels – cere-b, phyt

2. Becoming one by expanding

Expansion, open, to be vivacious, helpful, to speak, to converse, communicate and to do good things, not for self but for others, benevolence, making plans which are useful. *Expanding and becoming open to everything and become one with everyone.*

Rubrics —

- Mind; Delusions, imaginations; body, body parts; enlarged – anh, phyt
- Mind; Delusions, imaginations; enlarged – **Anh,** carn-g, phyt
- Mind; Delusions, imaginations; enlarged; he is – anh, phyt
- Mind; Delusions, imaginations; enlarged; objects are – **Anh**
- Mind; Plans; important and useful – cere-b
- Mind; Deeds; desire to perform – cere-b
- Mind; Deeds; desire to perform; useful – **cere-b**
- Mind; Merging of self with one's environment – anh

3. Alternation of states

The alternation of states can also be seen as a feature in this subclass.

Rubrics —

- Mind; Indifference, apathy; alternating; activity, with – sarr
- Mind; Cheerfulness; alternating with; sadness – lapa
- Mind; Cheerfulness; alternating with; moroseness - lapa

Here are the main orders of the Caryophyllidae with some remedies.

Caryophyllidae
Caryophyllales — • **Amaranthaceae:** Achy, Paro-i • **Cactaceae:** Anh, Cact, Carn-g, Cere-b • **Caryophyllaceae:** Agro • **Chenopodiaceae:** Aphis, Atri, Chen-a • **Nyctaginaceae:** Boerh • **Portulacaceae:** Peti, Phyt, Phyt-b
Polygonales — • **Polygonaceae:** Fago, Rheum, Rumx
Plumbaginales — • **Plumbaginaceae:** Plumbg
Nepenthales (Trapped & Released) - • **Droseraceae:** Dion-m, Dros • **Sarraceniaceae:** Sarr

Subclass 4

Dilleniidae

Typical of the Dillenidae is the remedy Bryonia alba. We see in it the aversion to movement, the desire for rest, the desire for a home, the fear of financial instability. The dynamic here is the need for stability and the sensitivity to be disturbed.

Dilleniidae	
Typical remedy	Bryonia
Common features	Home Comfort Cosiness Obstacle Barrier In and out Must cross the barrier Disturbed Rest, wants to retain the same position Home wants to stay in or leave the home Go out
Sensation	Averse to change or desire for change

(*Continues*)

(*Continues*)

Dilleniidae	
Perception	Comfort Obstacle
Dreams/fears	Loss of stability
Response	Stay in comfort Move out
Energy pattern	Stillness Disturbance
Pleasure	Comfort Rest Quiet Undisturbed
Music	Relaxing Comforting
Example	Door (protection and block)
Situation	Woman held by her children
Pathology	
Modalities	>rest <movement
Other features	Disturbed easily
Symbol	Resort
Words	Disturbed Routine Same Home Stability Held Obstacle Cross the obstacle Flow Stagnated Door
Animal	Mammals Sloth
Mineral	4th row
Plant	Gymnosperms
Nosode	Medorrhinum

1. The home, family and comfort

The home represents a place of comfort. It is where you can rest and gain respite. The home is also a shelter it keeps out the elements and keeps us safe. Similar feelings are provided by the family, they offer us protection and comfort and represent safety. So, one of the main feelings we see in this subclass is the *need for home. Home means comfort, family, money, what is familiar to them.* When away from this place, he feels that *he has lost or is losing his position of comfort.* Their *adaptation is to find and to retain this place of comfort, of stability, of feeling settled.*

Rubrics —

- Mind; Bed; get out of, wants to; home, go and – **BRY**
- Mind; Dreams; house, houses, of – brass, **Bry,** kola, salx-f
- Mind; Dreams; house, houses, of; find house where he wants to go, cannot – kola
- Mind; House; amel – cycl
- Mind; Dreams; family, of; own – choc, kola, paeon, salx-f
- Mind; Dreams; death, of; family, in – paeon
- Mind; Dreams; family; own, losing his – choc

2. Strange and familiar

Familiar is well known from long or having a close association and strange is unusual or surprising, not previously visited, seen or encountered. There is the need to stay with the familiar, the routine and avoid any change.

Rubrics —

- Mind; Delusion, imaginations; strange; land in a – bry
- Mind; Dreams; cities; strange – kola
- Mind; Delusion, imaginations; strange, familiar things are - choc
- Mind; Delusion, imaginations; strange, familiar places are – salx-f

3. In and out

To be inside the home, place of comfort is *one side* of the Dilleniidae. At times, this position of comfort becomes stagnant, monotonous, like water which is not flowing, or has met a barrier. At some point, there comes a stage where they need to go beyond this, and move out. But here the need to go out is a short lasting one, with the need to return to the place of stability

Rubrics —

- Mind; Home; go desires, to; go out, when they – **Bry**
- Mind; Anxiety; house or room; agg; entering, on – **Rhod**
- Mind; Escape, desires to; house, wants to get out of – elat
- Mind; Home; leave, desires, to – **Bry**, elat, salx-f

4. Doors

The door is an opening by which one goes from inside to outside. They are held indoors by their own attachment, need for security, love, affection, care. Indoors is smooth, undisturbed and comfortable. But the door can also become an obstacle or a barrier which they are kept in where it can feel like it is stagnating.

Rubrics —

- Mind; Dreams; doors – salx-f
- Mind; Dreams; doors; closing – salx-f

5. Change

Change reflects the need to move out. Again, because *inside is comfortable but stagnant.* It is the process of staying inside, in comfort or moving into new reality.

Do you want to stay in comfort OR do you want to get out? *And at some point*, there is a need to come out. But there can also be an aversion to change, they don't want any change to the status quo as this can cause discomfort. Therefore, they seek change, but only with a firm foot in their place of stability.

Rubrics —

- Mind; Change; desire for – **BRY**, **Salx-f**
- Mind; Dreams; changing; places often – led
- Mind; Monotony, overwhelming sensation of - brass

Here are the main orders of the Dilleniidae with some remedies –

Dilleniidae
Dilleniales: • **Paeoniaceae:** paeon
Theales: • **Theacaeae:** Thea • **Hypericaceae:** Hyper
Ebenales: • **Ebenacaea:** Diosp-k
Malvales (Attached, clingy): • **Cistaceae:** Cist • **Dipterocarpaceae:** • **Malvaceae:** Abel, Goss • **S**terculiaceae: Abroma-a, Cac, Choc, Kola, Theob • Tiliaceae: Til
Primulales: • **Primulaceae:** Cycl, Hott, Lysim • **Myrsinaceae:** Emb
Cucurbitales (Disturbed): • **Cucurbitaceae:** Bry • **Violaceae**
Ericales: • **Ericaceae**
Salicales: • **Salicaceae**
Capparales (Obstruction, flow): • **Brassicaceae** • **Capparidaceae**

Subclass 5

Rosidae

A typical remedy of the Rosidae is Rhus-tox and this can be used to understand this subclass. We see in the dynamic of Rhus-tox the opposite of Bryonia (4th Subclass), namely restlessness, the need to go out.

Rosidae	
Typical remedy	Rhus Toxicodendron
Common features	Tight Tied Squeezed Constricted Oppressed Pressure outward Get out Bound, band, stiff Domestic violence <in room >movement >stretching Restless Change desire Travel amel

Sensation	Cannot move Claustrophobic Can't breathe Can't take tight clothes
Perception	Suffocated Stuck
Dreams/Fears	Stuck
Sensitivity	Stiffness
Response	Get out Move
Energy pattern	Stuck, movement
Pleasure	Going out Moving
Music	Movement
Example	Trap
Situation	Wife of a violent drunkard
Pathology	Joints
Modalities	>movement
Symbol	Sportsman
Words	Holding Tight Tied Squeezed Stuck Bound Desire change Stiff, rigid Can't move
Animal	Mollusc: Cephalopods Spiders Insects Lac equinum
Mineral	2nd row right hand side 5th row
Nosode	Tuberculinum Carcinosinum Leprominium

1. Pressing outwards

There is pressure and pains which are extending outwards. Everything is *outwards because inside* there is the *sensation of being caught, tight, stiff and stuck.* The pressure is so much that the *movement is outwards*

Rubrics —

- Nose; Pain; pressing – **Astra-e,** bos-s, **Euph,** gran, **Laur,** manc, melal-l, mez, myric, prun, ptel, raph, rhus-v, **Ruta,**
- Nose; Pain; pressing; bones – laur, prun
- Head; Pain, headache; pressing; extending, to; outward – anac, ang, cedr, daph, euph, galph, guai, hyper, indg, **laur, Meli, Meli-a,** merl, **Mez,** passi, phys, **Prun,** ptel, rat, **RHUS-T,** rhus-v
- Head; Pain, headache; pressing; brain; outward – daph, guai, indg, laur, **Meli, Meli-a,** phys, Rhus-t, rhus-v
- Generalities; Pain; pressing; glands, liver, spleen etc, extending; outward – Rhus-t
- Generalities; Pain; pressing; upper limbs; extending; outward – Anac
- Chest; Pain; pressing; extending; outward – ang, gran, **Ruta**, seneg
- Abdomen; Pain; pressing; extending; outward – anac, ang, euph, gran, guia, mez, Prun, Rhus-t
- Eye; Pain; pressing; extending; outward – bapt, **Com,** daph, euph-pu, **Guai,** guare, iber, laur, meli, meli-a, merl, **Mez, Passi, Prun,** Rhus-t, **Seneg**
- Ear; Pain; pressing; extending; outward – guare, prun

2. Violence at home

Domestic *violence* occurs at home which is supposed to be your *place of comfort.* So as a result of this the *natural reaction* here is to *get out*

Rubrics —

- Mind; Delusions, imaginations; danger; world is dangerous – rhus-g
- Mind; Delusions, imaginations; enemy; surrounded by – **Anac**, bani-c
- Mind; Delusions, imaginations; injury; injured, of being; everybody has injured him – rhus-g
- Mind; Delusions, imaginations; murder; family, that she will, her; hatchet, with a – jab

3. Stiffness

Other words for stiffness are *caught, tight, band, plug, hoop, squeezing, bound. Squeezing* is to *press firmly* from all sides, compress. When you squeeze you *make tighter.* A *plug* is something that *fills a hole very tightly.* A *hoop* or band obstructs, fixes and *does not allow you to move.* There is constriction, both internally and externally. There is constriction, tightness, band, plug. All the above words denote the *feeling of being stuck and unable to move. The reaction is to move, to get out.*

Rubrics —

- Mind; Dreams; bound, being – **Bapt**, Citl-l, coca,
- Mind; Dreams; fights; generals, with six or seven black, who garrotted him and bound him with ropes, causing agony of mind – coca
- Mind; Dreams; ropes, chains, rings; chained to bed – **Bapt**
- Mind; Dreams; encircled tightly, being – ruta
- Mind; Delusions, imaginations; trapped, he is – anac, com, latex, mangi, rhus-g, rhus-t

4. Room aggravates

Room means *inside.* Inside there is the *experience of being caught, stuck, trapped* and most importantly unable to move. *Violence* is experienced *inside the home.* That is why they are worse inside and there is *desire to move out* and go in the open.

Rubrics —

- Chest; Oppression; room, in warm – anac, phyll-a, trif-p
- Chest; Pain; pressing; room, in; agg – laur
- Chest; Room, in; agg – anac, Laur, **Mez,** phyll-a, **RHUS-T,** saroth, **Seneg**, trif-p
- Mind; House; agg – anac, enal-c, laur, **RHUS-T,** ruta
- Mind; Room, in; agg – anac, merl, **RHUS-T**, ruta
- Head; External; room, in, agg – cist, indg, **Laur,** ptel
- Head; Pain, headache, room, agg – bos-s, coca, com, croto-t, euph, jatr, laur, merl, mez, ptel, rhus-t, **SENEG**, sin-a, Sin-n, Tong
- Vision; Room, in, agg – croto-t

5. Open ameliorates

Open means *outside.* Outside there is *freedom. Not caught, not trapped* and they can *move.* Inside the pressure is too much and it forces them to go out. An example is the Leguminosae family, like peas in the pod. Inside there is a lot of pressure. It is closed and eventually the *pressure builds up* so much that they *explode* and the peas *come out.*

Rubrics —

- Mind; Anger; air, open; desires – anac
- Mind; Anxiety; air; open, in; amel – anac, **Croto-t**, Laur, **RHUS-T**
- Mind; Fear; air; open; amel – **Croto-t,** Rhus-t
- Mind; Restlessness, nervousness; air, open, amel – latex, laur
- Mind; Self-control; loss of; air, amel. In open – caj
- Head; Fullness; air, in open; amel. – spirae
- Head; Noises, air, open, amel. - indg

6. Restless, move must, motion amel

Reaction to the pressure that is felt inside, the feeling being caught, stiff, bound, in a band and unable to move causes immense restlessness, need to walk and move. Movement is the *opposite of being inside and stuck.* Movement is *freedom.*

Rubrics —

- Mind; Walk, walking; must – caj, lepi, mez, paull-p, rhus-t, ruta, spirae
- Mind; Delusions, imaginations; die; about to; moves, unless he – rhus-g
- Mind; Anxiety; driving from place to place – anac, coca, **Rhus-t,** ruta, seneg
- Mind; Anxiety; motion; amel – rhus-t, saroth, seneg
- Mind; Anguish; motion, amel. – saroth
- Mind; Dreams; journey, travelling – aza, bani-c, bros-g, croto-t, galph, glyc-g, hura, hyper, **Indg,** linu-c, Mangi, Mez, pot-a, **RHUS-T,** rob, sin-a, Xan
- Mind; Wander; desires to – bapt, oxyt
- Vertigo; Motion; amel – com

7. Suffocation/oppression/respiration difficult

The suffocation and oppression occurs inside *because of the pressure* and inability to move.

Rubrics —

- Chest; Pressure; agg; clothes, of – ail, **CROTO-T**, gran, meli, meli-a, mez,
- Respiration; Difficult; clothing agg – glyc-g, manc, meli, meli-a, mez, pyrus
- Respiration; Difficult; room; closed, in – mangi
- Respiration; Difficult; restlessness, with – **Meli,** prun
- Respiration; Oppression, from; abdomen, in – mez
- Respiration; Oppression, from; throat, in – guia
- Chest; Fullness; oppression, with – Croto-t, prun, ruta
- Chest; Oppression; air, open; amel. – anac, **Bapt,** phyll-a, trif-p
- Chest; Oppression; clothing agg – gran, meli, meli-a, mez
- Chest; Oppression; motion; amel – rhus-t, **Seneg**
- Chest; Oppression; rest, during – **Seneg**
- Chest; Pain; pressure; agg; clothing, of - ail

Here are some of the orders of the Rosidae with their main sensation and some remedies —

Rosidae
Rosales (Compressed from all sides, suffocated) • **Crassulaceae:** Cot • **Hydrangeaceae:** Hydrang • **Rosaceae:** Agri, Crat, Laur, Prun-c • **Saxifragaceae:** Saxi-g
Myrtales • **Combretaceae:** Term-a, Term-c • **Lythraceae:** Cuph • **Myrtaceae:** Caj, Eucal, Syzg • **Ongaraceae:** Oeno • **Thymelaceae:** Daph, Mez
Fabales (Bursting out, Splitting apart) • **Mimosaceae:** Mim-p • **Caesalpiniaceae:** Cop, Haem • **Papillionaceae:** Alf, Bapt, Dol, Lath, Meli, Phys, Rob, Tama

Rosidae
Malphigiales • **Caricaceae:** Cari • **Erythoxylaceae:** Coca • **Geraniaceae:** Erod, Ger • **Krameriaceae:** Rat • **Linaceae:** Linu-u • **Malpigiaceae:** Bani-c, Galph • **Oxalidaceae:** Oxal • **Passifloraceae:** Passi
Euphorbiales (Tied, Tight Bound) • **Euphorbiaceae:** Croto-t, Euph, Hura, Manc
Sapindales (Stiff, Tight, Tense, Can't move) • **Anacardiaceae:** Anac, Com, Mangi, Rhus-t • **Hippocastanaceae:** Aesc • **Meliacaea:** Aza • **Rutaceae:** Ang, Jab, Ptel, Ruta, Xan • **Simaroubaceae:** Cedr • **Sapindaceae:** Neg • **Zygophyllaceae:** Guai
Rhamnales • **Rhamnaceae:** Rham-cal • **Vitaceae:** Vitis
Cornales • **Cornaceae:** Corn
Santales • **Santalaceae:** Santa • **Viscaceae:** Visc
Celastrales • **Celastraceae:** Euon

Subclass 6

Asteriidae

This rather large group includes remedies like Arnica, Ignatia, Cicuta, Belladonna among others. When we try to see what the common thread or dynamic in these remedies can be, we can see that all of them have the idea of trauma, shock, terror, attack, violence, convulsions, etc. This gives us the dynamic of the 6th subclass, namely violence.

Asteriidae	
Typical remedy	Stramonium
Common features	Sudden large impact Violence Rage Convulsion Injury Blow Shock Attack Fear, terror Escape, run, hide Alert

(*Continues*)

(*Continues*)

Asteriidae	
	Rapid Exhilaration Impulsive Shameless
Sensation	Paralyzed Violent Escape
Perception	Attack
Dreams/fears	Terror Violence Attack
Response	Fight & Flight
Energy pattern	Terror Panic
Pleasure	Thrill Adrenaline rush Horror movies
Music	Thrilling Exciting Fast
Example	Tiger
Situation	Big attack
Pathology	Convulsion
Other features	Shocked Injured
Symbol	Rollercoaster
Words	Big impact Attack Injured Violent Terror Fright Convulsion Blow Shock
Animal	Reptiles Lac leoninum
Mineral	Heavy metals: 6th row
Nosode	Syphilinum

1. Violence

The response is *fight* or *flight* either *escape* or *aggression*

Rubrics —

- Mind; Destructiveness; clothing, of – **Bell,** hyos, **Ign,** nux-v, **Stram**
- Mind; Vehemence; rage leading to deeds of, agg – **BELL, Chin,** cic, con, **HYOS, Ign, Led, Lon-p,** lycrpr, **Nux-v, STRAM**
- Mind; Rage; fury; strength increased – **BELL,** Hyos, lob, Stram
- Mind; Insanity, madness; escape, desire to – **Bell,** dig, nux-v, stram,
- Mind; Escape, desire to; delirium in – atro, **BELL,** cic, dat-f, dig, dubin, eup-pur, **Hyos,** hyosin, nux-v, oena, oper, past, sol-m, **Sol-n, STRAM,** val
- Mind; Escape, desire to; delusions during – **BELL, Hyos, Sol-n**
- Mind; escape, desire to; jumps suddenly up from bed – Atro, **Bell,** chin, cic, dat-f, dig, **Hyos,** hyosin, **Nux-v,** oper, past, sol-m, **Sol-n, Stram**

2. Fear with clinging or paralysis

Rubrics —

- Mind; Fear; fright – bell, **Ign,** olea, **Stram**
- Mind Fear; Mania, in; fright agg - **Ign, Stram**
- Mind; Fear; insanity, of losing his reason; fright, fear agg – **Ign, Stram**
- Mind; Forgetfulness; sudden and periodical, pain, from fright – bell
- Mind; Fright, fear agg, ailments from – abrot, aego-p. aeth, **Agn, Arn, Art-v,** atro, **BELL,** bell-p, calen, **Caps,** card-m, **CHAM, Chin,** Chrysan, **CIC, Cina, COFF,** coff-t, **Con,** corn, **Cycl, Dig, Dulc,** erig, **Euphr,** frax, **GELS,** gins, grin, **HYOS,** hyosin, **IGN, Ip,** jac-c, led, meny, mimul-l, mit, nic-r, **NUX-V, Oena,** olea, onos, **Plan,** sol-n, spig, **STRAM,** stry, sumb, tab, teucr, unc-t, valer, verb
- Mind; Fright, fear agg, ailments from; anger, with – **Ign,**
- Mind; Fright, fear agg, ailments from; children, in highly excitable, nervous – hyosin
- Mind; Fright, fear agg, ailments from; fear of fright still remaining – bell, olea
- Mind; Fright, fear agg, ailments from; grief, with – **Ign**
- Mind; Fear; speak, cannot – Acon, arn, Gels, hyos, Ign
- Mind; Fear; alone, being; light and company, wants – **Bell, Gels,** hyos, **STRAM**

3. Alert/rapid/quick to act

We will see alertness, wakefulness and quickness as there is always the need to be ready in case an escape from violence and trauma is required.

Rubrics —

- Mind; Thoughts; rapid, quick – bell, cham, chin, **Coff, Hyos,** ign, nic-r, onos, **Valer**

4. Restlessness

Restlessness is the need to move, as an escape reaction to the intense attack and fear they are perceiving

Rubrics —

- Mind; Runs about; room in – bell, **Coff,** hyos, spig-m
- Mind; Delirium; walk about, must – **Absin,** art-v, cham, cina

5. Sleeplessness

Rubrics —

- Sleep; Sleeplessness; tobacco, after abuse of – gels, nux-v, plan, scut
- Sleep; Sleeplessness; women, especially; excited – cimic, coff, coffin, hyos, senec

6. Convulsions, injury

Rubrics —

- Female; Abortion; convulsive, spasmodic – cham, **Hyos**, **Ip,** tanac
- Mind; Excitement, excitable; convulsions; before, epileptic – **Art-v,** bell, coff, stram
- Generalities; Convulsions, spasms; excitement, emotional, agg – **Art-v,** asaf, **Bell, CHAM, Cic, Cina, Coff,** con, **Gels, HYOS, IGN, Ip, NUX-V, Oena,** sol-n, **Stram,** stry, **Upa**
- Mind; Rage, fury; convulsions; during – **Bell,** cham, hyos, nux-v, Stram
- Mind; Fear; struck by those coming toward him, of being – **ARN,** bell, ign, stram

7. Mania

Rubrics —

- Mind; Mania, madness; anger, vexation, after – bell, **Hyos,** ign, nux-v
- Mind; Mania, madness; runs; about – bell, con, hyos, spig-m, stram
- Mind; Mania, madness; wild – bell, hyos, senec, **Stram**
- Face; Distortion; rage, in maniacal – **Bell,** hyos, nux-v, **STRAM**

8. Sexuality

Shamelessness

Remedies —

- Origanum – hysteria, sexual irritation from excessive
- Stramonium – Insanity, madness, erotic, sexual
- Conium – Hysteria, sexual excitement from suppression of
- Lamiales – has to do with pleasurable excitement

Rubrics —

- Mind; Lasciviousness; erections; without – agn, caps, **IGN,** meny
- Mind; Naked, wants to be – **Bell,** cham, **HYOS,** lycpr, **Stram**

9. Exhilaration, loquacity, Dancing, Singing, Laughing, Lively, Active

Rubrics —

- Mind; Exhilaration; mania, in merry – bell, cham, gels, hyos, ign, **Stram,** valer
- Mind; Dance desires to – **BELL, Cic,** con, dat-f, ign, ilx-p, sant, **STRAM,** Tab
- Mind; Loquacity – abrot, absin, aego-p, aeth, agn, arn, atro, **BELL,** cham, Chrysan, **Cic,** cich, cina, **Coff,** coff-t, Con, cyna, dat-m, dig, **DULC,** eup-pur, **GELS, Hydrc, HYOS, Ign,** ip, lact, lob, lycpr, mand, meny, nabal, **Nux-v,** oena, onos, oper, parth, past, physal, plect, pyre-p, sol-t, **STRAM, Stroph,** Tab, **Tarax, TEUCR, Thea,** thymol, thymu, **Valer,** Verb

10. Confusion & Intoxicated

Rubrics —

- Mind; Confusion of mind; paroxysms of pain, during – apoc, **Cham, Coff,** dulc
- Clinical; Catalepsy; fright, fear agg – art-v, bell, **Gels,** ign
- Mind; Confusion of mind; intoxicated feeling; carousal, after a – **NUX-V**
- Mind; Confusion of mind; intoxicated feeling – **Bell,** cent, **Chin, DIG,** dulc, grin, hyos, ign, lam, led, Leon, mand, mill, Myos-a, **NUX-V,** olea, phel, valer

11. Beauty

In China, we see beautiful colours, sense of beauty, artistic. Beauty is the opposite of black, ugly, scary. Beauty and the Beast.

Rubrics —

- Mind; Delusions, imaginations; beautiful, wonderful - Absin, **BELL, Coff,** dat-a, nic-r, tab

Here are some of the orders of the Asteriidae with their main sensation and some remedies —

Asteriidae
Apiales (Umbellifers) **(Sudden big blow/knife/attack without warning):** • **Araliaceae:** Aral, Gins • **Apiaceae:** Aeth, Asaf, Cic, Con
Solanales **(Terror, Fright):** • **Solanaceae:** Atro, Bell, Caps, Dulc, Hyos, Stram, Tab • **Convolvaceae:** Convo, Ipom • **Menyanthaceae:** Meny • **Hydrophyllacaea:** Erio-c
Gentianales **(shock):** • **Apocynaceae:** Apoc, Olnd, Rauw • **Loganiaceae:** Cur, Gels, Ign, Nux-v, Spig • **Asclepiaceae:** Asc, Cund • **Gentianaceaea:** Canch

Scrophulariales (Separation seen as trauma/fear): • Acanthaceae: Just • Orobanchaceae: Epip • Oleaceae: Jasm • Scrophulariaceae: Dig, Euphr, Scroph, Verb
Plantaginales: • **Plantaginaceae:** Plan
Rubiales **(Alertness):** • **Rubiaceae:** Chin, coff, Ip
Lamiales **(Thrill, sexuality):** • **Boraginaceae:** Borag, Onos, Symph • **Lamiaceae:** Oci, Orig, Teucr • **Verbenaceae:** Agn, Verbe-o
Dipsacales **(Suffocation):** • **Adoxaceae:** Adox • **Valerianaceae:** Valer
Campanulales: • **Lobeliacaeae:** Lob
Asterales **(Injury):** • **Asteraceae:** Abrot, Arn, Bell-p, Calen, Cham, Cina, Eup-per

SECTION THREE

Superclass comes after Subclass

Having discovered the main dynamic of the six subclasses in the dicotyledons of the plant kingdom, I began sharing this with colleagues from across the world.

There was a group of Brazilian homoeopaths at The Other Song. I thought the best way to convey the six subclasses was to do a small experiment. I asked them to think of Mumbai city and how they would describe it in a few words and what was their response to it. I was hoping that each one would give a different perception and response and such responses would illustrate the six subclasses.

Of course, perceptions and reactions vary from person to person. One can say, "I want to withdraw and be safe inside," for instance. Another would say, "I do not want to deal with it right now; I want to block it out". A third one would say they desire security because they feel unsafe, while a fourth person would say it is highly restricting. The fifth would reply, "I want to get out. It is too suffocating." The sixth would say, "It is too traumatic and dangerous."

It was observed that all of the responses could be narrowed down to the six dynamics that were mentioned. And it happened exactly like that. The first six people who volunteered to share their experience could clearly be seen to fit the dynamic of the six subclasses.

Later, when I went home, I got a question in my mind. Each of the six participants who shared their experience fitted into one of the six subclasses of plant kingdom. I wondered, then, how it could be that there are just plant perceptions. Animals and minerals should also be present, so where were they? This was illogical in every way.

Then it occurred to me that the dynamic of each of the six subclasses was not restricted to the plant kingdom, and that they share this dynamic with a certain group of minerals and animals.

The realisation that the dynamic we discussed in the subclasses of plants is not exclusive to plants was my "Eureka!" moment. Additionally, minerals, plants, and animals exhibit similar traits at the level of the dynamics. The concept of Superclasses originated in this situation. When there is a blurring of the lines between minerals, plants, and animals, you can see a certain collection of plants, animals, and minerals under the same dynamic. And I came up with the moniker "Superclass" because it seemed to be a logical extension of the 'subclass' idea.

Numerous experiments were conducted during this phase. In particular, the WISE processes were crucial. Occasionally, we would take 500 people at a time in groups. They would undergo an experiment from us. Asking what their fundamental experience is would reveal their perception and response. This would allow us to understand the dynamic. Each time it was discovered, it fit into one of these six categories. This shows that there is not a seventh classification or dynamic. At this point, it was obvious that the Superclass paradigm was a key one. This is because it classifies dynamics in a very broad way.

A note on the WISE: Witnessing Inner Song Experience

W-WITNESSING	• Observing from a distance • Withoutjudgement • Withoutlikes/dislikes,wants/ don'twants • Observe in most minute details (called Saakshi Bhaav in Sanskrit)
I-INNER	The wholedrama isinside, notoutside.
S-SONG	There is a pattern, a melody that is playing within us, across all our different situations. Irrespective of the situations, this melody remains thesame.
E-EXPERIENCE	That pattern is an experience, not just a thought, not an emotion, not an image.Itisa sensation,an energypattern whichis anexperience. It is beyond the mind, beyond logic and reason; felt in the body as well as themind at thesametime.

The WISE processes are something that I have been developing in the last few years. They have proven to be an incredible therapeutic tool in themselves, as well as tremendously assisting in the case taking and analysis processes. In a way the Superclass and the WISE processes have come about together and through each other we have a better understanding of both. In the case examples given in this book we will demonstrate the use of the WISE processes. However, it will not be the main focus of this book, if you wish to gain a deeper insight into their use and practical applications I would refer you to my book, "*From Shadow to Light*" which deals with this topic comprehensively.

Studying these dynamics resulted in a significant discovery. While perception and action are two sides of the same coin, as are Sensations and reactions. However, the reaction is more illustrative or obvious. In contrast, there may be some ambiguity what the perception actually is,we were not always able to determine which dynamic it belonged to. However, when we observe the reaction, for instance, if he withdraws, it must fall within the first dynamic. If one is sensitive to anything frightful or terrifying, dig deeper. Any of the dynamics could be behind it. All Superclasses are capable of experiencing dread. But what characterises the dynamic and establishes the Superclass is the response to the dread. If you go a little further and sharpen your perception some more, it will reveal the precise dynamic. Practically speaking, this can lead to uncertainty. In order to avoid identifying the dynamic based solely on perception, we need to look at the exact response. Response-related dynamics are much more obvious and reliable.

The three kingdoms are not the only places where dynamics and accompanying Superclasses exist. It is also possible to classify nosodes and sarcodes into specific Superclasses. This also holds true for additional categories of plant remedies, such as the Monocotyledons, Gymnosperms, etc. It is also possible to classify unrelated groups like Fungi. We are still in the early stages of evolution of this classification. At this stage the classification and definition of everything are neither complete nor precise, particularly when discussing remedies that do not belong to one of the six subclasses of the dicotyledons. In these subclasses the perception and reaction are very apparent. It is also obvious how each subclass fits into a higher Superclass. We have been able to further specify the characteristics of the Superclasses because the subclasses are so clear to us. As a result, the subclass description is very similar to or parallel to the Superclass description. To comprehend the Superclass, we can use the knowledge from the corresponding subclass. This area has the most clarity. This is significant because it can be challenging to comprehend animals. Bivalve, gastropod, and cephalopod are a few examples of molluscs. Each group within the mollusc has a unique perception and reaction. You cannot define one Superclass for all the molluscs.

Why is it like this that the Subclass gives us the flavour of the Superclass?

The Superclass represents the dynamic response. The dynamic response is a response to a certain perception, sensation, or experience. What do we mean when we say the dynamic response of the 6th Superclass is Violence or 'fight or flight'? We are implying that the perception or sensation is one that would elicit this response. i.e. one of threat, terror, danger, or violence. In the 4th Superclass we say the dynamic response is to find a position of stability. The perception is that the position is unstable, disturbed, or changeable. The response to this perception or sensation is best seen in the plant kingdom. In the mineral and animal kingdoms this response and perception are definitely present. They are overshadowed often by the features of the kingdom. Such as survival and competition in animal kingdom. Lack or loss of structure in the mineral kingdom. The kingdom co-ordinate in some sense is more prominent in the animal and mineral kingdoms. Among the kingdoms, the plant kingdom sensation and response defines the Superclass quality most clearly. More recently , I found that the superclass quality is expressed in an even more pure form through the understanding of specific Neurotransmitters. We will discuss this later. For the moment the 6 subclasses of dicotyledons are much more explored and known. So, we can use that knowledge to understand the respective Superclass better.

Originally, we had defined the main words of each Superclass. From that point we could jump into the understanding of the Subclasses of the dicotyledons. This was where we were able to refine the various defining features. Whether it was an atypical remedy, a dream or a fear. Through these we tried to understand the entire Subclass. These are only broad hints and should not be taken literally all the time. It is important to understand the deeper aspects and to use these as pointers. We had created a plant chart which defined the characteristics of the Subclasses. It is used to understand the characteristics of the corresponding Superclass. This chart and its founding paradigm have been tested over many cases. It is very helpful, demonstrating the importance and utility of this new classification.

The idea and use of the Superclass is like an atlas. For example, if I asked you to find a brown building you would want to know where is its location. The place to start is on which continent is the brown building. This can be compared with the Superclass. The next classification we will need is the sub-continent. In homeopathy we would think of the kingdom. The next information is the country, and this is the Subclass. Going from the country we would then look for the state. In homeopathy this would be the order. Having the location of the state, we could narrow it down to the city (the family, in Homeopathy). We would then need to know location of the building according to the street. This is comparable to the specific remedy. Once in the right street, the correct building is determined by the qualities of the building, such as it is a brown double story building, this would be the source qualities of the remedy we are looking for. This is a systematic classification and analysis used in conjunction with our knowledge of materia medica which ensures our accuracy and confidence in the remedy prescribed.

ATLAS						
Asia	South Asia	India	Maharashtra	Mumbai	17, Joseph Street	Brown Building
Continent	Subcontinent	Country	State	City	Street number	Qualities of the building
Superclass	Kingdom Class	Subclass	Order	Family	Remedy	Source
Basic Dynamic	What kind of ...(Class) sensitivity, survival Or structure issue?	What type of... (Subclass) issue within that?	What quality of that issue?	What shade of that quality?	What specific features within that shade?	What connects to the source?

There is a second way the Superclass classification can be used. It can show a similarity between a certain animal group with a certain plant group or with a certain mineral group. This gives a much broader understanding of the relationships of remedies. For example, if we are thinking of a particular mineral we could also think of a corresponding plant or animal in that Superclass.

Thirdly this is a paradigm by which we can understand the world we live in. We can have a perspective to see how people are, how the world is. It is not just limited to finding a homeopathic remedy.

The Superclass paradigm is a natural companion to the WISE processes, helping us gain a deeper understanding. Knowing the Superclass also helps keeping us grounded while exploring the patients' deepest experiences.

It is important that these ideas presented in this book should not be used superficially. The assignation of the Superclass should only be done when the patient reaches the depth of their experience. We know we are in the deepest experience of the patient when it is confirmed from different angles. The Superclass also becomes apparent at that level. It doesn't need guess work or thinking. It should come from a place beyond logic and thought. The homeopath doesn't need to classify people when their central pattern emerges. It becomes quite obvious.

The features of the superclass/subclass mentioned in this book should correspond with the words and expressions of the patient. No theorising is needed on the part of the homeopath. But one needs to make sure that the words come from a deeper place. Each word of the patient should not be taken at face value.

For example, if a person says I like to fight, it should not be automatically classified into the 6th Superclass. One needs to understand that expression in its totality and in depth and look to see what is happening at the deepest level of the patient's experience. That is where the patient will automatically put themselves into the correct Superclass. We will not have to put them anywhere, the information from the case will classify itself.

We should also keep in mind that there will be some overlap of qualities from the different Superclasses. In general, the patient from a certain Superclass can have also some features of the Superclass before and after the Superclass of the patient. In a case of the second Superclass, we may see overlap with the first Superclass. You may see the dynamic of withdrawal. We may also see some of the features of the 3rd Superclass in terms of a feeling of being limited or restricted. Though we may see the features of these other Superclasses, the main emphasis of the case will be the dynamic of the second Superclass.

Sometimes the whole of a certain plant or animal group may not fit into one Superclass. A simple example are the Molluscs. They are divided into 3 Superclasses. The bivalves go into Superclass 1. The Gastropods go to Superclass 2 and the Cephalopods to Superclass 5. Different mammals also go to different Superclasses. While Lac Leoninum is Superclass 6, Lac equinum is in Superclass 5, and Lac humanum is in Superclass 3. The Monocots may also spread across the various Superclasses. There are still many remedies and groups which are not located in the Superclass chart. This is a work in evolution. It may also happen that a certain remedy or group that is in a Superclass now, may move to another one if clinical observations suggest this. Many remedy groups and remedies need to be still assigned to specific Superclasses. What is offered here is a broad outline.

Superclasses and the remedy groups

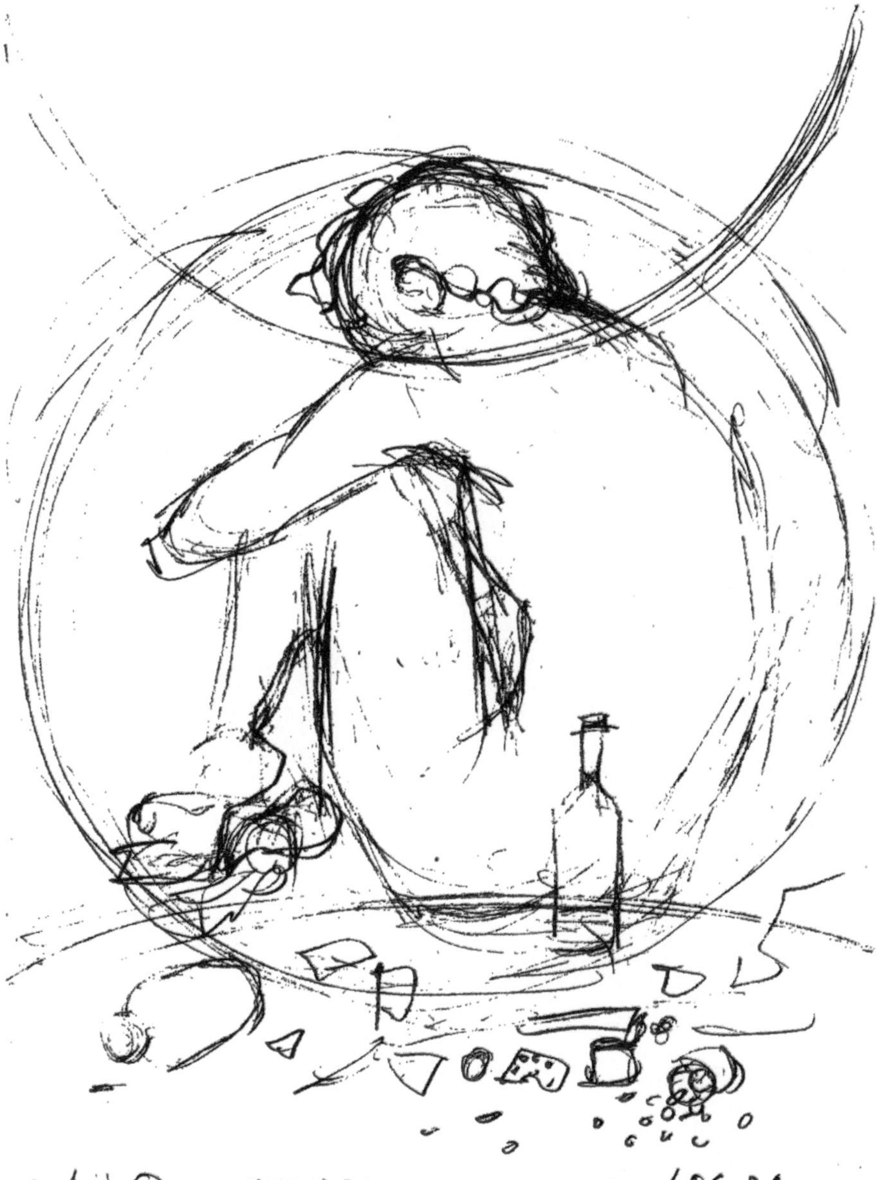

SC 1.1 ⊖ MONICA & MOMCHIL STOYANOV / 06.21

Superclass 1

The basic dynamic of this Superclass is shutting the world out. You go into your own little world where things are safe and familiar. It is as if there is no cover or protective skin. As if you are exposed and everything is felt very sensitively or acutely. Every little thing is felt in an exaggerated way. And all you want to do is go into your cocoon or shell where the outside world doesn't affect you.

If this is the dynamic, then let us look at where we can spot this dynamic in the different kingdoms. In the animals we will see this in the bivalves (molluscs), they go into the shell. In the plant kingdom we can see this in Opium, which is like an anaesthetic. You can also see it in Helleborus or Nux mos, these belong to the 1st Subclass. And where can we see this in the mineral kingdom? If we see each row of the periodic table as representing a certain stage of human development, we can think of the 2nd row which represents foetal life. The need for the womb can be seen in the remedies Lithium, Beryllium and Boron.

The mind-altering substance which would correspond to this dynamic would be morphine, which numbs you. The corresponding neurotransmitter would be the endorphins. The name 'endorphin' being the contracted form of endogenous morphine.

Thus, you can understand the different groups from various kingdoms have this kind of dynamics. You can see the similarities.

Below we see the groups of remedies which belong to the first Superclass. What is shown are the Animal, Mineral and Plant representatives of this dynamic.

SC	Dynamic	Animal group	Mineral	Dicotyledon	Other Plants	Neurotransmitter	Nosode	Drug
1	Withdrawal & CHnglng	Bivalves	2nd row: LHS	1st subclass	Mosses	Endorphins		Opioids

Taking all these representative groups, we have studied the features and common reactions of the remedies. We can see how they fit in. From the Animal kingdom there are the Bivalves. Here are remedies like *Mytilus edulis* and *Venus mercenaria.* We see the characteristic shutting off and closing out in response to stress. We can hypothesise that the Endorphins would be the hormone that represent the first Superclass. They show remarkable similarities to the effects of opioids. From the Mineral kingdom there is the left-hand side of the second row of the periodic table. Remedies such as *Lithium, Beryllium* and *Boron*. Here we can see the features of returning to the womb, not feeling capable to face the world and clinging to safety. Looking at the characteristic rubrics of Borax, we can see the dynamic of oversensitivity and the return to a womb-like state;

- Mind; Clinging
- Mind; Contented; himself, with
- Mind; Holding; held, or being; desire for
- Mind; Quiet; wants to be
- Mind; Sensitive, oversensitive; noise, to; slightest
- Mind; Starting, startled; easily
- Mind; Stupefaction, intoxicated as if

From the Dicotyledons of the plants we will have the first subclass, where there is an extreme sensitiveness. It is almost as if they have no skin. The sensitivity is to pain and suffering. The response would be to withdraw, benumb or anesthetize themselves. Common remedies from this group are *Nux moschata* and *Opium*. Here again we can see the idea of withdrawing like in *Opium* which goes into a catatonic state. The same is in the dreamy state of *Nux moschata.* They are completely confused and withdrawn from reality.

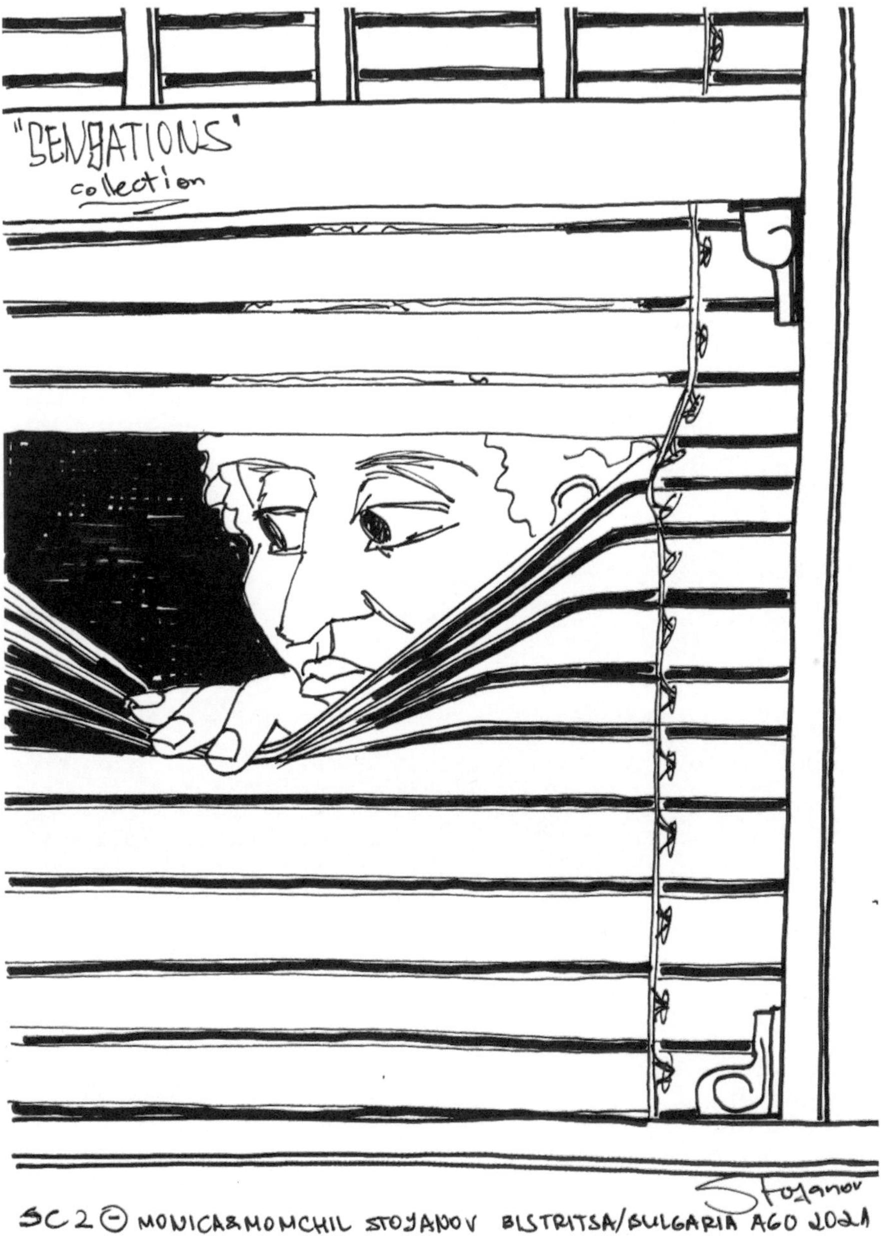

SC2 © MONICA&MOMCHIL STOYANOV BISTRITSA/BULGARIA AGO 2021

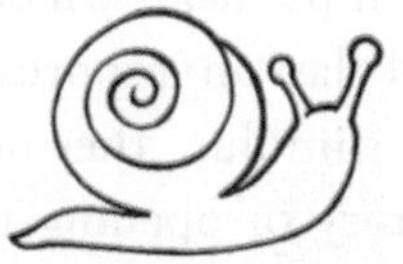

Superclass 2

The dynamic of the second Superclass is that of opening and shutting. A common example could be the window. We look through and see amazing sights. If something is disturbing then we can close the window and hide ourselves away.

Below we can see the remedy groups which lie in the second superclass. They represent this dynamic of opening and shutting.

SC	Dynamic	Animal group	Mineral	Dicotyledon	Other Plants	Neurotransmitter	Nosode	Drug
2	Open & Shut	Fishes Gastropods	Carbon	2nd subclass	Ferns	Endorphins		Cannabis

Studying the remedies which fall into this superclass, we can get a better understanding of the dynamic. For example, the gastropods will come under the second Superclass. This group are the snails, and we can see that their survival strategy is one of coming in and out of the shell. When there is danger present the snail will withdraw into the protection of the shell. After waiting a little while it will then come out again and begin to investigate and explore.

In the example of Carbon, we can again see the idea of withdrawing and coming out again. In the periodic table it lies in the second row which is representative of foetal life and the birth process. Carbon is stuck in the middle of the two sides. It is not quite ready to be born as the outside world can seem very dangerous and frightening. Yet it cannot remain in the womb which can become suffocative and ultimately just as threatening.

We would also hypothesise that Serotonin would be the hormone which corresponds to the second Superclass. Studies have shown the link between Serotonin syndrome and Cannabis toxicity. There has also been some research showing a connection between snails and Serotonin. This may be used in studying the effects of SSRIs on the heart which has recently come to light.

When we study the 2nd subclass an important remedy is Cannabis indica. It has an emphasis on sensory stimulus. They desire food, music, and colours which represents the exploratory or opening nature, but they do not leave the safety of the home for it. They want to sit on the couch all day watching television. The television is an incredible stimulus for them. It gives them the sensory stimulation. This is without the danger of the external world. This is the idea of open and shut. They are open to the sensory stimulation and pleasant experiences. They have completely shut themselves off to the reality of life around them especially the danger and unpleasantness it represents.

> *The Cannabis person feels unequipped to face the world directly and hence observes the world from within the safe confines of a "glass cage". Cannabis indica is the one who is locked inside the house. This is not an ordinary house but a palace. Thus, although he is very well provided materially, he is lonely. There is a total lack of any kind of stimulus within the confines of this house, but he fears to step out of it, since he feels it is risky to do so. So, he stays within this house, fearful of the dangers outside, and he makes up for the lack of stimulus by building fantasies and viewing things in a far more exaggerated form than they appear in reality - his sense of perception becomes exaggerated.*

If the reader would like to learn more about this, I would refer them to my book *The Soul of Remedies* where this extract has been taken from.

The following rubrics found in Cannabis show this dynamic.

- Delusion, deserted, forsaken.
- Delusion, is leading a vegetable existence.
- Delusion, injury, is about to receive.
- Delusion, beautiful visions.
- Fear, dark.
- Laughing, immoderate.
- Laughing, constant.
- Theorizing.

In the second Superclass we have also placed the remedies from the Fishes here. This is a hypothesis which we have based upon the study of Materia medica and provings. We can give a short summary below –

Being given a new vision by God, I was in a dark place, like a theatre. I was facing a large gray wall, like a curtain on a stage. On the upper right-hand corner was a window cut out. Somehow, I floated up and sat on the edge. We were sitting on the edge of a window. Into this new world colours, lights, movement. Objects were startling, gorgeous, kind of like an animated film. When I went into it, it was almost as if I were on a Ferris wheel, or some kind of carnival ride, and I was with a girl.

Here we can see from the proving of Seahorse the idea of the window and its use to provide sensory stimulation. This sensory stimulation is comparable to that in Cannabis Indica. There is Delusion of beautiful visions and Delusion he is in heaven.

In the proving of Salmon again this theme of the window was present.

Dream: I was looking in the windows of my neighbour's house. She saw me and presumed that I had come to visit for the first time. Her house seemed to have a lot of windows and light coming in, despite the windows being very small on the outside.

Also, we saw in Salmon the connection with Cannabis

Very strong desire to take recreational drugs, speed (amphetamines). Want to change my state of mind. Actually, took cannabis on two occasions. Had never taken this before.

"SENSATIONS"

collection

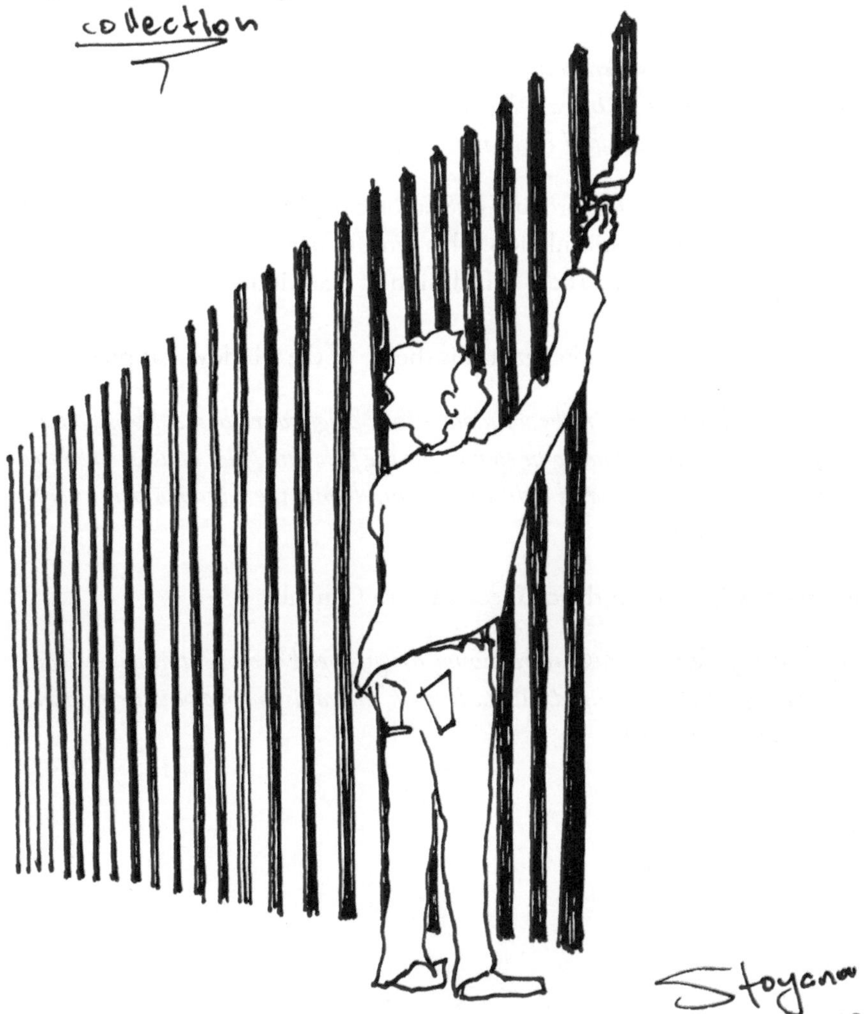

SC3 MONICA&MOMCHIL STOYANOV, LEIGHTON BUZZARD UK, SEP 21

Superclass 3

The third superclass is defined by the dynamic of limiting and expanding. Where a boundary is created so that no one can enter, but also then you cannot leave. This idea of the boundary or of limiting is fundamental to understanding the third superclass. When we see it in the light of the remedies of the third superclass then everything becomes much clearer.

Below are the groups of remedies which lie in the 3rd superclass;

SC	Dynamic	Animal group	Mineral	Dicotyledon	Other Plants	Neurotransmitter	Nosode	Drug
3	Limit & Expand	Bird Lac humanum	3rd row	3rd subclass		GABA & Glutamate	Ringworn	LSD Mescaline Alcohol

Here we can see the animal remedies belonging to the 3rd superclass are the birds. The larger birds of prey like the falcon and the eagle we know very well as remedies. They have issues of freedom. But we can also see especially in the falcon how the freedom or lack thereof is self-imposed. They have put their own limits upon themselves. The falcon is allowed freedom and not kept in an enclosure all the time. It is allowed to fly free but due its own limitation it returns to the arm of the captor every time. So, it has the protection of the captor but due to the limitation there is the loss of true freedom. When we look at the rubrics of falcon, we can see the idea of limiting and expanding as well as the freedom aspect;

- Mind; Delusions, imaginations, hallucinations, illusions; diminished
- Mind; Delusions, imaginations, hallucinations, illusions; small; he is

- Mind; Delusions, imaginations, hallucinations, illusions; enlarged
- Mind; Delusions, imaginations, hallucinations, illusions; space; expansion of
- Mind; Delusions, imaginations, hallucinations, illusions; division between himself and others
- Mind; Delusions, imaginations, hallucinations, illusions; separated; world from the, is
- Mind; Delusions, imaginations, hallucinations, illusions; trapped, is
- Mind; Dreams; cage, wired
- Mind; Dreams; captured, being

From the mineral kingdom we have the 3rd row of the periodic table and a remedy like Silicea is a very good example. Silicea feels the need to maintain a certain image of themselves. They have set a limit on their behaviour and appearance, and they must live up to this image. All their sense of self-worth is gained from living up to this image. Likewise, it is completely lost if they do not maintain this image. So, they are completely bound by the limit or boundary which they have set themselves. No one has imposed this image upon them or demanded the upkeep of it, it is completely self-imposed.

From the Dicotyledons we can see the Caryophyllids, with remedies like the Cactus. The set limit or boundary has a clear physical manifestation in the shrinking and expanding sensations of remedies belonging to this group. The limit and boundary can also be seen in the mental symptoms. There is a big issue with being limited. And the great desire for expanding beyond the limit of human consciousness in Anhalonium.

It is very interesting to see which Superclass *Lac humanum* belongs. When we study this remedy and the essential nature of human beings, we see that the human being is a social animal. She needs to be a part of the group. She needs to belong to society. She also needs to be a part of her family. Human beings need care and nourishment longer than any other animal. And for this she needs to conform, and act as per the norms and expectations of his family/group. She has freedom within these boundaries. To step out of these boundaries is an adventure, a risk. It is for this 'dynamic' that I would place Lac humanum in the 3rd Superclass

The Nepenthales (carnivorous plants e.g., Drosera) seem to have the qualities of both, the 3rd, and the 5th Superclasses. They have the need for nourishment and care like in the 3rd Superclass. They also have the trapped feeling and the need to get out like in the 5th Superclass.

The basic response of the 3rd SC is to shrink, to limit oneself. Once we say that then the basic experience is fear, but a fear of what? Fear that the attack is imminent. Something is going to happen. A lot of anticipation. Alertness. Now I am going to get cancer! This is the aspect we need to understand a bit more.

In the first superclass, there is so much fear they become numb or even faint they don't want to face it. They want to remain inside an anaesthetised space, like an oyster or a foetus. In the 2nd Superclass there is an opening. If I am safe, I can open, if unsafe I can shut it. And in this 3rd Superclass they actually come out into the open. They don't have this opening and shutting kind of mechanism. For the first time they are exposed. They are out there in the open. No anaesthesia, no open and shut. This is where they anticipate the attacks. Their mechanism is to shrink, to go into a limited space, to huddle up.

When you go out and someone tries to beat you up and you shrink so that your exposure is minimised. It is the most exposed in some sense. Because when you go into the fourth Superclass, you find stability. So only when there is a loss of stability is there fear. Like a loss in business in Bryonia makes you unstable. The anticipation is of the loss of stability

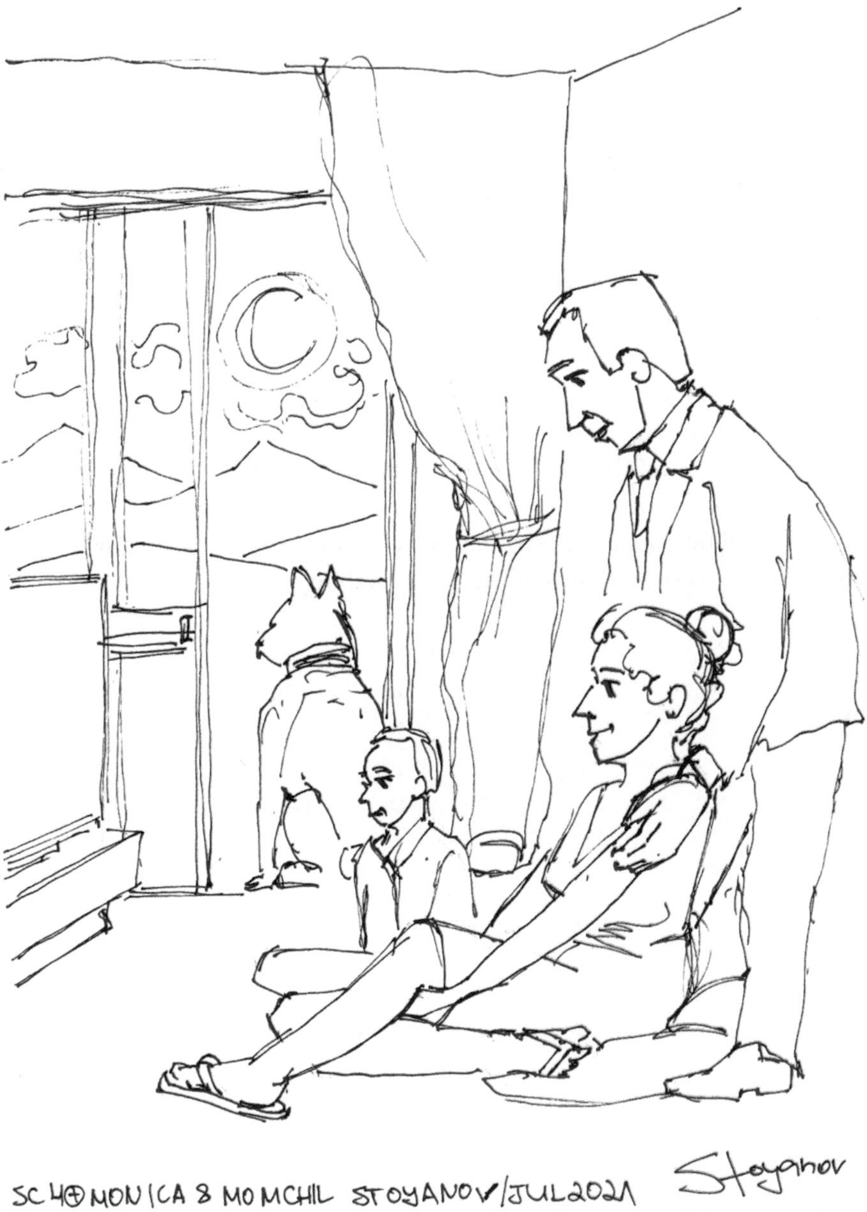

SC40 MONICA & MOMCHIL STOYANOV/JUL2021 Stoyanov

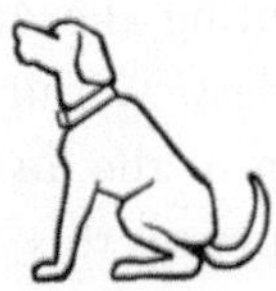

Superclass 4

The 4th Superclass is defined by the dynamic of stability and security and the need thereof. This is the attempt at finding some security and regaining the feeling of stability. They feel they are losing this or have already lost it.

Below, we can see the remedy groups which best represent this dynamic of security and stability.

SC	Dynamic	Animal group	Mineral	Dicotyledon	Other Plants	Neurotransmitter	Nosode	Drug
4	Stability & Security	Lac caninum	4th row	4th subclass	Gymnosperms	Acetylcholine	Medorrhinum	Diazepam

In the mineral kingdom, we can look at the 4th row of the periodic table. The entire row is related to the theme of security and either the need to gain it, maintain it or the feeling of losing it. If we take the example of *Calcarea carbonicum* which we know very well. We can talk of how Calc carb has the huge need for security and stability. From the source we can see how calcium provides for the security and stability of the body through the skeletal structure.

The vital expression of the Calc carb patient is the need for protection. Especially from the people surrounding him and this is shown in the many fears of the Calc carb patient. This is clearly the dynamic of the 4th superclass. But we can also see this dynamic from the other side of the same row in a remedy like *Arsenicum album*. The vital expression is that of the loss of the security. Ars alb feels weak and defenceless and that thieves are all around him waiting to take advantage of him. This is the other side of the dynamic as *Calc carb* where the main reaction is an attempt to gain security and stability.

For the dicotyledons representing the 4th superclass we will study the Dilleniidae. This is the 4th subclass. Within the Dilleniidae we can see the remedy *Bryonia alba.* The feeling of the loss of stability is very clear in the symptomatology. The patient expresses this as better for rest and aversion to disturbance.

We have also seen Lycopodium as part of the 4th Superclass. This is confirmed by study of materia medica and clinical cases. The main idea of Lycopodium that emerged is of seeking to put down one's roots in a new place so as to find to find stability. The spores of Lycopodium are carried to distant places by the wind. They need to latch on to a new surface where they have no roots. Then they have to develop roots and make their position firm. The sensitivity is to facing new situations, strangers, new job, etc. Initially they are very hesitant and underconfident. Then they slowly put down their roots and establish their position. Some rubrics give an indication of this idea in humans:

- Mind; Dreams; boats; foundering (11)
- Mind; Dreams; trees, of; growing on fences without ground under them (1)

The need for an anchor, for roots, gives a clue that Lycopodium belongs to the 4th Superclass. This is borne out by many cases.

Looking at the remedy group of the Gymnosperms we can again see this dynamic. The vital sensation is that of fragility and fear of being shattered. The symptom in Thuja delusion: *she is made of glass,* is evocative of this sensation. This sense of fragility comes from dynamic of stability and security. This dynamic is recurrent through all the gymnosperm remedies such as *Gingko biloba.* Gingko is representative of old age. Again, the dynamic of loss of security and stability can be seen in the symptoms of Ginkgo.

As we have mentioned earlier the animal groups can be bit trickier. The behavioural patterns within the same subgroup can differ so largely. This is well demonstrated within this Superclass where some of the mammals lie. We can look at remedies like Lac caninum and Lac defloratum. We see how they correspond to the 4th superclass. There is the need to belong to the group to maintain their security and stability. There is an acceptance of their lower place in the hierarchy, since it provides a comfort zone he doesn't want to leave. Lac caninum can sacrifice his independence or dignity for the sake of comfort and stability. However, some of the other mammals such as lions and tigers would have a different dynamic.

The Nosode *Medorrhinum* also fits into this dynamic. *Medo* is the central point of the sycotic miasm. which is the feeling of something being wrong with oneself. There is a feeling of inner weakness that must be covered up. This covering up which is so central in *Medo* can clearly be seen in terms of the 4th superclass dynamic. Here are some characteristic rubrics and symptoms of Medorrhinum –

- Fear change of
- Desire for familiar surrounding
- Change of weather agg
- Delusion everything is strange
- Fear happen something will— something will be changed
- Fear of misfortune
- Walking in open air amel— opposite pole

We know the following about Medorrhinum -

- There is always the feeling of avoiding risk, avoiding commitment
- Avoiding work
- Many ideas but uncertain of execution.
- Non-committal
- Aversion to responsibility
- Postponing
- Not someone who will step out and take a risk, he will stay where he is and avoid things

We can see the same dynamic through different symptoms in Calcarea carbonica

- Fear something will happen
- Fear something will happen to him or his family
- Fear public spaces
- Home desire to go
- Financial loss

Interestingly, if we look at the rubric 'Thunderstorm agg" we find remedies of the 3rd and 4th Superclasses. These Superclasses are generally risk-averse.

Amel from thunderstorm shows the risk-taking quality of the 5th superclass. Remedies in this rubric are largely from the 5th Superclass, such as Cobalt nitricum, Rhus radicans, Sepia, Carc and Tub.

CR19 - **Generalities; Weather; thunderstorm; amel.** (15) : bell-p.FoDM, beryl.ScJa, calc.GeAl, Carc.SCD, caust.FarH, Cob-N.StJa, ignisEiNu, lyc.ClJH, mang.JaGHG, nat-p.MorRo, phos.RiBo, Rhus-R.PhSR, Sep.HaSa, thuj.JoCh, tub.GeAl

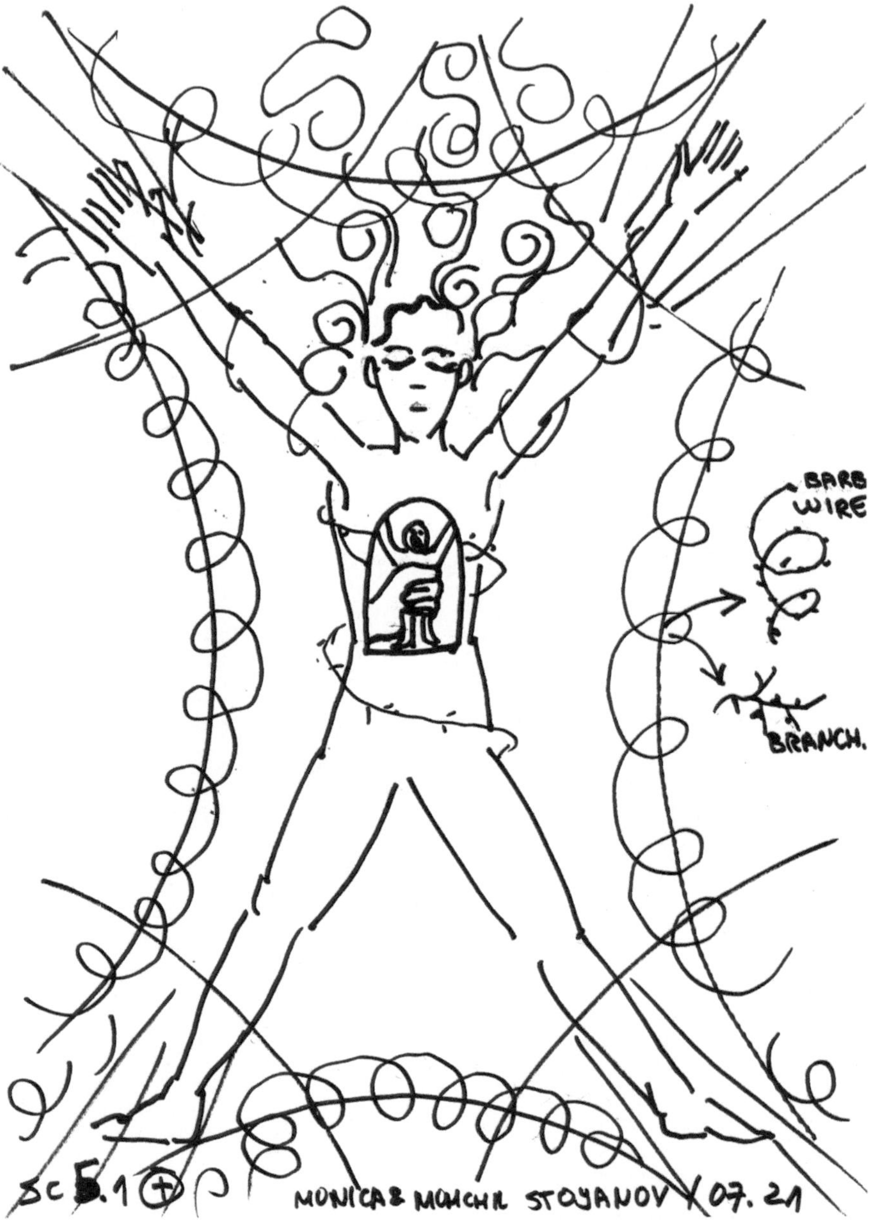
BARB
WIRE
BRANCH.
SC 5.1
MONICA & MOMCHIL STOYANOV
07. 21

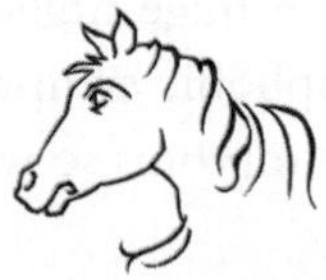

Superclass 5

The dynamic of the 5th Superclass can be seen as restlessness and the feeling that one must get out. The example of this would be to imagine yourself locked up in a tiny box where there is not enough air. The feeling would be of claustrophobia being caught and trapped. There is the urgent need to get out where you are able to move and be free.

Below can be seen the remedy groups which have this dynamic and belong to the 5th superclass;

SC	Dynamic	Animal group	Mineral	Dicotyledon	Other Plants	Neurotransmitter	Nosode	Drug
5	Restless & Must get out	Cephalopods spiders Insects Lac equinum	5th row & 2nd row: RHS	5th subclass		Histamine & Dopamine	Tuberculinum Carcinosinum Leprominium	Cocaine

Studying the 5th superclass through the remedy groups within it, we can see that animal groups which fall into the 5th superclass are the spiders, insects, and the cephalopods. For the spiders the intense restlessness and need to move and feeling of being trapped and caught is a clear illustration of this dynamic.

Even in a remedy like Sepia from the cephalopods we can see this same dynamic represented in the rubrics. Such as desire to escape from one's family. Sepia also has the desire for movement and dance. These activities ameliorate. They reduce the feeling of being trapped caught or stuck.

When we look at remedies in the second row of the periodic table on the right hand side are remedies like Nitrogen and Oxygen. These remedies represent the part of the birth process where the foetus is coming out of the womb. There is the feeling that they can no longer stay in the womb or they will suffocate and die. There is a huge urgency and need to "get out". We can also see this in the claustrophobic symptoms in these remedies and the nitrates. These claustrophobic symptoms so well represent the features of this dynamic.

Looking at the dicotyledons we have the 5th Subclass the Rosidae which includes families like the Anacardiacaeae. The feeling of stuck, stiff and cannot move sensation is very clear in remedies like Rhus tox. This is ameliorated by movement and exertion. This again clearly shows the features of the 5th superclass.

There are two important aspects of the 5th superclass.

1. Creative, out of box thinking, performing, innovation.
2. Claustrophobic, constriction, suffocating and the need to get out.

I have found that these two are found together in most of the 5th superclass remedies. Creativity and claustrophobia seem to go together. Claustrophobia is associated with a sense of danger. In the 5th Superclass they are preparing for facing a dangerous situation as well as trying to find a way out of it, often in a creative way. At the same time speed seems to be of the essence here. You have to find a way out quickly. All these elements, claustrophobia, restless, creativity and performance seem to be closely interconnected.

A typical example is Argentum nitricum. You have the high performance and the claustrophobia all in one. In the mineral remedies the performance and ability will be more emphasised than the claustrophobic element. While in the plant remedies it will be the other way around. However, if we study a remedy such as Coca, we will see high performance.

If we look at the neurotransmitter *Dopamine* it seems to have these two aspects as well. It is associated with achievement as well as the aspect of being prepared for danger.

When we study the nosodes of the 5th Superclass it is particularly interesting to see the similarities between Carcinosinum and Tuberculinum. Some interesting common rubrics between them:

- mind; ESCAPE, desire to (172)
- mind; ACTIVITY; desire for (100)

- mind; ADVENTUROUS (11)
- mind; ANGER; temper tantrums (85)
- mind; ANGER; children, in (39)
- mind; AUDACITY (75)
- mind; AUTHORITY, refusal to accept some one's (39)
- mind; CHANGE; desire for (47)
- mind; CHEERFULNESS; thunders and lightens, when it (11)
- mind; COUNTRY, desire for, to go into the (45)
- mind; CRUELTY, brutality, inhumanity; animals, to (14)
- mind; DEVELOPMENT, mental; arrested (59)
- mind; DOMINATION by others agg.; father, by (22)
- Mind; Escape desire to (172)
- mind; FEAR; narrow place, in, claustrophobia (73)
- mind; FEAR; narrow place, in, claustrophobia; vaults, churches and cellars, of (14)
- mind; FIGHT; wants to; rebellious (13)
- mind; MUSIC; amel. (46)
- mind; RECKLESSNESS, temerity (37)
- mind; TRAVEL, desire to (77)
- mind; TEARS; himself, herself (22)

One side of Carcinosinum which is well known is that of control and obedience. A picture of perfection. There is also a lesser known side where he feels dominated and doesn't want authority and wants to be free from that.

- Carcinosinum is seen in the rubric love animals. As well as cruelty, brutality, inhumanity for animals
- Like Anacardium- where the two sides are seen. One of obedience and the other side of cruelty.
- Similar also to Tuberculinum who wants to break free from domination, authority
- Both Anacardium and Tuberculinum come in the 5th superclass
- Feeling of being crushed by authority and wanting to fight back
- mind; MILDNESS; violence, masking the
- mind; FIGHT; wants to; rebellious

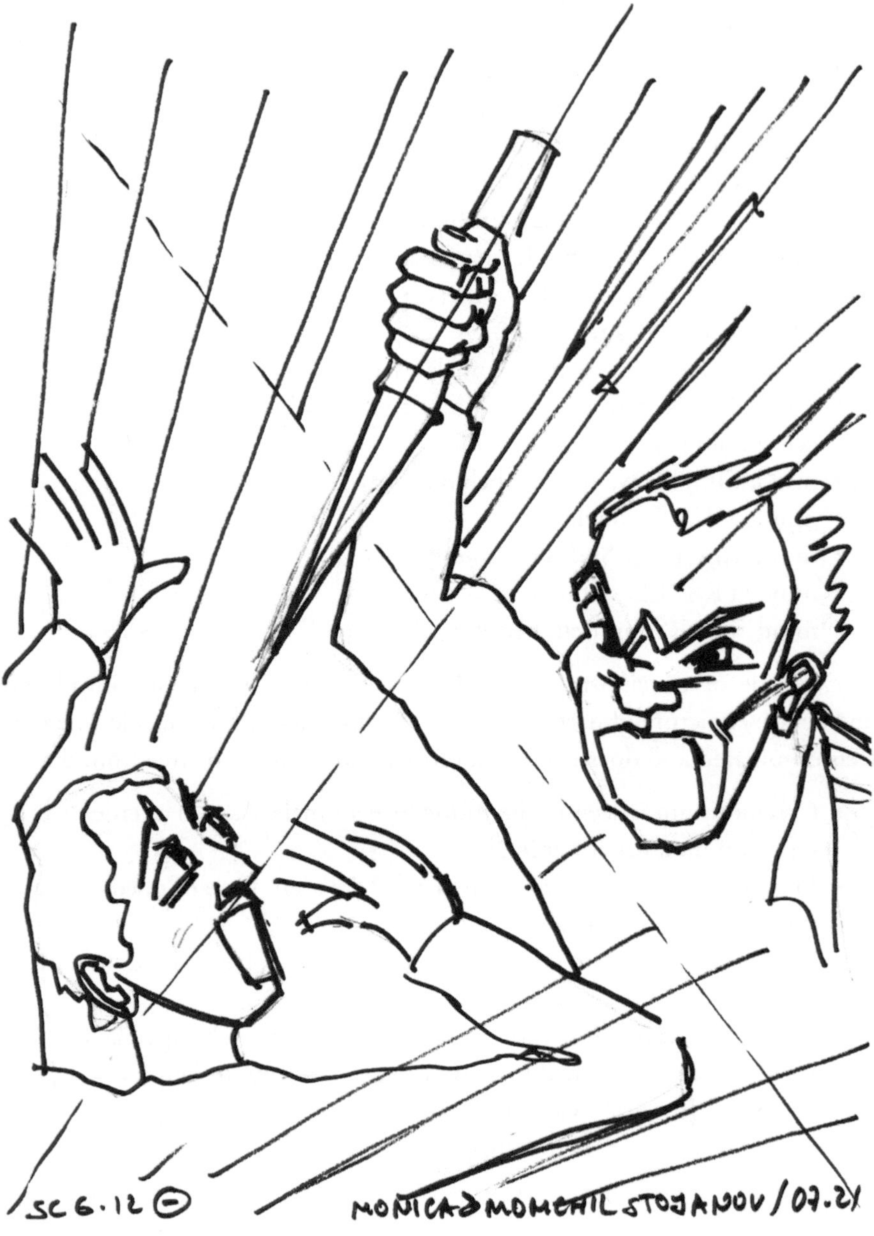
SC 6.12
MONICA & MOMCHIL STOJANOV / 07.21

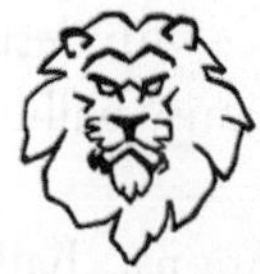

Superclass 6

The 6th Superclass is defined by the perception of danger all around. And having to fight to the finish.

Below, we can see the group of remedies which belong to the 6th superclass;

SC	Dynamic	Animal group	Mineral	Dicotyledon	Other Plants	Neurotransmitter	Nosode	Drug
6	Fight & Flight	Reptiles Lac leoninum	6th row	6th subclass	Fungi	Noradlrenaline	Syphilinum	Methamphetamine

In the 6th superclass from the animal group, we can see the reptiles. We can see in the snakes see this idea of enemies and danger. They must attack and destroy their enemies. There is no other option or half measures in the characteristic themes of the snake remedies. When we take the most well-known snake remedy Lachesis and look at just a few rubrics we can see this perception and reaction quite clearly;

- Mind; Delusions, imaginations, hallucinations, illusions; enemy; behind him
- Mind; Delusions, imaginations, hallucinations, illusions; Injury; receive, is about to
- Mind; Dreams; knife, knives; keeping them ready for use
- Mind; Dreams; revenge

Studying the mineral group from the 6th superclass we can see this dynamic within the 6th row of the periodic table. This is very evident in a remedy like *Mercurius* where we have the following rubrics;

- Mind; Anticipation; evil, sensation of impending
- Mind; Anxiety; night; escape, with desire to
- Mind; Delusions, imaginations, hallucinations, illusions; enemy; surrounded by
- Mind; Delusions, imaginations, hallucinations, illusions; pursued, being; enemies, by
- Mind; Destructiveness

From these rubrics we again see this same idea of being in danger with enemies all around. The only possible way to survive is to fight or flee.

In the dicotyledons we have the 6th Subclass, namely the Asteriidae. We can see these features in families like the Solanaceae or Compositae. There is this perception of danger and fright and a huge injury. All the families in this subclass can clearly show this dynamic. Think of the Umbelliferae with the characteristic "sudden, violent attack".

Neurotransmitters serving as the Superclass's central node

As I continued to work on the Superclasses, I discovered something quite intriguing. What is the connection between neurotransmitters, hormones and Superclasses, I wondered? For the sixth Superclass, I could readily see its similarity to adrenaline. It is the fight-or-flight hormone. If we compare the effects of remedies like Belladonna and Stram to the effects of adrenaline, they are remarkably comparable. The heart beats faster as the sympathetic nervous system becomes active. This is a relatively common response.

If the neurotransmitter associated with the sixth Superclass is adrenaline, then we need to determine which neurotransmitter might be associated with the others. There is some experience with Histamine which shows similarity with the fifth Superclass. It is extremely eager, agitated, and vigilant, as if something is about to happen. Histamine cases show these qualities. So we started to understand how histamine relates to the fifth Superclass.

In the wake of this, we also learned about Dopamine, a neurotransmitter. The hormone for success is Dopamine. When compared to Cocaine, which is also a member of the fifth superclass, Dopamine effects resemble Cocaine in several ways. Additionally, the fifth row's performances are high-achieving, much like Cocaine. They are also artistic individuals. Histamine and Dopamine may both belong to the fifth Superclass.

Then, some intriguing investigations took place. Even the sixth Superclass persons are performers. In terms of their output, they are also achievers, including Nux vomica, Aurum, and others. Dopamine's role as adrenaline's precursor is interesting. We can infer that the fifth Superclass is getting ready to face an assault. One must be prepared and awake. The attack might come at any time. In the sixth Superclass the response is as if it is happening to you in the moment. As a result, we can observe how the sixth Superclass' response of one who is actively being attacked differs from the fifth Superclass response of being prepared. Dopamine's role as an adrenaline precursor is another instance of this. We have histamine and dopamine in the fifth Superclass. Having stage-fright or jumping with a parachute releases dopamine, which is also a hormone. Before a significant occurrence, there is some sort of readiness. This is seen in remedies like Arg-Nit. The Dopamine impact is what gives you that sense just before a crisis.

We then started researching the first superclass in the wake of these discoveries. We were hunting for a hormone that functions similarly to Opium, one that induces either numbness or withdrawal. It was simple to relate this to endorphins. Endorphins can give you this sensation of pleasure, anaesthesia, and lack of pain. Consequently, we can tie the first superclass to endorphins. They have a painless sensation and are also known as the happy hormone. They are quite similar to Opium. It is interesting to note that the name "Endorphin" is a contraction of "endogenous morphine". This is really intriguing to us and supports our theories.

I then began learning about the second superclass. I knew that Cannabis has many pleasurable experiences, I was looking for a hormone with a similar effect. Serotonin is the hormone that is most similar to cannabis and most difficult to distinguish from its effects. It is a joyful hormone as well.

I then began hunting for hormones and neurotransmitters similar to the dynamic of the third and fourth Superclasses. I initially believed that the third Superclass neurotransmitter should resemble the remedies from the third row of the periodic table. You have remedies like Magnesium and Natrum and Phosphorous. They all have something to do with love, sympathy, and bonding. Therefore, oxytocin came to mind because the hormone that promotes bonding is oxytocin.

Oxytocin is produced by the pituitary gland. Hormones originate from glands called endocrine glands. Each endocrine gland makes a difference because they make hormones that perform a certain role. Like prolactin, which produces milk. Growth hormone promotes growth, while insulin regulates sugar metabolism. The endocrine glands that produce these hormones are responsible for a number of extremely specialised bodily tasks.

The hormones of response, however, are neurotransmitters. These are produced by nerve cells. When there is a threat and noradrenaline is secreted.

To elicit a response, it engages a variety of different organs. Since, each Superclass represents a specific type of response we must focus on the various neurotransmitters and see which one is related to which Superclass.

Terminal nerve cells secrete neurotransmitters which operate in two distinct ways. They either stimulate or inhibit a function. This also functions well for our Superclasses which has two polarities of effect. How do we go about identifying a specific neurotransmitter for the third Superclass?

We require a neurotransmitter that is active while the decision to take a risk is being considered. Are you going to grow, or are you going to stay the same size? After researching every neurotransmitter, I discovered GABA, or gamma aminobutyric acid and Glutamate. Together, these two neurotransmitters complement one another. Inhibitory GABA complements Glutamate which is an excitant. Glutamate will encourage you to move forward, but GABA will inhibit you from doing so. And research demonstrates that these neurotransmitters play a role in taking risks. They complement one another, much like Yin and Yang.

We now come to the fourth Superclass. How can I locate a neurotransmitter for the fourth Superclass? I discovered that histamine, dopamine, and adrenaline are all sympathomimetic; they stimulate the sympathetic nervous system. This means that they keep you prepared for danger, an unexpected incident, or a catastrophe.

In the case of the fourth Superclass we need to look for a neurotransmitter that stimulates the parasympathetic nervous system. The sympathetic and parasympathetic nervous systems function similarly to Yin and Yang. Additionally, parasympathetic activity affects the neurological system while you are resting. You may say it represents "Relax and digest." Where the sympathetic represents "Fight or Flight". "Feeding and breeding" is another way of describing the effect of the parasympathetic nervous system.

Therefore, you might say that the parasympathetic nervous system is active when you are at rest. The sympathetic nervous system is what is active while you are alert. I began my search for a neurotransmitter that increases parasympathetic nervous system activity. It must be dopamine's or noradrenaline's opponent. I thus searched for one that was the polar opposite of this and found acetylcholine. This neurotransmitter is the primary one that activates the Parasympathetic Nervous System

Let us summarize what we have learnt so far about the connection of the neurotransmitters to specific Superclasses. The first would be endorphins, which promote calm and painlessness. The second, serotonin, is associated with joy and enthusiasm. The third, GABA/glutamate for risk-aversion and risk taking, The third, GABA/glutamate for risk-aversion and risk taking. The fourth corresponds with Acetylcholine, for relaxation and sleep. The fifth one would relate to histamine and dopamine with the qualities of alertness. The sixth would relate to noradrenaline, the hormone associated with flight and fight. These six are the neurotransmitters must be in the centre of the Superclass since Superclass defines a classification of the type of response.

A neurotransmitter is to the superclass what a nodose is to the miasm—it is the very centre. If we can determine the person's primary neurotransmitter, we can get a fairly accurate idea of his dynamic response.

Related to neurotransmitters are also mind-altering substances some of which actually enhance neurotransmitters. It would be interesting to see if we could relate specific substances to specific Superclasses. Opium and its derivatives, such as morphine, would be in the first superclass, this is easy to derive. Cannabis would be the second superclass. LSD and mescaline would be in the third. Mescaline is another name for Anhalonium. This is the substance that makes Anhalonium active, and mescaline and LSD have a lot in common. They are the ones who seek out daring adventures and desire to step beyond their comfort zones. I thought of benzodiazepines when I thought of the Fourth Superclass. If you want rest, you take benzodiazepines. Cocaine is obviously the fifth Superclass. Methamphetamine is the drug of the sixth Superclass. Under their influence, individuals become violent and hostile. They refer to it as "crystal meth" on the streets.

These substances stimulate these neurotransmitters, as you will discover if you investigate them. Dopamine and histamine have a lot in common with cocaine. Cannabis and serotonin share many similarities. Opium and endorphins have a lot in common. People who express particular genes in the dopamine system frequently exhibit traits such as creativity, spontaneity, curiosity, and mental flexibility. They enjoy novelty and take risks. People with high serotonin levels are more gregarious and eager to fit in (as are those who take SSRI antidepressants). All these observations fit in well with our Superclass paradigm.

Modern medicine views the neurotransmitter as an aetiology. It postulates that you require levodopa for Parkinson's because you have very little dopamine. They administer selective serotonin reuptake inhibitors (SSRIs). Consequently, your serotonin levels will rise. They make an effort to increase or replace the neurotransmitter, thinking that excess or lack of it is the issue.

In Homoeopathy (and our understanding of Superclasses) we do not believe that an excess or deficiency of a specific neurotransmitter is the root of the issue. We believe it to be a result of the issue. We research the personalities of endorphins, serotonin, and dopamine. We do not claim that this "X" hormone is the issue.

We see that disease is something that affects the whole person. This affection affects the release or absence of a specific neurotransmitter. We therefore claim that depression causes you to secrete less serotonin, not the other way around. Of course, giving them a serotonin boost will make them feel better. However, since that is not the cause, the effect will only last a short time.

In this sense, it becomes clear that each Superclass will represent either an excess or a deficiency of the related neurotransmitter. Therefore, there are either too many or not enough endorphins in the first superclass. Consequently, either extreme pain or excessive painlessness results. The second is either too little or too much serotonin. So, either incredibly happy and thrilled or introverted and unhappy. Too fearful to get outside or exceedingly risky in the third superclass. You can comprehend the polarity of the superclass by comparing glutamate to GABA. A Diazepam user is either completely peaceful or extremely anxious.

If we comprehend the neurotransmitter, then we comprehend the Superclass's overall underlying dynamic exactly.

	Neurotransmitter	Drug
1st Superclass	Endorphins – pleasure (peace?) & Painlessness	Opium
2nd Superclass	Serotonin – pleasure & excitement	Cannabis
3rd Superclass	GABA/Glutamate – Risk taking vs Risk averse	LSD/Mescaline
4th Superclass	Acetylcholine – Rest & digest	Diazepam
5th Superclass	Histamine/Dopamine – alert, motivation & drive	Cocaine
6th Superclass	Noradrenaline – Fight & Flight	Methamphetamine

It is important to understand that a remedy will have all the shades of all the remedies of the same Superclass. Then it will have its own keynotes, peculiarities, and source qualities. The common feature or dynamic response of the Superclass will be found in all the remedies. That common feature will be most emphasised in the neurotransmitter. So, the neurotransmitter will be at the centre point of the Superclass. What a neurotransmitter is to a superclass is what a nosode is to an miasm. Every remedy of a miasm will have some similarity to the nosode.

Pulsatilla, a sycotic remedy, will have avoidance and anticipation at its centre. But what will it avoid and anticipate? This will depend on which kingdom and subkingdom it belongs to. Since Pulsatilla is a plant remedy belonging to Ranunculaceae, it will be sensitive to and therefore avoid the slightest insult and hurt. So, its avoidance and anticipation will be related to its extreme sensitivity (first Superclass).

Gelsemium is also a sycotic remedy. It is found in the 6th subclass or Superclass. Here, the avoidance will be of a big trauma or big shock of a sudden big bad news, these being the features of the 6th subclass. So there the sycotic miasm expressed in relation in the 6th subclass.

However, consider a patient who shows avoidance and anticipation across the field in all aspects, when avoidance and anticipation is his main experience. Then he would need the nosode (Medorrhinum) itself.

Similar, is the case with neurotransmitters and Superclasses. All remedies of a given Superclass will have a dynamic which is best represented by the corresponding neurotransmitter.

All remedies of a given superclass will have features or shades of all other remedies. In all 6th Superclass remedies you will find shades of Lachesis, Merc, China, Stram, etc. Yet each remedy will have features of the kingdom and subkingdom to which it belongs. Each remedy will demonstrate the features of its family. Each remedy will also exhibit its own generals, peculiars, keynotes, mental essence, pathological symptoms and source qualities. All this will help differentiate from other remedies.

Hormones and the Superclasses

What is the basic difference between hormone and neurotransmitter?

Firstly, a Neurotransmitter is secreted by neurons. The hormones are secreted by endocrine glands. Secondly Neurotransmitters are quick acting and short lasting. Hormones have a slow release and longer lasting effect. The Neurotransmitter has more of a local effect. An hormone is distributed through the blood stream. Its effect is more global. A Neurotransmitter is more of an acute response. A hormone is more of a longer lasting response.

One example is Cortisol and Noradrenaline. Noradrenaline is a neurotransmitter and Cortisol is a hormone. Cortisol is found in chronic stress. Noradrenaline is found in acute stress situations.

We are currently working on investigating which Neurotransmitter corresponds with which hormone. E.g., Noradrenaline and Cortisol. This is very much a work in progress and this remains a working hypothesis.

Testosterone seems to be the long-term hormone for aggression. 90% of criminals are males. 99% of dictators are males. Aggression is associated as a male quality. This aggression corresponds with Dopamine. Aggression can also be manifest as desire for achievement, risk-taking and ambition.

This is useful in differentiating Nat-mur and Sepia. While Nat mur has the issue of keeping in limits or taking the risk (3rd Superclass), Nat mur would have more of an oxytocin quality. Whereas Sepia (5th Superclass) has more of a testosterone quality. It has male-like features, indifference to children, ambitious, wanting to move out. The Acute manifestation of Sepia could exhibit a dopamine like effect, the chronic would be a testosterone like effect. When the situation becomes even more acute, then Sepia may go into a Nux-v state. The Dopamine like state (5th Superclass) becomes an adrenaline like state

(6th Superclass). It has been noted by earlier Homeopaths that Sepia and Nux vomica are very closely related.

With these observations we are starting to see a feminine/masculine spectrum across the Superclasses. We could see that the from the 1st to the 3rd Superclass there is an emphasis on the feminine qualities. Starting in the 4th and going to the 6th Superclass the Masculine qualities are more emphasised. This is not to say that only males will need remedies from the 6th Superclass.

Rather, these remedies would correspond with what we traditionally call as masculine qualities. When we start to study the basic feminine principle vs the basic masculine principle, we can see that the feminine has a more of an inward or centripetal dynamic while the masculine which is more outward or centrifugal in its dynamic.

Thyroid (T3) can be associated with Calcarea carb. Calcium metabolism is an important function of the thyroid. It is also a hormone which is greatly involved with regulation in the body. When functioning normally it maintains the metabolism and other functions in the body at a stable rate. When it goes out of control either hyper or hypo, we see a great loss of stability in our metabolic rates. There is abnormal functioning of the body.

Oestrogen has a big impact on the mood. We can see this related to the changes in mood. Oestrogen acts as an SSRI. It is a female hormone which also goes with our understanding of the feminine principle being more emphasised in the first 3 Superclasses.

	Neurotransmitter	**Hormone**	**Drug**
1st Superclass	Endorphins – pleasure & Painlessness	Melatonin	Opium
2nd Superclass	Serotonin – pleasure & excitement	Oestrogen	Cannabis
3rd Superclass	GABA/Glutamate – Risk taking vs Risk averse	Oxytocin	LSD/Mescaline
4th Superclass	Acetylcholine – Rest & digest	T3 (triiodothyronine)	Diazepam
5th Superclass	Histamine/Dopamine – alert, motivation & drive	Testosterone	Cocaine
6th Superclass	Noradrenaline – Fight & Flight	Cortisol	Methamphetamine

Colour and the Superclasses

Is there a connection between colours and Superclasses? The colour red is usually associated with violence and danger. Thus, it seemed to fit well with the 6th Superclass. Red is one end of the spectrum of the 7 primary colours. We wondered if one could work backward. Could we see if yellow and orange are connected with the 5th Superclass and violet, indigo, blue and green with Superclasses 1, 2, 3 and 4 respectively. We found some confirmations of this in patients as well as in remedies. For example, Thuja from the 4th Superclass, has a connection with the green colour. In the materia medica there is a symptom in Thuja that it sees the colour green. Tarentula and Theridion from the 5th Superclass have affinity to orange colour. The connection between a specific colour and a specific Superclass is still in the realm of hypothesis. We feel it deserves mention so that it can be further tested by colleagues.

SECTION FOUR

The '5 finger method'

If one needs a strong grip on anything, one needs to use all five fingers of one's hand and bring them together to get a grip. Similarly, if one wants to get a firm grip on a case, one needs to bring five aspects of the case together.

These five aspects are

1. Superclass
2. Kingdom and subkingdom
3. Miasm
4. Characteristics
5. Keynotes and source qualities.

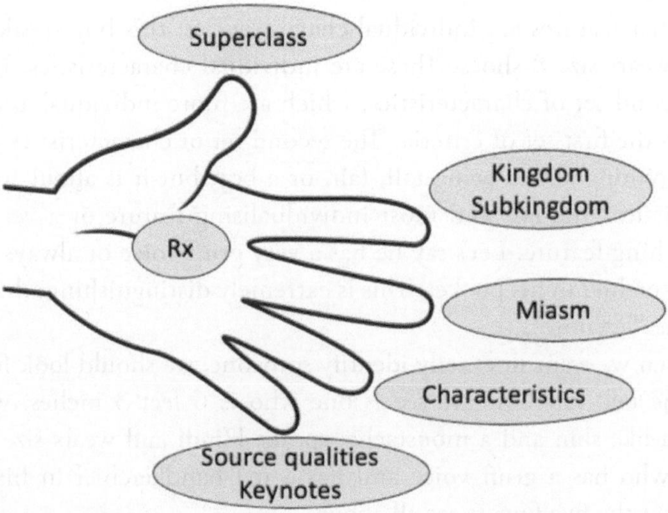

I'd like to illustrate the '5-finger method' with the idea of identifying someone.

When we identify someone, e.g., when we go to the airport and get this person. You are not given a photograph; you are given a description. How do you describe this person?

You are told that the person you have to bring back is a tall, fair boy.

When someone says this, they are describing three dimensions.

1. Height
2. Skin colour
3. Gender

So, when you go to the airport, you will look out for these 3 dimensions: somebody who is tall, somebody who is male, and somebody who is fair-skinned. This will narrow your search to a very small group of people. So, on that shortlist, how do you know who is exactly the one we need?

Here we come to characteristics. In the characteristics, there are two types of characteristics. One is a characteristic that describes details of the qualities of the three dimensions of the tall, fair boy. E.g., we can say he is 6 feet 3 inches, he has a moustache, he has short hair, and then his skin colour is fair, like a Caucasian. What are we describing here? We are describing the tall, fair boy in factual terms: the moustache depicts that he is a boy, 6 feet 3 inches depicts that he is tall, and skin like a Caucasian depicts that he is fair. So, we are now giving more factual information about the three dimensions.

The other features are individual characteristics; this boy speaks Hindi; this boy wears size 8 shoes. These are individual characteristics. Now you have a second set of characteristics, which are more individual and do not pertain to the first set of criteria. The second set of characteristics does not denote anything about being tall, fair, or a boy, but it is about individual characteristics. The last and most individualising feature or a very special distinguishing feature. Let's say he has a very gruff voice or always carries a red handkerchief in his pocket. This is extremely distinguishing; this is what we call the "keynote".

So, when we want to exactly identify someone, we should look for which among the tall, fair boys we see is one who is 6 feet 3 inches, who's got Caucasian-like skin and a moustache, speaks Hindi and wears size 8 shoes, and one who has a gruff voice and has a red handkerchief in his pocket. This is what the five fingers are all about.

Five fingers describe three dimensions tall, fair, and boy, which describe height, skin colour, and gender. Similarly in homeopathy, the three dimensions are superclass, kingdom (and sub-kingdom), and miasm. You shortlist the remedies that are needed according to these three.

Then you will have characteristics symptoms; some of these characteristic will describe the miasm, kingdom, sub-kingdom, and Superclass and will describe more individual symptoms such as headaches worse from the sun, desire for salt, etc. The totality of the characteristic will represent the fourth finger.

The last finger will denote the keynote, which will be very specific for this particular remedy, e.g., Thirst for large quantities of water at long intervals or great confusion of identity, etc. This is how our whole identification process gets precise. And we will get the right person home from the airport.

The Superclass idea adds the most recently discovered dimension to the others previously used. In fact, it gives the most powerful grip on the case just like the thumb gives the most powerful grip to the hand.

It is also possible that you might see someone in the airport with a prominent red handkerchief in the pocket. However, before we decide that this is the person we want, we need to be sure that he is a tall, fair boy and that he has the other characteristics we know. Similarly in Homeopathy, if we see the patient has a keynote symptom of a remedy, we need to see that the remedy also matches the patient's Superclass, Kingdom and Miasm.

To take an example, If Pulsatilla is the remedy of the case, the five 'fingers' of the case would need to match Pulsatilla

1. Superclass - 1

With features of withdrawal, clinging, sensitive to external stimuli etc.

2. Kingdom – Plant. Subkingdom - Ranunculaceae

The perception of sensitivity and reactivity. We would see the sensation and its opposite.

3. Miasm- Sycotic

Pulsatilla, as we know, would serve as the meeting place of the Ranunculaceae and sycotic miasm.

4. The characteristics such as

- Worse warm room better open air
- Aversion to fatty/oily food
- Thick green discharges
- Pain in the eyes as if the eyeballs are pulled backwards.

5. Keynotes –

Extremely sensitive and weeps easily and at everything. Thirstless with a dry mouth.

Earlier it was proposed that we could analyse a case according to 8 boxes. This has now been simplified to 5 fingers. In the latter, we have added Superclass and have put physical, general, and mental characteristics under one heading rather than having separate headings as in the 8-box method.

Either method of analysis is useful and can be used interchangeably but we have found this 5-finger idea to be fairly simple. It also incorporates the idea of the Superclass, which like the thumb is the most important finger for having a good grip. The Superclass aspect needs to be seen in sync with the kingdom, subkingdom, miasm and the characteristic symptoms and the keynotes/source qualities.

When working with the idea of the Superclasses we have asked ourselves what the main difference between animal, plant, and mineral kingdoms is. And how would these be expressed in cases?

The key to this is:

I – Something – Someone – It

"I" – is related to the Mineral Kingdom
"Something" – is related to the Plant Kingdom
"Someone" – Is related to the Animal Kingdom
"It" – is related to the Nosodes.

"I" denotes what I have or what I lose or lack. If this is the main emphasis in the case, then we can classify it as the Mineral Kingdom.

"Something" happens, and I need to react or adapt to it. Then we would classify it as the Plant Kingdom.

"Someone" is there, who is creating a problem and I need to face that with my survival strategy. This is classified as Animal Kingdom.

"It" is hectic/out of control/destructive etc. Here the experience of the perception is at the centre of the Miasm. Everything is expressed in terms of the pace and depth of the miasm.

First Superclass

In the first Superclass the main theme is withdrawal -

Mineral Kingdom: I need to withdraw because I do not have the resources to face the situation. I need something into which I should withdraw as I do not have it. I need to have the womb. That is what I lack.

Plant Kingdom: I need to withdraw as something out there is too much for me to bear. So, I need to in some sense, desensitize myself or anaesthetize myself, as it is too much to bear - that is my adaptation.

Animal Kingdom: I need to withdraw as something will come to attack me, so I need to create a shell to survive. This is my survival against the other.

Second Superclass

In the second Superclass, the main theme is 'in and out' -

Mineral Kingdom: I don't know if I am capable of coming out. Whether I should stay in or do I have the capability to come out and face the world?

Plant Kingdom: The inside is so grey and dull. So, my adaptation is to come out for some time and feel some sensory stimulation.

Animal Kingdom: When it is dangerous if I am going to be threatened by something, then I will go into a shell. When nobody is threatening me, I can come out.

Third Superclass

In the third Superclass the main theme is to be limited –

Mineral Kingdom: I need to stay within the border. I am not capable of providing my care and nourishment. Therefore, I stay within the border that provides it to me.

Plant Kingdom: I feel as if I am within some borders. I feel a sensation as if something is shrinking me and I want to expand.

Animal Kingdom: I feel someone has put me in a cage and I need to fly out. The cage is good; the one who is putting me in a cage, gives me care and nourishment but I also feel controlled, and I don't like it. It is an ambivalent feeling.

Fourth Superclass

In the fourth Superclass the main theme is stability -

Mineral Kingdom: I need stability and security. I must get it through home, job, family, money, etc. I need this. I need to find it. I lack it and I should not lose it.

Plant Kingdom: I am very sensitive to instability and change. When there is any change, it disturbs me.

Animal Kingdom: As long as I am under somebody, I would feel stability and security (like a dog)

Fifth Superclass

In the fifth Superclass the main theme is to get out –

Mineral Kingdom: I need to now develop my resources to come out. Whether it is coming out of a narrow place or a routine idea. I need to find a new idea, I need to find resources, ability, and skill. I need to come out of the box.

Plant Kingdom: Something makes me feel like I am being held tight and I feel suffocated, and I need to move. I feel stiffness in my body. I feel tied up; I feel constricted. Something in the situation feels constricting or renders me immobile.

Animal Kingdom: Somebody is suffocating me, restricting me, holding me tight.

Sixth Superclass

In the sixth Superclass the main theme is fight or flight -

Mineral Kingdom: I am needing a lot of power; I need the ability to lead. I need the ability to defend myself against almost murderous attacks.

Plant Kingdom: It feels like something is threatening. A situation is very threatening. I need to fight or flee. Something is injuring me, and I need to respond.

Animal Kingdom: Somebody is doing that to me (like a snake or lion). A murderous attack by somebody.

This is the difference in the kingdom perspectives between each Superclass. I, Something and Somebody/Someone. In each case, we need to see where the emphasis lies. Is it in having or not having resources? Is something happening and I have to adapt? Or is someone doing it to me? The language will be similar, but you have to see where the emphasis is.

If the emphasis is on capacity and capability: Mineral Kingdom

Sensation and reaction: Plant Kingdom

Me versus somebody else: Animal Kingdom

Subkingdoms

Once you understand which kingdom it is that the person falls into then you need to see which subkingdom it is.

For example, if the patient is in the Mineral Kingdom, then we need to see you will need to see which row the patient falls into in the Periodic Table. I see the Periodic table as a kind of map of human development with each row representing a certain stage of development. In the first row, we have the theme of conception with the issue of do I exist or not? The second row corresponds with the foetal development beginning with needing the safety of the womb and later the birth process unfolding as the womb is no longer the place of safety but becomes constricting needing the foetus to come out. The 3rd row deals with the development of Identity and issues of care and nourishment. The 4th row has themes of either the need for or loss of security. In the 5th row, we see the development going beyond the routine tasks of the 4th row to themes of creativity and performance. The 6th row represents the development of responsibility and leadership.

In this way by looking at the main issues of the patient we can place them into a specific row. From left to right in the 18 columns you can see a gradual building up of something and then from column 10, we see a decline of that quality. This is the summary of the mineral kingdom.

In the plant kingdom we have delineated the 6 subclasses of the dicotyledons and there we have the individual orders and families, each with a specific sensation within the dynamic of each subclass.

As far as the animal kingdom is concerned, we have different classes like molluscs, insects, birds, spiders etc. and each has its survival strategy. For example, Spiders are highly restless, and sensitive and trap others.

Miasms and Nosodes

Each nosode represents the main qualities of each miasm. For example, Medorrhinum would represent the sycotic miasm. In Medorrhinum we have all the sycotic features as the central characteristics of the remedy, such as avoidance, acceptance, and anticipation.

Miasm	Quality	Corresponding nosode
Psoric	Optimism and struggle	Psorinum
Ringworm	Struggle and Acceptance	Ringworm
Sycotic	Avoidance, acceptance and anticipation	Medorrhinum
Tubercular	Hectic oppression and getting out	Tuberculinum
Cancer	Beyond your control	Carcinosinum

Leprosy
Despair
Leprominium

Syphilis
Hopelessness
Syphilinum

Characteristic Symptoms

Characteristic symptoms are usually seen as rubrics in the repertory. These symptoms include –

Pathological symptoms
Physical symptoms
Local symptoms
General symptoms
General modalities
Mental symptoms - including fears, delusions and dreams

Keynotes and Source Qualities

The fifth aspect (after Superclass, Kingdoms/subkingdoms, Miasms and Characteristics) is Keynotes and source qualities.

Each remedy, especially our well-known ones, will have keynotes. These are symptoms which are highly characteristic and are found in many cases of the remedy. They are in some way central to the remedy.

For example, the mild yielding weeping disposition of Pulsatilla. Or aggravation from least motion in Bryonia.

In some cases, you will have qualities which represent the source of the remedy. Usually, these come up when you go very deep in the case. The patient sometimes mentions or describes something completely illogically about a certain shape, texture, colour or consistency of something. These seemingly extremely strange descriptions can be understood sometimes as qualities of the source of the remedy.

For example, a patient needing the carnivorous plant remedy Dionaea muscipula (Venus flytrap) can, in the course of the narration, almost exactly describe through gestures or words how there is a trapping mechanism where two parts come together and interlock.

This does not happen in all cases, yet when it does it is a very powerful indication and confirmation of the remedy.

Using the '5 finger method' In Practice: A few short cases

Aurum –

This is the case of a man with diabetes, which was accidentally discovered in October 1969; he was asymptomatic. Then he had chest pain and was diagnosed with myocardial infarction and hypertension. Subsequently, he developed a diabetic ulcer on the right foot that wouldn't heal.

Diabetes is now controlled but there are no pulses on foot. He went into left ventricular failure during the angiogram. Later angiogram showed the occlusion. Chest X-ray showed an enlarged heart and CHF.

With the ulcer, the right foot toes were involved, and amputation was recommended. The attending internist felt he was too high risk for surgery. The surgeon was saying if you don't operate you die and the internist said if you do operate you die. So, he came to us.

We saw him in September 1986.

He had grey hair and clipped speech. He developed his first myocardial infarction as he was discharging his official duties in Delhi and was hospitalized for six weeks.

He gives dates, sequence and progression. The way he says it is the fundamental issue of the case: He says it happened in the course of discharging my official duty. He is an income tax officer known to be extremely conscientious, honest and hard-working.

He was in search of some tax evaders and he raided the premises of someone whom he thought was evading taxes. He found the vital documents and then the next morning the documents were stolen from his desk. So, someone in his office was involved. He moved heaven and earth and the next day he found the documents.

He used to lose his temper and become very angry.
The tone of his voice is strong and powerful.
Religious aspect and high desire for music.

Approaching this case we can apply the 5 fingers –

Superclass: in this case, we could see the great leadership and responsibility of the patient. There was the idea of a fight to the finish, come what may he was going to get back those documents. We can also see in his nature his confrontational attitude, there was no fear in taking on his superiors. In fact, he mentioned to us that even his bosses were afraid of him as he would put them in their place if needed. This is the 6th Superclass.

Kingdom: in this case, there are soft hints at the mineral kingdom just from his presentation alone. The way he narrated his case was very organised and matter of fact this can be a defining feature in mineral kingdom cases. The subkingdom was very clear as we could see all the issues of the 6th row. These were features of –

Conscientious
Duty bound
Rigid
Hard and determined
High-performance and high value
High morality

Miasm: There is high destruction of bones, heart and blood vessels. This gives us hints of the syphilitic aspect (high destruction). His desperation when he lost the papers also indicates this Miasm.

Characteristics:

	Aur.	Sep.	Thuj.	Carc.	Ign.	Jade	Kola.	Aur-m-n.	Aur-s.	Lsd	Merc.	Nat-m.	Posit.
Total	17	11	10	9	8	7	6	4	4	4	4	4	4
Rubrics	5	4	4	4	4	4	4	4	4	4	4	4	4
Kingdom													
CR19 - Mind; Delusions, imaginations; neglected; duty, his(32)	4				1	1	1	1	1	1			
CR19 - Mind; Industrious, mania for work(244)	4	4	3	3	3	1	3	1		1	1	1	1
CR19 - Mind; Injustice, cannot support(86)	1	2	1	2	1	3	1	1	1		1	1	1
CR19 - Mind; Religious affections(167)	4	4	3	1	3	2			1	1	1	1	1
CR19 - Mind; Music; amel.(46)	4	1	3	3			1	1	1	1	1	1	1

	Aur.	Calc.	Hep.	Merc.	Nit-ac.	Puls.	Con.	Lach.	Lyc.	Ph-ac.	Ruta	Ars.
Total	12	12	12	12	12	12	11	11	11	11	11	10
Rubrics	4	4	4	4	4	4	4	4	4	4	4	4
Kingdom												
CR19 - Skin; Ulcers(579)	4	4	4	4	4	4	4	4	4	4	4	4
CR19 - Skin; Ulcers; deep(89)	4	4	3	4	4	4	3	4	4	3	3	4
CR19 - Generalities; Abscesses, suppurations; bones(123)	3	3	4	3	3	3	3	2	2	3	3	1
CR19 - Generalities; Abscesses, suppurations; denuding, bones(21)	1	1	1	1	1	1	1	1	1	1	1	1

Aurum met 200 healed the ulcer within 2 months. There was a miraculous regeneration of the bones as well.

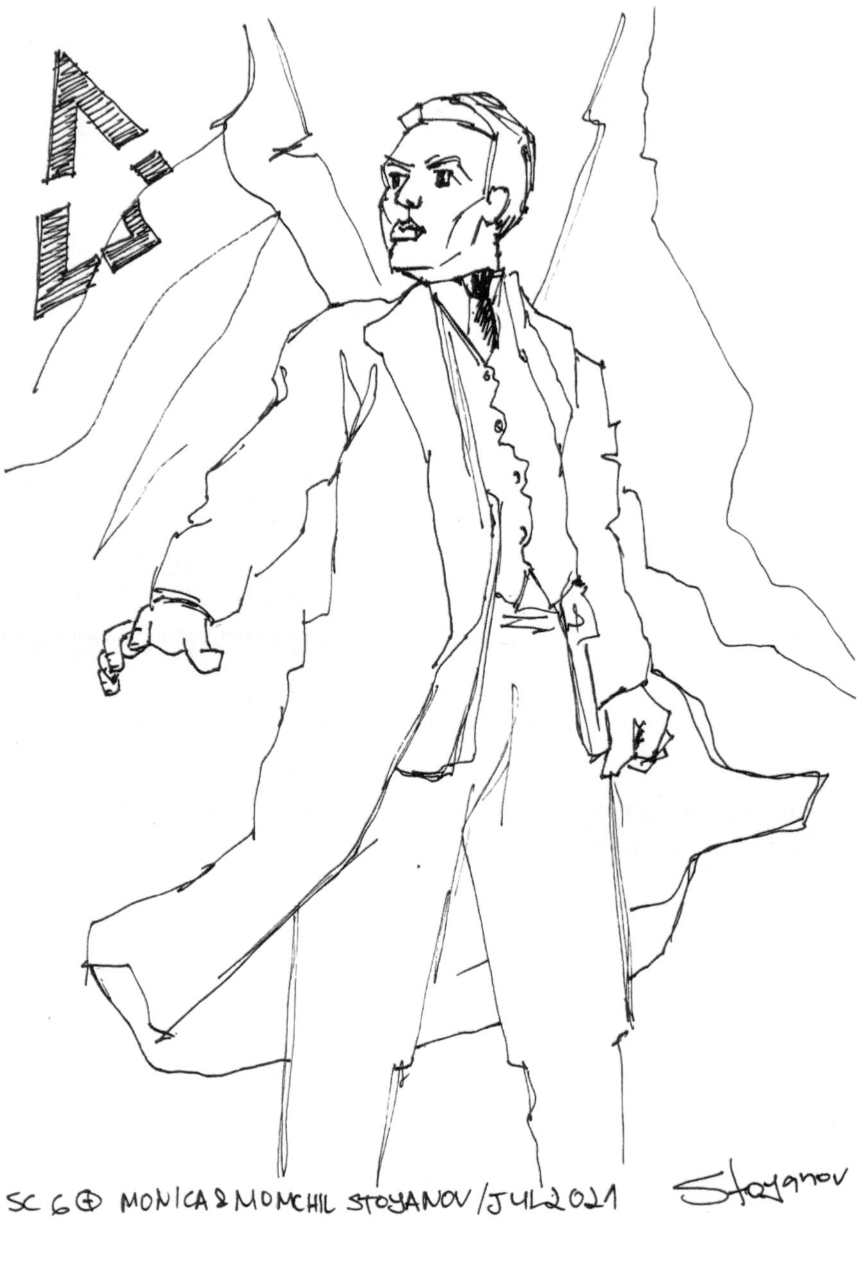
SC 6 © MONICA & MOMCHIL STOYANOV / JUL 2021
Stoyanov

Thuja –

A seventy-year-old male was brought for consultation on 14.08.2001, by his two sons. He had been diagnosed as having cancer of the prostate with metastases in the bones. A surgery to remove the testes had been done, following which he had stopped passing urine, and could only do so with a catheter. Attempts to de-catheterize him had been so far unsuccessful, and the doctors were looking at the possibility of a second surgery if he was not able to pass urine normally.

When asked about his problems he mentioned the difficulty in passing urine. He also mentions that he is suffering from constipation. There is pain passing urine like a needle. When passing stool it does not come out and he has to force it, there is severe itching. The skin is very delicate and soft, the stool is hard and rubs the skin till it comes off. The patient also has poor memory and cannot even recall who he has just spoken to on phone calls. He also has cataract but he doesn't want to get it operated on (avoidance) and when asked why he describes cases which can go bad (anticipation).

The patient describes how he feels sorry for himself with his complaints but is not able to express himself to others. He cites the fear of displeasing others if he expresses himself so he just keeps quiet. At this point, he mentions that he has not laughed for thirty to fifty years. When asked why he says that due to his age, he should appear sober otherwise he could be criticised by others. This is the same feeling he had when he feels that he cannot express himself to others. When we take this experience deeper he talks about how the family should not split up (he gives a HG) but should stay together (gives another HG) here we can see the same delusion of fragility and feeling of split that he has in his complaint with the rectum.

Using the 5-finger approach we can see the following –

Superclass: this is the 4th Superclass as we see the need for stability and for maintaining the status quo in the family.

Kingdom: There is a situation to which he is sensitive leading to a sensation and reaction. This is the plant kingdom. For the subkingdom, we can see all the features of the Conifers which are –

Delicate
Fragile
Easy to split

Miasm: the patient is constantly anticipating and trying to avoid situations, this is the sycotic miasm.

Characteristics:

We have the following rubrics which confirm Thuja which is at the meeting point of the 4th Superclass, Plant kingdom, Gymnosperms (conifers), Sycotic miasm –

synergy	Thuj.	Ars.	Alum.	Am-c.	Aur.	Ambr.	Tub.	Con.	Sabal.	Sep.	Cadm-p	Ion-rad.	Hep.
Total	5	5	2	2	4	3	3	3	2	2	2	2	1
Rubrics	3	2	2	2	1	1	1	1	1	1	1	1	1
Kingdom													
CR19 - Mind; Smiling; never(11)	[illegible]	4	[illegible]	[illegible]	4	3	3						[illegible]
CR19 - Male; Cancer; prostate gland(55)	[illegible]	[illegible]	[illegible]	[illegible]				3	2	2	2	2	
CR19 - Mind; Delusions, imaginations; body, body parts; delicate(1)	3												

Keynotes: this all points to the remedy Thuja which we know has the keynote - Delusion he is made of glass.

The patient was followed up for three years. His retention was relieved immediately and his PSA came back to normal. The best part of the follow-up was that his smile came back in a very good way.

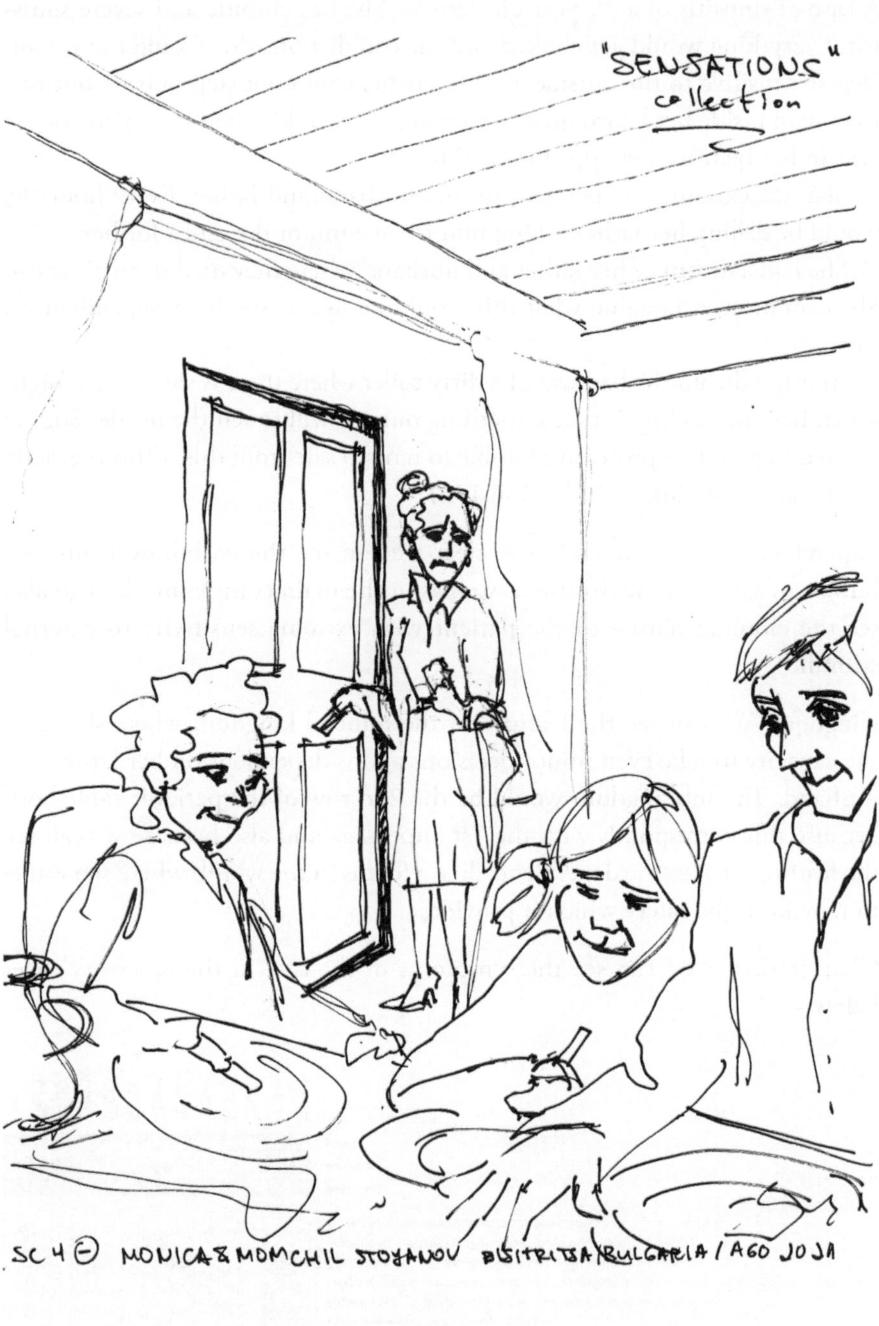
"SENSATIONS"
collection
SC4 © MONICA & MOMCHIL STOYANOV BISITRITSA/BULGARIA / AGO JOJA

Beryllium –

A case of sinusitis of a 25-year-old female. She has chronic and severe sinusitis. Everything would get choked and she couldn't breathe. Could not get air. Was so sensitive to the outside world that she could not step outside but had to remain inside her bedroom covering up. She would spend large parts of the year in her bedroom wrapped in a quilt.

She was extremely dependent on her husband and father. Every hour she would be calling her father asking him to take minor decisions for her.

She had a dream of her father and husband where they died in an air crash. She cannot even imagine what this would be like as she is so dependent on them.

Another dream she had was of a dirty toilet where there is shit which might touch her. The feeling is that something outside will touch the inside. So, she wanted to go into a protective bubble to remain safe from this. (This is exactly what was happening with the sinusitis.)

Superclass: the first superclass is clear we can see the withdrawal into the bubble of safety in the dreams as well as in the main complaint. We can also see the clinging nature of the patient with extreme sensitivity to external stimuli.

Kingdom: We can see the features of the mineral kingdom where she lacks the capacity to take even minor decisions and is dependent on her father and husband. The subkingdom would be the 2nd row of the periodic table both because this corresponds with the 1st Superclass and also because we can see the features of extreme dependency like a foetus in the womb where she wants to remain in the safety which it provides.

Characteristics: we can see the symptoms of the case in the repertory sheet below –

synergy	Beryl.	Haliae-lc.	Lyc.	Hoch.	Bar-c.	Ign.	Kali-c.	Med.	Staph.	Ozone	Argo.	Germ.	Lsd
Total	7	7	3	3	5	5	4	2	2	2	2	2	2
Rubrics	7	3	3	3	2	2	2	2	2	2	2	2	2
Kingdom													
CR19 - Mind; Confidence; want of self; inadequate, feels(51)	1	1	1	1	1			1	1	1	1	1	1
CR19 - Mind; Confidence; want of self; support, desires(7)	1						3						
CR19 - Mind; Death; ailments from, agg.; parents or friends, of(39)	1	2	1	1		4	1	1	1			1	
CR19 - Mind; Delusions, imaginations; child, children; again, he is a, and acts like a(20)	1										1		1
CR19 - Mind; Delusions, imaginations; diminished; small, he is(5)	1												
CR19 - Mind; Fear; freedom, of(2)	1												
CR19 - Mind; Indecision, irresolution; acts, in(35)	1	4	1	1	4	1				1			

Beryllium is not a well-proven remedy, yet we are still able to find some characteristics in the repertory which can corroborate the symptom with the system.

On this basis the remedy Beryllium was prescribed with which the patient did amazingly, recovering from her physical complaints and also becoming far more independent in her personal life.

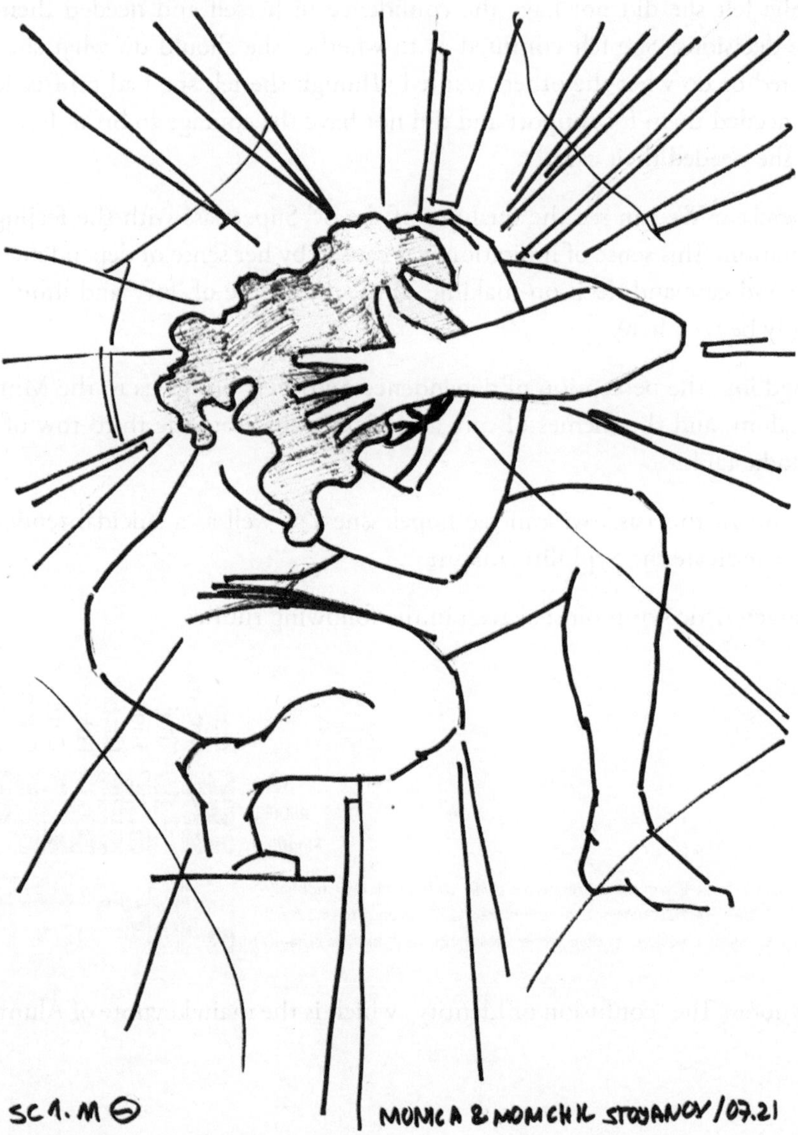

Alumina

This is the case of a 26-year-old married woman, the mother of a 3-year-old child, who came to me with depression and had attempted suicide. She felt that she had no freedom. While she felt dependent on the support of her in-laws, she felt that they gave her no freedom of choice. She felt like she was a doll whose remote control was in their hand, and she had to do exactly what they told her to.

She felt she did not have the confidence in herself and needed them to take decisions. She felt confused as to whether she should do what she felt wanted or do what the others wanted. Though she felt she had no freedom, she needed them for support and did not have the courage to break free. She felt she needed their care.

Superclass: We can see the qualities of the 3rd Superclass with the feeling of limitation. This sense of limitation was caused by her sense of dependence for love and care and decision-making. Thus, the theme of 'love and limit' can clearly be seen here.

Kingdom: The perception of dependence on others brings us to the Mineral kingdom, and the themes of care and identity indicate the third row of the periodic table.

Miasm: In this case, we can see hopelessness as well as a suicidal tendency. These indicate the Syphilitic miasm

Characteristic symptoms: as seen in the following rubrics

synergy	Alum.	Nat-m.	Thuj.	Ther.	Lach.	Falco-p.	Cypra-e	Cann-i.	Cann-s.	Betul.
Total	5	2	2	3	1	1	1	1	1	1
Rubrics	3	2	2	1	1	1	1	1	1	1
Kingdom										
CR19 - Mind; Confusion of mind; identity, as to his; own, as if it were not his(6)	1	1	1		1	1	1			
CR19 - Mind; Delusions, imaginations; head; belongs to another(6)	1	1	1	3				1	1	
CR19 - Mind; Delusions, imaginations; sees things as if through others(2)	3									1

Keynotes: The "confusion of Identity" which is the main keynote of Alumina.

The remedy Alumina healed her and brought back her self-confidence over a period of time and consequently her perception of limitation and dependence disappeared.

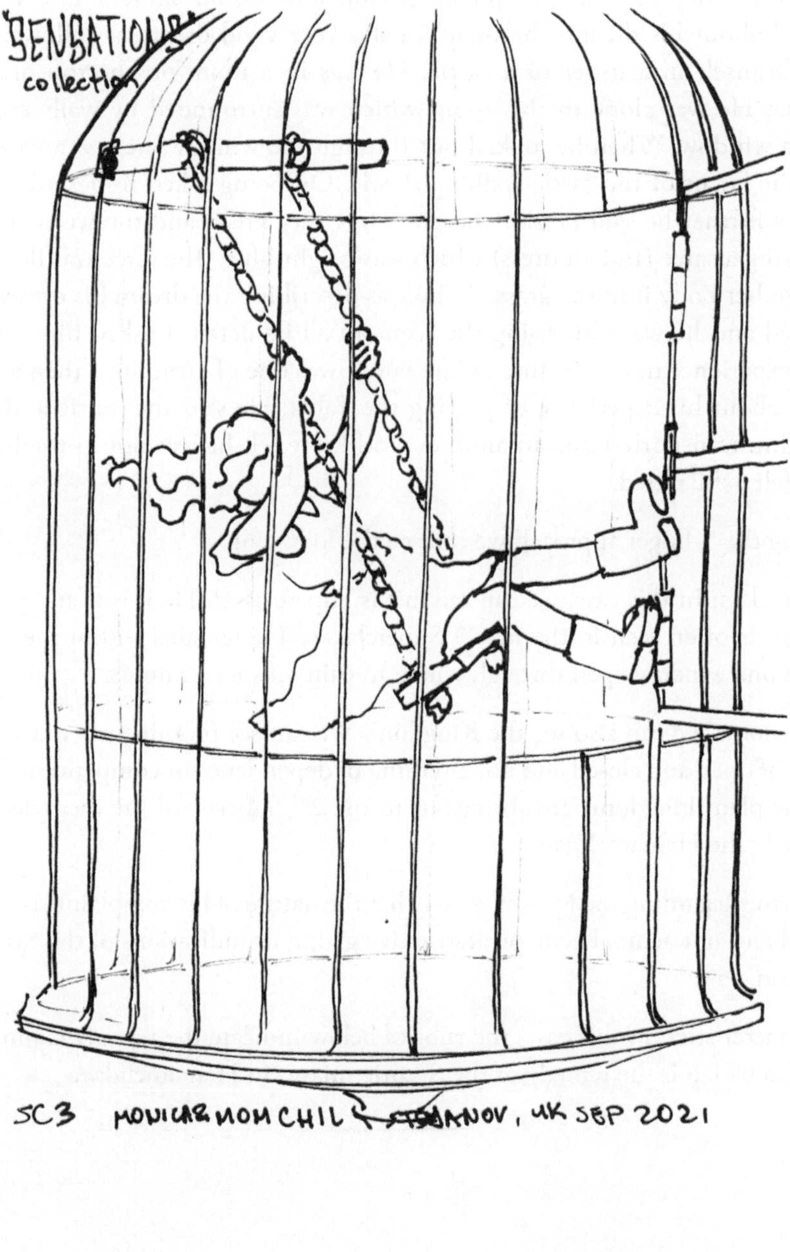

Cannabis indica –

A 40-year-old male patient came with several complaints including hypertension. He was a well-known player of the percussion instrument called *the Tabla*.

By nature, he is a soft-spoken person and would smile a lot. When asked about his dreams, he mentioned a very vivid dream as follows: He saw himself in a tower of a castle. He was in a room on the top of this tower. He was alone in this room which was surrounded by walls except for a window. When he looked out through the window, he saw a woman on the lawns of the castle walking slowly. On being asked to describe this scene further he said he saw the grass was very green and the woman was wearing a saree (Indian dress) which was bright blue. The saree was flowing down her body into the grass. As he was describing the dream his eyes were closed and he was visualising the scene in all its detail. I asked him about the experience in the dream, and he said it was one of great joy. I then asked him about his experience of playing the Tabla. He said the music and the rhythm transported him to another world. He felt he was not in the body. He felt exhilarated.

Using the 5-finger approach we can see the following –

Superclass: In this case, we can see this is Superclass 2. He is soft and gentle which is often seen in the first 3 Superclasses. He remains within the walls with one window open through which to gain sensory stimulus.

Kingdom: We can also see the Kingdom. We can see prominently the sensation of open and closed and not anything of dependence or competition. This is the plant kingdom. This brings us to the 2nd Subclass of the dicotyledons namely the Hamamelidae.

Miasm: Regarding the Miasm we see that the nature of his complaints is more fixed and not acute, hectic or destructive giving us indications of the Sycotic Miasm.

Characteristics: in this case, the rubrics below indicate the remedy Cannabis Indica which is the remedy of the Sycotic miasm in Hamamelidae.

synergy	Cann-i.	Lach.	Coca	Germ.	Lsd	Bell.	Coff.	Sulph.	Op.	Phos.	Agar.	Nic-r.	Fic-sp.
Total	14	16	9	4	4	11	10	9	8	8	7	5	5
Rubrics	9	6	4	4	4	3	3	3	3	3	3	3	3
Kingdom													
CR19 - Mind; Delusions, imaginations; beautiful, wonderful(35)	3	3	1	1	1	4	3	4	2			1	1
CR19 - Mind; Delusions, imaginations; music, hears; melody, a; sweetest and most sublime(3)	1	3											
CR19 - Mind; Delusions, imaginations; outside of body(38)	1			1						1	1	2	2
CR19 - Mind; Delusions, imaginations; space; carried into, that he is(7)	1	3	3	1	1							2	
CR19 - Mind; Delusions, imaginations; transferred to another; world(1)	1												
CR19 - Mind; Delusions, imaginations; walls; around her(3)	1												
CR19 - Mind; Dreams; beautiful; scenes(6)	1	1											
CR19 - Mind; Dreams; vivid(288)	1	2	2	1	1	3	3	4	2	4	3		
CR19 - Mind; Exhilaration(188)	4	4	3		1	4	4	1	4	3	3		2

Source qualities: We can also see as the source quality in this case, the effects of Cannabis as a drug substance which has the feeling of exhilaration and exaggeration of sensory inputs.

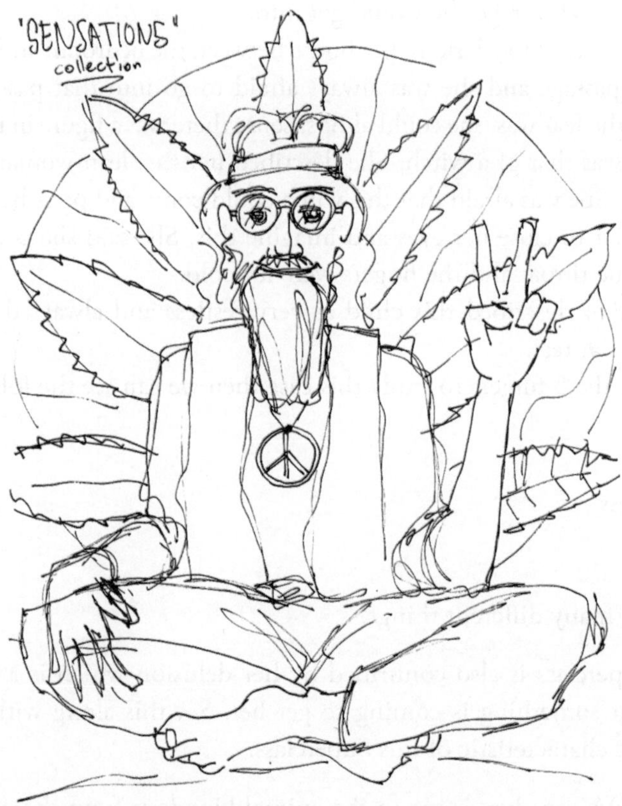

Cantharis –

This is the case of a young girl of about 13 or 14 years old. She had come to me with an acute urinary tract infection. Not only acute but recurrent. It was very severe and had to take antibiotics each time. Having gone through this they decided to come for homeopathy. The symptom was extremely severe burning while urinating. Sharp cutting pains. Urine was passed drop by drop with tenesmus. Would go to the corner of the room with her legs crossed tightly as each drop of urine would burn so much she would shriek and shout with the pain.

Her parents described her as a very ambitious girl, always coming first in class. Also ambitious in sports and extra-curricular activities. She was very competitive and wanted to do better than other children. The mother described that if someone went ahead of her she would get very angry. In anger, she would get violent impulses. She wanted to take the head of the other child and smash it against the wall. She never did anything like this but this was the kind of rage she would get into.

Her fears were of the dark. In her house between the bedroom and washroom was a dark passage and she was always afraid to go into that passage. When asked what the fear was, she could almost sense there was a figure in the passage. This figure was that of a witch. She described her as a lean woman with very long fingers. She was afraid that this witch could come and press her throat.

I asked her to close her eyes and imagine this. She said she could feel the fingers on the throat and the fingers were icy cold.

The mother described this child as very restless and always doing something. Never at rest.

If we use the 5 fingers to study this case then we can see the following -

Superclass:

She is restless
Ambitious
Active
Involved in many different things.

The 5th superclass is also confirmed by her delusion which is a threat perception that something is coming to get her. So, this along with the other qualities are characteristic of this Superclass.

Kingdom: We can then come to the animal kingdom from the comparison, anger and jealousy

When considering the Sub-kingdom, in the animal kingdom in the 5th Superclass we have insects, spiders and cephalopods. There is not the deceitfulness of spiders and not the escape impulse of cephalopods. But there is the rage and high activity along with smarting burning pain. These are the qualities of insects.

Miasm: We can see the tubercular miasm with the hectic pace.

Characteristics: As far as the characteristics are concerned there is a prominent infection of the urinary tract. There is burning smarting pain. Passing drop by drop with shrieking.

synergy	Canth.	Berb.	Nux-v.	Apis	Cop.	Chim.	Sulph.	Acon.	Petr.	Prun.	Puls.	Staph.	Thuj.
Total	20	6	12	10	9	7	6	5	5	5	5	5	5
Rubrics	5	4	3	3	3	3	3	3	3	3	3	3	3
Kingdom													
CR19 - Bladder; Pain; burning, smarting; neck; extending through urethra(2)	4					3							
CR19 - Bladder; Pain; burning, smarting; neck; urination; during(21)	4	1	4	3	3		1	1	3	1	1	1	1
CR19 - Bladder; Pain; burning, smarting; urination; during(63)	4	1	4	3	3	1	1	1	1	1	1	1	1
CR19 - Bladder; Pain; urination; during; drops passing, after a few(6)	4	1											
CR19 - Bladder; Urging to urinate, morbid desire; constant(159)	4	3	4	4	3	3	4	3	1	3	3	3	3

Then you can go to the mental symptoms. Hyperactive, violent. And the delusion of being choked by icy-cold hands.

The mother also said she is a very proud, haughty person.

The characteristics of Cantharis are all found in the following rubrics -

synergy	Canth.	Nux-v.	Hyos.	Bell.	Lach.	Phos.	Lyc.	Aur.	Stram.	Chin.	Calc.	Ign.	Arn.
Total	23	21	25	21	21	16	22	19	19	16	15	13	11
Rubrics	13	9	8	8	8	8	7	7	7	7	7	7	7
Kingdom													
CR19 - Mind; Activity; hyperactive(70)	2	1	1	3	1	3		1	1	3	3	1	1
CR19 - Mind; Anger; violent(191)	3	4	3	4	2	3	3	4	2	2	3	3	1
CR19 - Mind; Cruelty, brutality, inhumanity(65)	1	1	3	3	3			3	3	1	3		
CR19 - Mind; Delusions, imaginations; choked, of being; ice cold hands, by(1)	1												
CR19 - Mind; Delusions, imaginations; images, phantoms, sees; night(42)	1	1		1		1	1			1	1	1	1
CR19 - Mind; Delusions, imaginations; seized, he is(3)	1		3			1							
CR19 - Mind; Delusions, imaginations; throat, someone takes her by the; hands, with cold(1)	1												
CR19 - Mind; Fight; wants to(114)	1	3	3	1	1	1		3	1			1	1
CR19 - Mind; Haughty, pride(118)	2	1	4	1	4	3	4	3	4	3	1	1	3
CR19 - Mind; Malicious, vindictive(167)	3	4	4	4	4	3	4	3	4	3	3	3	1
CR19 - Mind; Shrieking, screaming, shouting; urination; before(15)	1	3			3		4						
CR19 - Mind; Shrieking, screaming, shouting; urination; during(15)	4						3						3
CR19 - Mind; Violence, vehemence; rage leading to deeds of, agg.(72)	2	3	4	4	3	1	3	2	4	3	1	3	

The keynote of Cantharis is the Urinary burning such as we see here.

The remedy helped her immediately and the recurrences of the Urinary infections stopped.

Croton tiglium –

This is the case of a lady of around 40 who used to teach dancing. She was 35 years. She was very passionate about Indian classical dancing. But was also interested in innovating within traditional dancing.

Her problem was that she would get acute attacks of asthma and her chest would become so tight that she could not take a breath in. It was very acute and would cause panic. She described the tightness that she feels not only in the chest but also in the whole body. The word bound was also very important and the whole body would feel bound not just in the chest. It was as if being tied with a rope.

The reason she dances is because she feels the complete opposite sensation as if free, loose. Any tight thing she could not bear.

While using the 5 fingers we can see she is an innovator and thinks out of the box. Wanting movement all the time and the experience of being stuck and wanting to get out. All this points to the 5th Superclass.

Kingdom: we can see there is a sensation and reaction.

In subkingdom, we can see clear features of the family Euphorbiaceae which is the sensation of being tied, bound, and tight.

Miasm: the attacks of the asthma were very sudden and would cause great panic in her. From this, we can see the aspects of the acute miasm.

Croton tig is the remedy in the acute miasm in the Euphorbiaceae family.

Characteristics: We have the following rubrics

synergy	Croto-t.	Brom.	Ars.	Phos.	Dig.	Lach.	Con.	Sep.	Cann-i.	Ail.	Calc.	Mez.	Op.
Total	24	16	16	13	12	10	9	9	8	7	7	7	7
Rubrics	7	5	4	4	4	4	4	4	4	4	4	4	4
Kingdom													
CR19 - Chest; Air; desire for, wants to fill chest with air(5)	4	3											
CR19 - Chest; Constriction(513)	4	4	4	4	4	4	4	4	2	3	4	4	4
CR19 - Chest; Clothing agg.(65)	4		4	3		4	3	3	2	2			
CR19 - Chest; Expand, as if lungs could not(95)	4	3	4	3	4				2				
CR19 - Chest; Pain; drawing; string, as by a, mamma towards axilla(3)	3	3											
CR19 - Chest; Pain; pulling; string, as of a, nipples; extending to back(1)													
CR19 - Respiration; Difficult; expand lungs, cannot(78)	4	3	4	3	3				2				

synergy	Croto-t.	Tax.	Bell.	Lach.	Plat.	Sep.	Ign.	Nat-m.	Tarent.	Agar.	Merc.	Lsd	Salx-f.
Total	14	6	14	12	12	12	10	10	10	9	9	5	5
Rubrics	6	6	5	5	5	5	5	5	5	5	5	5	5
Kingdom													
CR19 - Mind; Dance, desires to(84)			4		3	3		2	4	3			
CR19 - Mind; Walk, walking; amel.(369)	3		4	3	3	4	4	4		3	3		
CR19 - Mind; Thoughts; persistent; himself, about; think of anyone besides, cannot(2)													
CR19 - Mind; Suspiciousness, mistrustfulness(187)	3		4	4		3	3	2			3		
CR19 - Mind; Selfishness, egoism(78)	3			3					3				
CR19 - Mind; Air; open; amel.(145)	3				4								

Keynotes: the Keynote of Croton Tig is the sensation of a string being tied to the nipples and drawn back.

The follow-up of this case is quite interesting. Within a few months she had significant improvement in her asthma. Her wheezing attacks did not come back. She felt much less anxious and the sensation of 'tied' and 'tight' during anxious situations also went away. When asked what the difference in her dancing was, she said that as a teacher of classical dance, it was customary to sit down and guide her students with the beat. But her desire to dance was so compulsive that she would get up and dance rather than teach the students to dance. She said that after the remedy, this compulsion went away and she could give her attention to teaching dance.

It was in the follow-up that I realized the beauty of the rubric:

CR19 - Mind; Dance, desires to; business, rather than attend to (1): croto-t.

Argentum nitricum –

This is the case of a 50-year-old man who came with the diagnosis of orbital haemangioma and who was advised of a very difficult and risky surgery.

He was an important executive in a multinational company, and it was his job to strategize and execute sales and other projects. His job required a lot of skill and out-of-the-box thinking and innovation. By nature, he was extremely well-organised and had a lot of anxiety before presentations. He had a very good reputation of being a top performer and it was very important for him to maintain this reputation. He was quite proud of his reputation. Among his hobbies was flying aeroplanes and other adventurous activities where one needed a lot of control and also which made him different from others. He had a great fear of narrow places. (You can find the details of his case in my book: Structure. And also, in the VitalQuest program included in the Synergy Homeopathic Software.)

When we look at it from the 5 aspects:

Superclass: Innovation, out of the box, claustrophobia, outstanding - 5th Superclass

Kingdom: Skill, Performance, Loss of position - Mineral Kingdom 5th Row

Miasm: Control, perfection - Cancer Miasm

Characteristics:

synergy	Arg-n.	Thuj.	Staph.	Lyc.	Calc.	Sil.	Lach.	Plb.	Sulph.	Plac.	Kali-c.	Nux-v.	Tax.
Total	12	7	6	10	9	9	6	6	5	5	3	3	3
Rubrics	4	4	4	3	3	3	3	3	3	3	3	3	3
Kingdom													
CR19 - Mind; Fear; self-control, losing(47)	3		3		3					2			
CR19 - Mind; Timidity; public, about appearing in(72)	4			3		4		4					
CR19 - Mind; Fear; narrow place, in, claustrophobia(80)	4			4	3					2			
CR19 - Heart & circulation; Tumors, bloodvessels, angioma, hemangioma(56)		4		3	3	4	4		3				

Keynotes: Claustrophobia, performance anxiety.

Within 3 months of the remedy, the Haemangioma was over 90% reduced in size and the patient felt better in all aspects.

We have ended this chapter by sharing three cases from the 5th Superclass. We can see the following commonalities in all three –

Restless
Ambitious
Innovative
Outstanding
Threatened
Caught
Egoistical

The difference between the three is that they each belong to a different kingdom and as such their perceptions would differ as follows –

the animal is innovative to be better. The threat comes from another (witch)
the plant is innovative to feel free. The threat is a sensation (tied)
the mineral is innovative to perform. The threat is a challenge to his ability.

This kind of interplay between the dynamic of the Superclass and the perception of the kingdom would be visible in all of the Superclasses. This chapter was only to serve to give a taste of these interactions between the various categories of information.

Following this chapter, we will be showing in-depth cases which would more greatly highlight the subtleties of the case-taking and analysis.

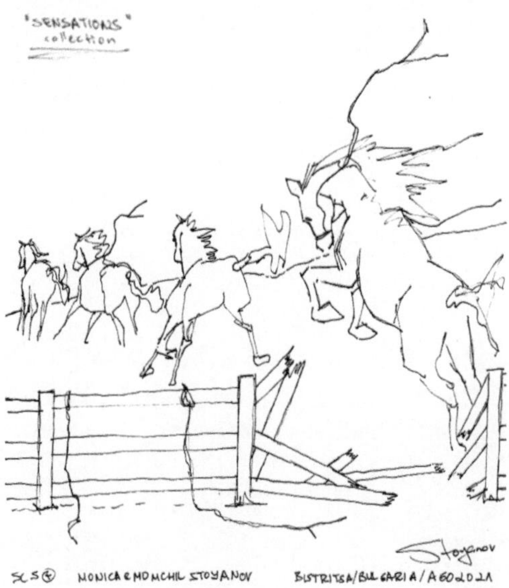

Case 1

To better display the features of the first superclass we will take up a Case example. This is the case of a 23-Year-old Female. She presented with complaints of headache and Dysmenorrhea.

The patient began the case narrating her complaint of headache.

> *I can get it every day. It starts 2-3 hours after waking in the morning and it carries on throughout the day. I get the headaches in the temples and occasionally they spread to the rest of the head.*
>
> *The pain can sometimes be very severe but in general it is bearable. It is a pressing and throbbing pain as if someone is pressing hard on the temples with some sharp object. It is almost like something is piercing, trying to cut through.*
>
> *The headache is worse from sun and strong smells. The only thing that helps is Pepsi as this causes eructation's which help to reduce the pain.*

The first question asked was "What is the effect of this pain on you?"

> *If its severe then I lie down, I feel tired and lethargic.*
>
> *I dislike noise or anyone talking to me or being around me at that time. But this occurs very rarely. In general, I have a high tolerance to pain. Even though I have the pain every day, it doesn't affect me and I go on with my work. People don't even come to know I am having the pain, unless it's very severe.*

The patient goes on to describe the dysmenorrhea.

> *I have had it for 10 years. Nowadays I feel it has reduced maybe because my tolerance to bear the pain has increased. It is a pushing type of pain, as if someone is trying to press very hard on the abdomen. When this happens I have severe back pains as well.*
>
> *It is worse lying down. And better when I sit with my legs close to the chest. While having the pain there is nausea. And during my menses the sight of milk can make me nauseous and I feel better after vomiting.*
>
> *I feel hot if the pain is severe, generally I feel very hot and I cannot tolerate heat.*
>
> *Since the past few months there has been pain in the lower abdomen between menses. It has occurred 5-6 times and lasts 5 days, I have to take Crocin. I want someone to sit with me and talk to me continuously to divert my attention otherwise I will keep thinking about the pain. I have high tolerance for pain anywhere in the body – except for abdomen pain so I would take Cyclopam. I would feel as if I am in a daze, very disoriented. Not giddy but just feel as if zoned out. If someone says something it doesn't register in my brain or things get jumbled up*

We now ask the patient to describe her nature.

> *I am very sensitive; I cry very easily when a close person hurts me. I feel very bad if there is fight with parents or close friends. If I am having an argument with my parents, even for small things then I start crying. I sweat a lot if there is a confrontation or an argument and my body becomes hot. I don't like to try new things. I have a fear of the unknown. I want to stick to what I know, for example, small things like trying a new flavor of ice-cream. I am stubborn and determined. I have rigid opinions about a lot of things.*
>
> *I like reading a lot of murder mystery, I read a lot in newspapers about plane crashes or terrorist attacks. I have always been an introvert, always in my own shell. I can't go out and party all day or meet friends all the time. I need my alone time. I like to be at home with my parents or to be with my friends. I keep getting crushed between what my peers do, what my family says and what I actually want. I feel guilty if I go against my parents. Since childhood I am very obedient. I am very particular about small things.*

We then ask the patient to describe her childhood.

> *I was very submissive. Anyone could say anything to me and get away with it. I would just cry or feel bad and go into a corner. People would take me for granted as I am being nice to them or trying to help them.*

Next, we ask the patient what she is afraid of.

> *Heights and rollercoasters and my legs feel shaky. If my father is going alone by flight, I have the fear that it will crash. If I am with him and we crash, there is no fear because then it won't impact me as we will be dead. I won't be alive to feel anything anyway. If he is alone then my mother and me will suffer. I also have the fear of losing family and close friends.*

The patient narrates some of the dreams she gets.

> *I dream of someone in my family being killed or myself getting killed. Robbery or Murder or even at times natural death. There is one where we are driving on the edge of the road and the car falls down the cliff.*

Then, we ask the patient to describe what she is sensitive to in movies and on TV.

> *Accidents or deaths in movies. When I was a child, I watched the movie Koi Mil Gaya and started crying when I saw the accident scenes. In general, I get very disturbed with violent scenes. I close my eyes and don't watch them.*

The patient was also able to give us some physical general symptoms.

> *Desires- food with many spices, cheese, ice-cream, pasta, pizza, burgers*
> *Aversion- meat*
> *Thermals- very HOT ++ I need the room to be very cold when I sleep*

At this point we decided to conduct a WISE process with the patient. We show her a picture of the first woman from the DEWISE calendar.

We ask the patient to not use their reasoning or logic. Only to use their imagination and to look at the picture and describe all that is happening there.

> *Someone is trying to hit her with a pole, and she is trying to resist that and protect herself. She is feeling helpless and powerless. Screaming, shouting*

for help, and crying. Afraid that she will be beaten with the pole and feels traumatized.

Feels the pain, sharp, like a needle prick. It will pierce through the skin cutting through making a mark, not a hole, not like it penetrates. Something that pierces through the skin and cuts through it.

What is the response to this kind of pain?

Running away from it or if he has the physical power will hit back, or else submit. It is a lot of helplessness

We then show her the second picture of the woman and ask her to repeat the process.

She is looking at something. She is surprised and shocked. What she has heard or seen is unpleasant, just takes you by surprise. You don't know how to react. Hands and feet become cold or sweaty, power in the limbs goes away. Legs feel shaky, difficulty in standing, loose feeling in hands and feet, no reflexes, just not able to react. Will not respond to any action.

— End of case —

Using the Atlas analogy which we discussed earlier, it becomes very easy to study this case. So first we need to find the continent or the superclass. Now the features of the superclass in this case are quite easily identifiable. We can see them as follows;

- Extreme sensitivity
- Weeps for slightest things (like Pulsatilla)
- In a daze, disoriented, doesn't register, jumbled up (like Nux moschata)
- When there is an argument, body becomes hot, starts to perspire (like Ranunculaceae)
- Murder, accident, killings, plane crash, terrorist, death (like Papaveraceae)
- The reaction is to go into a corner, or be in her own shell or zone out

We can see that these are the basic reactions. These belong to the first Superclass. The subcontinent or the kingdom is also quite easy to identify. We can see that patient is very sensitive to everything. With each sensitivity there is a reaction. This is the feature of the plant kingdom. So, the subclass is the Magnoliids. This becomes even more clearer when we study the key themes of the Magnoliids (Section Two).

We then need to look at the orders of the Magnoliids. As discussed earlier once the themes of the subclass were refined it was much easier to understand the qualities of these orders. As they will all have the features of the subclass. Their experience of the basic reaction will differ subtly.

So, in this case which we are studying can we identify the order? If we review some of the key points, the order then becomes clear to us…

- Chief complaint is pain, almost every single day from morning till night.
- She says in general I have a high tolerance to pain
- With the pain she feels zoned out, nothing registers in the brain.
- Likes reading about murder, plane crash, terrorist attacks
- Fear if father is going alone by flight – fear that it will crash. If I am with him and we crash, there is no fear because then it won't impact me as we will be dead. Won't be alive to feel anything anyway.
- Dreams of death, murder, car falling from the cliff
- Sensitive to accidents or death in movies
- Disturbed with violent scenes and again the reaction is to close her eyes and not watch it

These key points make it clear that the indicated order is the Papaverales. The sensitivity is to pain and suffering. This is also made clear when we did the WISE process with her.

Process 1 –

- Helpless
- Beaten and traumatized
- Pain – sharp pain, pierce through the skin and cuts it
- Response to the pain is to run away from it

Process 2 –

- Shock
- Don't know how to react, hands and feet cold or sweaty, power in the limbs goes away. Legs feel shaky, difficulty in standing, loose feeling in hands and feet
- No reflexes, just not able to react. Will not respond to any action.

The Miasm of the patient can also be identified in the way the patient has an emphasis on avoidance. We can see this when her response to pain is to run away. And when she discusses the accident scene, she says she closes her eyes. This gives us the confirmation for the sycotic miasm.

By now we have a lot of information to help us find the remedy, we know the kingdom, the subclass, the order and the miasm. The next step to finding the remedy is through the characteristic symptoms. These are listed below;

The headache –

synergy	Sang.	Nux-v.	Lach.	Ign.	Bell.	Sep.	Carb-v.	Acon.	Nat-ar.	Calc.	Bry.	Nat-m.	Ther.
Total	18	15	15	12	15	13	13	13	13	12	12	11	11
Rubrics	6	5	5	5	4	4	4	4	4	4	4	4	4
Kingdom													
CR19 - Head; Pain, headache; morning; agg.; evening, until(13)	4	3				3				1		1	1
CR19 - Head; Pain, headache; eructations; amel.(13)	3		3	1			3				1		
CR19 - Head; Pain, headache; noise agg.(169)	3	4	3	3	4	3	3	3	4	4	3	3	4
CR19 - Head; Pain, headache; odors; strong, from(34)	3	1	1	3	3			3	4				
CR19 - Head; Pain, headache; sun, exposure to; agg.(98)	1	3	4	1	4	3	3	4	1	3	4	3	3
CR19 - Head; Pain, headache; temples(702)	4	4	4	4	4	4	4	3	4	4	4	4	3

Further confirmatory rubrics –

synergy	Sang.	Gels.	Nat-m.	Lyc.	Puls.	Kali-c.	Sil.	Arn.	Ars.	Calc.	Phos.	Stram.	Aloe
Total	10	14	14	13	13	12	12	11	11	11	11	11	8
Rubrics	6	5	5	5	5	5	5	5	5	5	5	5	5
Kingdom													
CR19 - Female; Menses; painful, dysmenorrhea(477)	1	3	3	3	4	4	3	3	3	4	3	1	1
CR19 - Stomach; Nausea; pain, with(225)	1	3	3	1	2	2	1	3	2	1	3	1	1
CR19 - Mind; Helplessness; paralyzed sensation, with(1)	3												
CR19 - Mind; Helplessness(128)	3	3	3	4	1	1	1	1	1	1	1	3	1
CR19 - Mind; Trifles; ailments from, agg.(359)	1	1	4	4	4	4	4	3	4	4	3	3	4
CR19 - Mind; Fear; falling, of(92)	1	4	1	1	2	1	3	1	1	1	1	3	1

All this information comes together and gives us Sanguinaria Canadensis. There are so many confirmations. With this step-by-step analysis we can prescribe with complete confidence and we know that it will help her.

According to the information gathered we can set out the atlas of the case as such;

Superclass	1
Kingdom	Plant
Subclass	Magnolidae
Order	Papaverales
Family	Papaveraceae
Miasm	Sycotic
Remedy	Sanguinaria

After receiving Sanguinaria Canadensis 1M the patient followed up with us after one year of treatment;

> *Pain in the head is better by 90%. It has almost gone. I hardly get it now. Intensity of pain has reduced significantly. The dysmenorrhoea is better by 80%. I can hardly feel it at all now. Mind and mood state is much more stable now. I am calmer than earlier. I don't react to things like I would before.*

Case 2

This is the case of a 45-Year-old Male who came with the main complaint of skin issues and some acidity.

The patient begins with his main complaints –

> *Boils coming on the chest. I used to take antibiotics. Pustular boils. Sometimes bleeding. Itching is worse in the evening before going to bed. This is for 4 years now. It came up suddenly. I took medicine it went away but now since it is coming back it is more recurrent. It comes back after 2-3 months. I used to get massages and maybe because of the oil they used this has started. Earlier I used to get the itching on the back of my head, and on the occiput. I am also having acidity issues over last 2-3 years. Sometimes there is growling in the stomach. Some kind of noise which comes from inside. Something is moving from above to downwards. It is worse in the afternoon 3-4 pm and it is better after eating. I also have acne, which is coming back, sometimes it bleeds. The skin also becomes red sometimes like an urticaria. It has been happening since the last 3 years. There is no swelling or itching though. It is worse in the evening between 8:00 and 8:30pm. I work quite late until 8:00pm so I notice it when I get back home. I also sneeze a lot, especially when there is a lot of dust. It is also worse from the AC. I am comfortable in cold climates but in the AC, I am not comfortable. If I sleep in the AC then in the morning, I have a running nose. If I go in cold climates, I don't have the same issues. There is also a history of corns on the feet, but I had*

surgery, and they went. They were very painful when walking. I have also had a deviated nasal septum since my childhood. It doesn't bother me so much I just tend to sleep more on the left-hand side as this is the side which is deviated more.

These are the physical complaints which the patient presents with. They are fairly non-individualistic so we will have to take the case to a deeper level. But from a retrospective point we can see that the patient is sensitive. It is small things which can make him worse or affect him. This is a quality of the first Superclass. In the initial case taking we won't allow ourselves to become prejudiced by this information. Later we can see how it all fits into the picture of the case and also corresponds with the superclass.

We ask the patient to tell us about himself. He begins by narrating his childhood and again there is an emphasis on how sensitive he is –

As a kid I used to be quite sensitive to anything emotional happening, I used to cry. In movies if there was some sad scene, like someone is dying, I used to cry. If somebody dies in the movie, whole atmosphere in the movie becomes depressing. Suppose there is death. Or kids don't do well with parents. Tough time for parents. Old couple have to live on their own. They will be shocked. Not expecting this and that happened to them. That age they would expect that sons would have taken care of them but that didn't happen. Suddenly force comes and takes you out of the comfort zone.

This now builds on the soft hint of sensitivity, which was discussed earlier. We can see it a lot more evidently here. It is very interesting to observe this in the context of the first Superclass. As we can see how similar this is to the remedies in the first Subclass. We had described them as having no skin or being raw and exposed and this is what it is like in this case. We allow the patient to take this a bit further and he describes a recent incident. We can see how this theme of sensitivity is still very much a core theme of his life.

The day before yesterday, I read about an actor who died. He has a 3-year-old son who is now alone. How will the kid grow? He doesn't have a dad. There is insecurity, limited resources. It is like a void or a gap. Something is missing in your life. You feel anxious. Now what will happen ahead?

We can see how he is projecting all his fears and worries of insecurity etc. on to the child. Hence the huge sensitivity to this story he read. We can see now how he connects this incident and this sensitivity with his own life.

> *Many years back when my kids were small, I used to feel what if something happens to me? What about their security, financial security. Do you have resources? Can you live a comfortable life? Who will take care of you? Am I living enough for the family? Did I save enough for them? This feeling was there in 2015. I transferred money to my wife's name.*

So, we can see how this is a continuous issue for this patient. But we should also bear in mind this is not the sensitivity and reactivity of the plant kingdom. Yes, there is huge sensitivity in this case yet, the patient is viewing everything through the perception of capability and structure. This is the mineral kingdom. There is the issue of resources and of capability. In this case, the 'sensitivity' is a quality of the first Superclass and not the kingdom.

We then ask the patient to tell us a little more about his childhood –

> *Both my parents used to work, I used to live with some other person. After 6th and 7th standard I started staying alone. From 16-20yrs of age I stayed in a hostel. There was no traumatic experience. Somebody teasing you. I was bullied and teased, called lot of names. There is low self-esteem. Not confident about yourself. In childhood there was low self-esteem. People use to tease you. I became shy person. I never use to play sports, there was a fear I would break my specs. I was comfortable in childhood. At ease. The opposite feeling is anxious, not knowing what will happen fear. Fear of the unknown. Like a bomb blast, flight crashing, tsunami in tourist place. You are dead. External variables which you don't have control on. External force which comes out of the blue. You didn't expect it, but it happened. In 2001 my mother was diagnosed with cancer. I was not married. Suddenly. Out of the blue.*
>
> *I was anxious, wanting to know what will happen ahead? What is the ending? Is it a happy ending or sad ending? Sad ending is death.*
>
> *Same thing happened in 2009 my dad had a cyst in his appendix. Doctor said we don't think he will live now. I thought I had lost him. Felt insecure. Void and gap. Somebody very close is no longer with me. I felt sad, dejected, depressed. Internally there is tension, nervousness.*

So again, we can see the sensitivity of the patient. Especially to things which happen unexpectedly. We can also see that emphasis of the things which happen is not about the violence, but the unexpectedness of it. This differentiates this Superclass from the 6th Superclass. We don't see any call for fight or flight but rather we see the patient's reaction is to 'become shy'. This is an introversion, going within oneself. A retreat, a withdrawing from the unexpected or unpleasant events. When the patient talks about bigger more traumatic events there is no emphasis on violence or running away as there would be in the 6th Superclass. However, there is the feeling of insecurity. The pattern we see is that when something unexpected happens, the patient becomes introverted and withdraws within himself.

Now when we take the patient to another area and ask about his fears we can see the same pattern here as well –

> *I am afraid of mosquitos because my son got dengue. It was harrowing experience for me. What can happen to the kid? I can lose him. It's depressing. A gap. A void. It is suddenly broken, no longer perfect. Things will never be the same. There is one person less. Full family is not together. I have fear of high places. Once I was in Macau and below my feet was a glass. So, I was extremely scared. I felt I will fall down. I avoided the glass completely. But after that I went to many other places, but I used to hold something. Fear of lizards. I just don't like that. Fear of rides, esp. when coming downwards. I don't do giant wheel. I startle from sudden loud noise.*

Now we can see the expression of the mineral kingdom very clearly. The patient puts everything in terms of the loss of a structure and lack of capability. We also get some very good rubrics. Such as the fear of heights, clinging, fear of downward motion and startling from sudden noise.

Thinking back to our atlas analogy, where we are in the case? We know this is from the first Superclass and from the mineral kingdom as well having some solid rubrics. This makes us much more certain in our analysis. Throughout our case taking we can map out very well where the patient is taking us.

We ask our patient what he is sensitive to in movies/tv and news –

> *Operations, inside the body, stitching, I can't see that. Even if someone WhatsApp forwards anything related to that I can't see it. I just shut myself off.*

Interestingly we again see some of the themes we discussed earlier. The first Superclass themes of penetrating are highlighted. This is what an operation represents to him ; something that penetrates and goes on inside. He speaks of stitching. When we visualise the act of suturing, we can understand his sensitivity. The suture penetrates the skin repeatedly.

The reaction of shutting oneself off is the most basic dynamic of the first Superclass. After asking the patient to tell us about a stressful incident in his life all the earlier themes are confirmed for us –

> *Younger son had pneumonia and was in ICU. And when my elder son had dengue. Dengue was more stressful. One of my school friends lost her husband because of dengue. She had two kids. Then there was no perfect family. Two kids had to study on their own. I am not complete. Complete means husband, wife and two kids. Struggle. How will she do everything? Challenges she will face. Financial insecurity. If you want to live a comfortable life you don't have that. Basic needs like food, shelter, education. Without this there is Incomplete feeling. Less privileged. Random event and your life is changed. If things are in normal, suddenly something comes up. It makes me anxious. What happens next? Why didn't you prepare for it?*

The perception of the mineral kingdom in this case is very clear to us. It is all about the loss of structure. The patient feels the family is no longer perfect with the loss of the husband. Along with the perception of the mineral kingdom, Superclass themes are also seen especially with the sensitivity to sudden unexpected events. This also reminds us of the acute miasm, the perception that something is very sudden and unexpected.

Once we see this case as one from mineral kingdom, and that it is the in the first Superclass, we can zero in on the 2nd row left side of the periodic table.

We don't take this for granted. We need to investigate and look for the confirmations of the 2nd row and the left hand side in particular. Throughout the case we have seen these confirmations. Especially in the issues which the patient talks about such as the basic needs for survival. This is a more primitive struggle than that of the 4th row with issues of task and duty. Here it is about basic survival. The sudden loss of those you depend on to survive, you are as helpless as unborn baby.

We can also see this fear of loss within the family as a fear of separation; the family must stay together 2nd row where would see the desire to get out due to the feeling of suffocation and claustrophobia. This patient wants to avoid this separation.

Then once we have a very good idea of where the remedy lies. In this case in the left hand side of the 2nd row we can go to the characteristic symptoms and keynote symptoms to confirm the remedy. Here the keynote symptom is the fear of rides and in particular the fear of downward motion. This is the very well known symptom of the remedy Borax which lies exactly where we need our remedy to be. There are other confirmatory symptoms of Borax such as the easy startling from noise which will give us even more confidence when prescribing the remedy.

From this case we can learn many things. There is the art of analysis, esp. on how to sort this information. We must be able to differentiate between what is representative of the Superclass, the kingdom, the miasm, the sensation etc. Often all this information is often given to us all mixed up.

This sorting out of the information becomes much easier with practice. It is very similar to driving a car. At first it can seem overwhelming. There are the gears, the clutch, brake, accelerator, steering wheel, indicator etc. There seem too many things to give attention to at the same time. After a while the process of driving becomes smooth and synchronized. So also, with case taking and analysis.

Superclass	**Kingdom**	**Row**	**Side of periodic table**
• Sensitivity • Sudden/unexpected events • Penetration • Shutting off = 1st superclass	• Loss of structure • Issues of Capability = Mineral Kingdom	• Basic survival • Issues of separation = 2nd row	• Fear of separation = Left side
Rubrics			
• Fear of downward motion • Clinging • Fear of heights • Startling from noise = Borax			

For this case we can sort the information as follows;

Superclass	**1**
Kingdom	Mineral
Row	2nd
Remedy	Borax

When we put all this information that we have sorted out together it points very clearly to the remedy Borax. The patient received Borax 1M and one can see how well he did in the follow up after almost 1 year of treatment:

> *Boils are less by almost 90%. There is no pus, no itching. The acidity is very less, has reduced by 70%. No bleeding acne. Tendency of sneezing is much less. The appetite is good, and I am sleeping well. Feeling much better in my mind state with a relaxed feeling and no anxiety.*

Through this case we are able to see how the study of the Subclasses has furthered the knowledge of the Superclasses. Using our previous knowledge, we were able to recognise the themes of the Superclass.

Case 3

This is the case of a 38-Year-old male suffering from Hypertension with an erratic pulse.

The case starts with the patient narrating his complaints —

> *Since one and half year my BP is high, and my pulse is staying high around 100-110 b/min, and I am taking medication for the same. My BP would stay in the range of 150 by 100. In latest blood report, my uric acid was high and each time if it is high, I get itchy boils on my body. Taking medication for uric acid too. Also, I have deviated septum and adenoids, hence my nose is blocked all the time, I have to breathe a lot from my mouth and so I get foul smell from my mouth. Saliva dribbling during the night. Snoring in sleep. Last 3-4 months due to my wife's health I am tense. I am getting disturbing dreams at night; don't remember them but not peaceful sleep due to those dreams.*

The patient mentions that he is getting disturbing dreams. This was spontaneous and gives us a good entry point into a deeper level of the case. We ask the patient to describe the dreams.

> *I do not remember any of them except one that I am playing with the dog in my house and by mistake I hit the dog on his mouth and the jaw comes out of its mouth and the dog runs away. Earlier I used to get dreams. In one I am somewhere in a public place and suddenly I realize that I am not wearing*

anything, and I am thinking what I should do now. How I should cover myself. In the other one I am running away from something, or I am chasing something, but I am not fast enough, so I am using my arms to move faster, like how an ape runs. My legs are not moving fast enough.

We need to understand a bit more, we ask for the experience in the dream without clothes —

I feel shy and ashamed. How I can go out like this? How this happened? Where am I? Why is all this happening? I get up suddenly. Usually when I have woken up, I have been sweating. A couple of times due to the fear of my wife's death. It is playing since long in my mind. I just feel that how will I be able to survive without her. We are very, very close to each other. We are 23 years together now. (Since college till now)

So far, the dreams have been very interesting. We need some more insight, so we ask the patient to tell us about the dream with the dog —

There is a common passage in the house, I am playing with a dog, he jumps over me, and my hand suddenly hits his mouth, and the jaw falls out of its mouth and breaks, in 4 pieces and the dog runs away. I was surprised that how come the jaw has completely come out and how precisely broken into 4 pieces. The lower jaw was actually symmetrically broken. Exactly from the centre; equal number of teeth on both sides. The jaw is normally U-shaped, and it is divided right from the centre that is how I saw it in my dream. And it was broken right in the centre exactly. It was like when my hand touched its mouth, the jaw fell out of its mouth. 4 pieces were lying there. Two pieces were like a pair; identical; with the same teeth combination. Piece A of lower jaw was lying down with piece A of upper jaw, and piece B of lower jaw was lying with piece B of upper jaw. They were not lying all in one place, they were scattered all over, so two pieces were together, and the other two pieces were together. And I could make out that these two were identical pieces and those two were identical pieces. Two similar looking, with probably very minute differences or almost no differences, almost the same. Difficult to differentiate one piece from the other; like mirror image. It is almost as if it has been two pieces casted from similar dye. There is no difference between 2 pieces at all, except that one is in one direction and the other is in the other direction which would mean that the pieces would fix together and make a shape.

This is a very strange part of the case, and it is difficult to know what to do with this information. However, that is the beauty of case taking; that we don't need to know. We can just keep going with the case taking and eventually we will be able to see the full picture and how it all fits in. So, for now, we leave this dream here, but make sure we don't forget it… we will come back to it.

We then ask the patient if there is any other dream he can recall, even from childhood —

> *Especially when I have headache; a huge crowd is chasing someone and I am a third person standing there, and this person comes running by me and this crowd comes onto me and it completely envelopes me, and then completely dissolves and then the whole dream is repeated. I need to move out of the way of this crowd as they are shouting, and they are angry so to keep myself safe and must find a way out of it. I am a bit afraid that if I am here, then probably I will get hurt but besides that….*

Here there is a word which interests us, 'envelope'. We ask the patient to tell us more about it —

> *It completely surrounds me; I am not part of that crowd, but the crowd has totally surrounded me (HG: making a circular space from front to the sides). I can see myself standing there and suddenly there are people all around me, above me, below me and surrounding me. I don't see flooring. I am suspended in the air. As if you are inside a cocoon completely enveloped in all sides (Hg) and nothing can be seen except people around you. I need to move out, but you cannot find a way. Within a few seconds the whole scene dissolves and I find myself again standing on the ground. And the whole scene starts again. I feel scared, and I want to get out, I feel afraid that I might get hurt if I do not move out. I have not paid much attention to that. I just feel afraid and my body tenses, but I don't know it is because I have headache, or it is because I am tense. I get spasm with my headaches.*

The patient had told the resident doctor that he experienced a feeling of peacefulness when he is inside. So, we ask about that now —

> *That was feeling in the cocoon, not related to the dream. In a cocoon when you are cut off from the world, it is peaceful; alone in your own world; peaceful (HG: Making a ball like space) But at the same time, you cannot interact with people, you would be lonely and that would be fearful.*

Honestly, I am an introverted person, I don't openly mingle with people, but I like to have people around me; once I am comfortable with someone... I have inhibition going and talking with people. I cannot meet a stranger and suddenly chat with them. I need time to get comfortable with someone, need time to know that person, and once I am comfortable, I want them to be around me. I don't have a big circle of friends; I only have 2-3 friends. But those friends are very, very thick. When I am with them, I really enjoy myself, and if I am not with them, I know that if I am going through a problem or anything I want to share the first people I think after my wife would be these friends. It makes me very happy, extremely happy to be with her, irrespective of whatever we are doing. Even if we are not talking, we are just sitting it is Ok, just being there with her gives my mind a lot of peace.

So now we are starting to get the hints at the Superclass of the case. Especially when we compare this with the features we highlighted in the previous two cases. We can see this idea of the cocoon and peaceful being inside. There is the idea of withdrawing when he doesn't know someone well.

We then go back to the dream without clothes. We see if we can understand it a bit further now that we have an idea of the Superclass in the case —

I am in a random room, I am confused. It is very uncomfortable. Just feels uncomfortable. I don't like that feeling at all. I feel why I am like that. How I managed to get here without clothes. There is nothing to cover up and I feel ashamed. There is not a cloth or a towel to wrap around myself. To hide my body. To just something around my body so that no one can see that I am wearing no clothes. So that no one can see it. Probably staying behind a curtain or something so that no one can see. When something is in a direct line of vision, it cannot be seen, if you put something behind a wall, table, sofa, curtain then you cannot see it. We close the curtains because we don't want anybody look into our room. We want our privacy.

We ask the patient to describe the word 'close' —

(HG: Closing) Close. I shut it (Same HG). It is like closing the gaps... Bringing 2 ends together (HG) closing together (HG) so that it shut you out from anything else; from the unwanted things. When you want to be left alone, you go into your room and shut the door so that any voice, people from outside cannot come in and disturb you. Similarly, when you want to be alone you shut yourself off, shut your mind off completely, distance yourself

from people so that they cannot reach out to you or disturb you. When in a room you want privacy or you want to change your clothes, you normally shut the windows (HG) so that the outside people cannot see. It just gives me the feeling that this is close, and I am secure, and nobody can see me. It is like I cannot be hurt, not affected, no one can see me no one can judge me, even if they judge or see it doesn't matter to me anymore because I shut myself completely and I am not concerned with what they say, what they do. I can channel my thought process much better; I can think much clearly of what I want to do what actions I want to take without the pressure of what the person will think. I can remain in that state for a while. I come back to normal; I have lot more clarity of what has to be done, I am back to being open, and I am absolutely ok then.

We ask him to tell us what is "open" —

Ready to interact, mingle with people and be with people. (HG: Opening the palms like opening a book) I am open to talk to people.

We ask him about the hand gesture he is showing —

It is about opening up (HG: opening). It is about removing the barrier. Barrier is like an obstacle (HG: wall in front) to put in front of you. A wall, a shield; something that will protect you from others or keep you away from others. An object that protects you from getting hurt

We ask him to describe the qualities of this wall/shield —

It is supposed to be strong enough to protect me; to keep me safe and keep me covered, and flexible enough that when I want to remove it, I can put it away until I need it again.

This dream has now confirmed what we were thinking. The features of the first Superclass are clear. We can see the language of mollusc behaviour. The bivalves put up a wall or shield so that they can protect themselves from the outside.

The patient had also been complaining about a type of restless leg syndrome. Now we ask him about this complaint —

When I am resting for longer period, especially on the bed, after a little while I feel restlessness especially in right leg like muscle cramping, it

> *cramps and releases, it cramps and releases (HG: half fist and opening; repeated)*

The patient immediately uses a hand gesture. It is somewhat similar to the process he was speaking about earlier. We ask the patient to describe this for us —

> *As if my muscle is tightening up (HG: closing fist), pulls completely from inside, tightening up (HG: fist) and then automatically releases on its own (HG: Opening up the palm); it again tightens up (Hg: closing the fist) and again it releases (Hg: opening up the fist) I am holding something in my grip and I am releasing it (Hg: closing the fist and opening); It is like something being constricted and released. There is something there which you are trying to press in and compact. (Hg: closing fist), and then again you release it (HG: opening the fist) It is trying to reduce the size or giving it a different shape or trying to re-mould it. Trying to change shape, when you keep pressing something which is soft enough you will change the shape. Something mouldable; like a clay; when it is wet you can press it (Hg: Cup shape!); you can mould it. You compress it (Hg: closing the fist) together to make a solid thing like a ball; all the particles are joint together (Hg: interlocking fingers); they are fixed together*

We ask the patient to describe this interlocking gesture which he makes —

> *All the particles are joint together (Hg), more solid. It is interlinking (HG: Same) When things are interlinked, they are stronger (Hg: Interlocking) Bringing two different objects they merge together, they join together, and they become stronger (HG) Stick two things together. Probably like this wooden coaster. The glass has been probably stuck (HG) in the wood, so when two things are stuck together, that is like 2 objects coming together. Like magnet attaching itself to iron; it connects with each other. Or two papers stuck together with glue (Hg: Attaching the fingers of two hands to each other)*

Everything that the patient is saying is starting to make sense. We can understand how he is describing the source of the remedy he needs. We are also confirming that it is an animal remedy he requires. At this level of the case he is not describing an issue of lack or capability or that of sensitivity and reactivity. This is a process of survival which he is describing.

Therefore, confirms that we would need an animal from the First superclass. This would be a bivalve.

We then ask the patient to describe the headaches he gets —

> *A dull pain starting from forehead, mainly around my temples and forehead with heaviness in my eyes, and slowly it will move upwards, and it will get focused on one side of my head; either on the crown or on one side. And it gets very unbearable, and I get spasmic feeling (HG: Flashing like!) As if there is a constant pain going on, and suddenly there is a spasm in my head, which radiates downwards especially to my eyes and back of my neck. Again, after some time I will get another spasm. My muscles tighten up, I can feel that shooting pain, it is usually on my right side. As if somebody has hit a nail on my head suddenly (HG). In a particular spot when it is hurting, I feel the pain has magnified uncontrollably and it does not stay in that area, but it moves downward and then it goes off. Somebody has hit on my head with hammer, or nail. You have to hit on the nail really hard so that it penetrates in the wall. Penetrate means going inside something. Entering something. Going inside something from outside. My muscles tighten up. My body becomes very alert that the pain will just come and probably to prepare to receive that pain. The muscles would contract. (HG: Fist) Squeezing in. Trying to fit something into a smaller place. When you try to put an elephant into a horse stable, fitting something in a smaller space, it doesn't belong there, that room is not fitted for its size.*

Through the symptom of the headache the patient gives us some of the sensation words of the bivalves. These are "penetrating" and "piercing." We also see the survival reaction to withdraw. We already know the sensitivity to penetration is a characteristic feature of the first Superclass. There is the animal reaction of a survival mechanism to withdraw and squeeze inside. We can see how it all points to the bivalves.

Now we should look at how we arrived at this point in the case. The patient had started off by giving us symptoms. But when there is something more prominent than symptoms you must follow that. In this case there were some dreams. Dreams are at the level of delusion and closer to the level of sensation than the symptoms. So instead of looking into the symptoms at this point we focus on the dreams. If we go deeper into the experience in this strange dream of the dog it starts to make more sense.

The important words are 'symmetrical' and 'identical'. They are of two opposite sides which have come together. In the dream, you find that those opposite sides are scattered apart but exactly cut in the middle! He is not able to say anything more but that these two opposite sides fit into together to form a larger shape. There is no feeling associated with it at all. When a person gives an exact description of something especially its colour, shape, size, texture, taste, smell, temperature, consistency, etc factually, this is often the language of the source.

At the sensation level there are 3 levels. A: Kingdom, B: Subkingdom and C: source. And you will not know what the source is unless you know the kingdom and the subkingdom. How would you know what these identical pieces are?

You don't need to guess. You have to keep this aside and go to the other dream. Through other information about Superclass, Kingdom, etc the source information will make sense. The source is the deepest level. You cannot push the person further.

In the other childhood dream he sees that a crowd is coming and it envelopes him. He is caught in the middle, and it is like a cocoon and there is the feeling that is safe and peaceful. Yet meanwhile it is lonely. You can see a duality in this cocoon.

Then there is the 3rd dream of nakedness that he has to cover up. He has to be behind another object so that the people neither can see him nor hurt him. He says that it is like a curtain which closes the gap. You are safe and secure. There is a barrier, obstacle, shield and a wall. A wall that you put up. A wall that is strong but flexible so that when you don't need it, it won't be there.

This is the survival mechanism of this particular creature. This creature is a mollusc. Molluscs are of 3 types, Bivalves, Gastropods and Cephalopods. Once we know the Superclass, kingdom, and the subkingdom, we know that it is a bivalve. You can now understand the dog dream with two identical pieces. Now the question is which bivalve?

The bivalve that opens when it feels safe and stays shut when it feels unsafe is the clam. The remedy is Venus mercenaria. Now we have to confirm it from all aspects of the case. You drop whatever you have and start again from another aspect and see if we get to the same place.

One symptom is restlessness of the legs. Restless legs has remedies like Zinc, Rhus tox, Medorrhinum and Tarent. Can you imagine a clam being so restless?!!

Each characteristic of the case should come to the same point. So, we need to go deeper into the restlessness. And he says that the restlessness is due to some sensation in the legs. It is like constricted and compact and then compressed. Squeezed in and compressed are one of the main words of molluscs.

Then he says that two objects are interlinked. So, we confirm here. So, we go to another area. In headache the sensation is penetrating which is one of the most important words of the mollusc. Another word they use is hammering. 'Soft' is a very important word of molluscs. Then he talks about something entering from outside. When this happens you tighten up. You contract so that you fit into the room which is closed and not an open space in which you can be seen. Whichever aspect of the case we look into, at the depth we come to the same place.

The Patient took Venus 1M and reported to us in his follow up at 8 months;

Feeling much better, feeling much fresher. The anxiety is not there.

My Headaches are non-existent, and the Blood pressure has reduced and is absolutely fine.

Superclass	1
Kingdom	Animal
Sub-Kingdom	Mollusca
Class	Bivalves
Remedy	Venus Mercenaria

Case 4

This is the case of a 21-Year-Old-female suffering with a major depressive disorder.

The mother begins with the narration of the complaints —

She gets attacks. Hands become cold, starts shivering. We have to control her. We have to hold her or else she will hold her own neck and we have to open her hands. She grips her neck very strongly. 5-6 people have to hold her. Once she made a fist so tight that her long nails got into the palms and the palm was bleeding. Intermittently she shrieks, stiffens her body, clenches her teeth. Every 2-4 minutes this attack comes, lasts for 1 hour. She stares at ceiling or down on the floor.

The mother then tells of an incident in the recent past —

Since last 6-8 months, she changed the way she used to dress. Earlier she used to wear fashionable clothes. One college professor touches other girls inappropriately and tells them that he calls them to teach a particular topic. She complained to a female professor. The female professor said to change her manner of dressing, so she did so.

The mother then tells of a second incident —

In July 2019, she had gone to birthday party of a common friend. Something was mixed in her drink. She was found in the swimming pool. Few friends said, she was swimming; few said, she was drowning. She had to be pulled out by her hair. Friends dropped her at home late, she did not come out of room until next day evening. She wanted to go to our guru, she wrote a letter to him. Since that day she decided not to smoke or drink.

The patient then shares her complaints with us —

I am suffering from depression, anxiety, suicidal and negative thoughts. There is sleeplessness due to overthinking. Eating too much or too little for no reason. I feel hot and cold at the same time. My hair is falling out. Have had chronic constipation since around 10 years - hard painful stools, I pass stools once in 3-4 days or sometimes once in 10 days.

Depression for 6-8 months. I cannot sleep due to too much thinking. I have negative thoughts of being alone, lonely, being raped by 4-5 people. I see their faces. Every night, I am waking up with jerks and feeling suffocated. Heaviness in the chest. Taking cold shower makes me comfortable. I get zoned out.

The patient shares an incident with us —

I was working on sewing machine at home at 2 am. My hand went into the machine and the needle went inside piercing my finger but for 2-3 minutes, I did not realize it. The needle was coming out from the other side of my finger. I was zoned out and felt numb.

The patient then describes a second incident she recalls —

While driving the car I was at a crossroads, there were two buses coming from opposite directions and I did not push the accelerator. A traffic policeman banged the car window then I realized. It was a feeling of being zoned out. I also cannot see menstrual blood.

I feel zoned out, like I am in a different world.

We ask the patient to tell us about the suicidal thoughts —

I tried choking myself. Hurting myself by cutting my wrist. I have punched the wall. Banged my head against the wall. I do this, so that I can forget the pain inside my heart. If I hurt myself, I get distracted. My mind will then rest for a while. Once I went to the bus stand and stood in front of the bus to die. I feel that if I die my mind will be in peace then forever.

I feel mentally exhausted, suffocated, helpless, worthless, feel like giving up. Feel guilty, unhappy, suicidal. I feel heavy, can't feel anything, numb. Confined to myself, confined to a room. Heaviness inside, like a big burden. Everything inside me is shouting, howling, crying but no one knows or can understand. I can't figure out myself what is going on.

I get 7 to 8 anxiety attacks in a day. Feeling cold in my hands and feet. Do not feel like living, choking myself, giving up, heavy from inside. I see a black room, few faces in front of me of very close people. Some family members try to hold me, put water on my face. Water is like blood. People are raping me; men are holding me. I react in a horrible manner. I don't want to live, feel worthless, hopeless.

We then ask the patient to tell us some of the dreams she gets —

I am in a black, dark, confined, cold room. There is a white spotlight. Water below me up to my ankles, slowly it is rising and suffocating me. I am drowning. There is no one to save me. I will slowly die being alone. Lonely, isolated, abandoned. Feel numb, lifeless, cold.

The patient tells us a second dream she gets –

I am being raped by 5-6 people in a dirty, shabby room. Initially it was 1-2 men, then there were 5-6 of them. I see their faces in front of me. I am tied with their belts; they are bashing me with their belts. I could see their faces distinctly. They are laughing and deciding who is going to rape me. They are smoking and inserting cigarettes into my vagina. Throwing blood on my face.

Very suffocating. Felt numb. I am crying and howling. I feel dirty and gross. Scrubbing every part of my body, removing their dirty touch. I start to feel hot and cold and heavy. I feel heavy, lonely, sad, abandoned, hopeless, worthless, guilty. Heat in hand, chest. Finger pains, cold sensation.

I want to feel happy, stable, at peace. Don't want to feel empty. Empty, lonely, sad, heavy, abandoned, unsatisfied, hopeless, guilty, worthless. Feeling heat in the chest, head (deep breathing). Hands pain and have a cold sensation

We ask the patient to describe the exact opposite of the experience in the dream —

Less heavy - Feel yourself, light, happy, jolly. Laughing, dancing, singing, painting, creating, designing. Fresh, bright sunshine, beach, waves.

Everybody part has been released of toxins. Positivity running through the veins. Yellow golden glow liquid flowing in my veins. Starting from fingers gradually spreading and enlightening the entire nervous system. Feeling happy - Hot and cold at the same time. Smells like sunshine – smells fresh – feel calm and composed. Little tingling. Can feel pores of my hands.

The patient then tells us of a third dream —

Someone very close to me, stabbed me in my back. My intestines, stomach popped out. Could feel the pain, burning in stomach. It is very cold out there, am dying. Soul comes out – body has no life. Soul has liberated (HG – hands widening). This happened in a very beautiful park.

We ask the patient to describe this hand gesture —

Opening to people, sharing. Feeling good, less heavy, relaxed. Small current from heart to the body parts - but I feel this very rarely. When things are not going ok – feel heavy sad, guilty. Everything is a mess. Feeling cold in hands, feet, numb, shivering, and stiff.

Don't want to live.

Whenever I get these dreams, I take a shower in cold water, even if I fall sick at times due to cold water. It makes me feel better. All these thoughts make me feel suffocated, hot, and cold at the same time.

The patient describes her fears —

Being abandoned, isolated. To die alone. Can't see blood, get zoned out Reptiles, crocodiles. Horror movies. Disturbing scenes – murder, rape

We ask the patient to describe her nature as a child —

Cheerful, playful, jolly. Bad memories of being beaten up by parents, aunt on different occasions when I had misbehaved or did not study well or when I was arrogant. Used to hate being at home. Confined to myself, to my room – paint, draw, watch movies. I would be alone.

We then conducted a WISE process with the patient —

Showing the picture of the first WISE woman, we ask the patient to just imagine the situation, scenery – what is happening to this person?

She is scared, trying to avoid something, push people, wants to be left alone. She is crying, sad. She is asking people not to touch her, stay away. She wants to be confined in herself. People are harassing her sexually, touching her. She is helpless, powerless.

Scared of being with people, scared of being raped, molested.

Scared of people – they will physically use her, hurt her. Beat, torture her, insert something inside her, stab her in abdomen. There is nothing she can do, she is helpless, crying and just scared.

How does she experience to be in this moment? How does she feel inside? —

There is nothing that she is feeling. It is very dark, very sad, hollow.

Describe dark and hollow bit more.

Very deep inside, once you start to sink inside, there is no end to it.

Describe dark, hollow, sink, nothing inside – describe the experience inside, what is the sensation?

It feels soft, touch is soft. There is cold air, temperature is cold. Once you start there is no end to it, you keep falling. It is breezy, you have cold temperature around. Gradually going deeper and you die.

Describe gradually going deeper and deeper?

There is no escape around, no way of getting out, hollow.

Describe hollow —

It is like a hole; it has no end to it. Once you go out you cannot come out. The door is closed, you cannot find it.

Describe this hole, you are doing very well —

This hole is dark, reddish, brownish, maroon, smells like blood.

What do you mean by smells like blood —

Sweet smell like blood, like fresh wound. It is dark, you have one source of light, that is very small source of light, this is way of escape, but it is not, it is dark hollow circle room.

What is circle? —

Circle is dark, circle I walk into, after it gets shut, circle, spherical room and small source of light, room is very cold.

How is the experience in this room, cold, dark and circle —

Feel suffocated and heavy inside. Breathless, want to come out again, finding that one hope, there is no way to it. No way to come out of room. Can't find any way to come out of it.

What is the experience when you can't come out —

Suffocated, breathless, chest is heavy, unable to breathe, stomach is heavy, entire thing sinking inside.

Describe sinking —

Like drowning. Going deeper and deeper inside. When you don't know how to swim…

You used the word soft, what is soft —

Pleasant which you like to touch. It is cozy, fluffy, silky.

You used words helpless —

Nothing she can do. Her hands are tied, she can't do anything. Makes me feel irritated and restricted.

Restricted – what would be feeling inside?

It feels trapped.

Describe word trapped, in general.

Not free.

What is the experience?

They feel worthless, helpless, they are trapped, cannot do anything. It feels suffocating again.

How does suffocating feel in body, head, chest, abdomen -

Feel like every body part is restricted, everything around me is restricted.

Like someone ties my hands with rope, feels restricted. Heart, chest feel so heavy that I can't breathe and feel suffocated.

Heavy? —

Heavier than stone, not heavy physically but inside it feels heavy.

What is the opposite of heavy —

Light feeling, relieved, relaxed. Feels like happiness running through my veins, feels like sunshine.

What is the sensation in head, chest, heart —

Tingling sensation, it feels good, there is warmth, and it feels light.

Describe light?

Light feels happy, jolly.

How does it feel inside the body?

Lighter, like a sunshine

We show her the picture of the second WISE woman and again ask her to use her imagination and tell us what is happening here —

She is from poor family background, she is tired of working, done too much work, wants to sit and relax. She is exhausted. She has worked the entire day, her legs are hurting, she wants to sit. She looks sad. Her eyes are sad.

What is the feeling in sadness?

She is sad about her situation. She is poor, has to work. She is an old lady; she must work to earn. She feels depressed, low. Feels like crying but she cannot cry.

Low means?

Don't feel like doing things you love. Mood is off.

How does it feel in the body?

Heavy. Chest and abdomen becoming heavier. It feels heavier than stone.

What do you mean by heavier than stone?

It feels like someone has kept huge stone on my chest. Feel breathless. I can't breathe normally. Feel suffocated (HG: two hands coming together)

Describe this hand gesture – what is this you are showing?

Clamping. Getting stuck

What means clamping, what is a clamp?

Things that join two things together. I feel stuck between two things.

What happens to you?

I am stuck, feels hurt.

What will be the exact opposite?

Free (HG: widening)

Show clamping and it's opposite and describe them.

HG (hands coming together) is uneasy, tied together. HG (hands widening) is free, breathing normally. HG (hands coming together) is stuck – can't breathe, can't move at all. When I do this HG (hands widening) person is free, opens up.

We ask about the patients interests and hobbies —

Painting, sketching, drawing. Paint flowers. I love colorful flowers. White and purple. They are very happy.

Why they are happy?

Because they are colorful. Flowers are colorful, jolly, they give happy vibes.

How does happy vibes feel?

Golden yellow sunshine going through my veins, feels liberating.

Describe liberating?

Flying. Away from all tensions, reality

What is the opposite of tension and reality?

Not feeling suffocated

Describe flying?

Breezy, soft air that feels on face and body

What is the experience of flying in your head, chest, abdomen. How would it feel to fly, what would be the inner experience?

Tingling sensation, all my pores are happy. Every single body part.

What things cause stress for you?

Thinking too much, I feel suffocated. I take cold shower.

How does it feel?

I feel the cold droplets on my face, makes me feel calm down, drops are very soft.

Describe cold droplets?

Makes my mind calm down, it is soft and smooth.

How does it feel when droplets fall on your face?

Calm, composed, confined.

Confined means?

To myself, wrapped myself, I clean the mess I created.

The mother shares about the patient's nature –

Happy child, we never thought she can get depression. Restless. Whenever she felt something wrong, she would rebel. When she gets scary dreams, she goes to bathroom and takes cold shower. Her energy is low, not much active, very less stamina.

Any situation that had deep impact on you?

I was not close to the family. Was close to one guy – had a breakup, since then I have fear of abandonment, became introvert. I am confined to myself, I feel lonely.

Describe lonely feeling?

I have no one to talk to, when I become comfortable, I open up. When people start judging me, I cut off. I block them. Cut all connections.

Describe block, cut connections?

Avoid, running away.

Running away where?

Inside you. In dark hole, inside me. Feel lonely, empty, hollow.

Opposite?

Being happy, loved, cared

You get some attack?

If I start thinking, I get unconscious, can't see. Tingling sensation in hands and feet, get cold. I try to choke myself.

Why do you do that?

If I choke, brain will stop thinking, I will have peace.

How does peace feel?

Calm, blissful. Like in heaven – white cloud, sunshine

How does heaven feel?

Warm, cozy, comfortable, peaceful

The Patients medication —

- Tolaz 2.5 mg/once a day
  (Anti-psychotic medicine - Used for Mania/Schizophrenia)

- Cipralec 10 mg/once a day
  (Escitalopram – Anti depressant / used for anxiety disorder)
- Softeron 1 capsule/day (Stool softener)
- Keragel Eva (for hair loss)
  The mother also mentions that the patient hasn't slept for 8/9 months without sleep medication.

This is not an easy case to analyse. But if we keep it simple and follow the central themes of the case the whole picture begins to emerge. We can gain a beautiful insight into this superclass.

What do we understand about this patient? Basically, there are two sides to this patient. The one side she was a cheerful happy person, then the other side is this depression.

She has these attacks which can be characterised by:

- She tries to choke herself and her strength is greatly increased.
- Suicidal and negative thoughts.
- Depression
- Constipation
- Feeling of hot and cold
- Feels better with a cold shower
- There is a delusion she is being raped, but in reality nothing like this has happened

She also gets these situations where she zones out. Often related to fear as well with just this zoning out.

To further characterise her case we can see a clear experience. There is a basic reaction in the experience –

- Zoned out - painlessness
- To withdraw - Needle going through finger but there is no pain.
- Go inside/Own world – Numbness
- Shut out the outside world – while driving zoned out as if she was not there
- Heaviness – I go into my own world

There is also this other side to her which is opposite to the experience and basic reaction –

- Laughing, dancing, painting, bright sunshine, yellow golden liquid flowing through veins.

- Everything is sensory – light, yellow, sunshine
- I feel my pores (Opens and closes in our skin)
- Someone stabbing – soul comes out
- Soul is liberated – out of the body

Before coming to the Superclass we can already see clearly the kingdom in this case i.e., the plant kingdom. She only speaks about her sensation and its opposite. We can see clearly the sensitivity and the reaction to situations.

We see the two sides namely open and shut and this brings us to the 2nd Superclass . Since we already know it is the plant kingdom it must be the second subclass namely the Hamamelidae. If we study the main sensation of the Hamamelidae from Section Two we can clearly see the features discussed in the case.

We can see in the case that the break-up affected her. The effect was that she went inside, introverted, confined to herself. We could see this pattern repeated again and again in this case. After the break-up we also see the reaction of cutting off, blocking out, cut off all connections.

In the Magnolidae the movement is inside of oneself. But in the Hamamelidae it is going inside and going outside. The inside feels lonely so they go outside to make a connection. In the animal kingdom the Magnolidae are like the Bivalves and the Hamamelidae are like Gastropods.

The case is very clear from the WISE processes. We can see in the first process –

> She says the inside surrounding feels soft. There is a breeze, you suffocate and die, feel heavy and breathless and want to come out again. The patient describes it as not feeling free, feeling trapped, restricted and clamped. There is heaviness as if a stone on the chest. We can see the initial response is to go in but then the inside becomes suffocative. You want to come out again. This is the clear distinction with the first subclass. This dynamic is confirmed again in the second WISE process. She again comes to the idea of heaviness and suffocation.
>
> When we start to see all this information in conjunction with each other the case becomes so much easier to understand. This classifying of information is such an important and useful tool. We can see the kingdom information and the Superclass information very clearly. This narrows down the remedy selection hugely. In this case there are also some peculiarities which will help us come to the exact remedy.

We can see some peculiar symptoms. There is amelioration from the cold shower and trickling of drops of water. We repertorize this information. If we limit the search to the parameters which we have defined earlier the remedy jumps out at us —

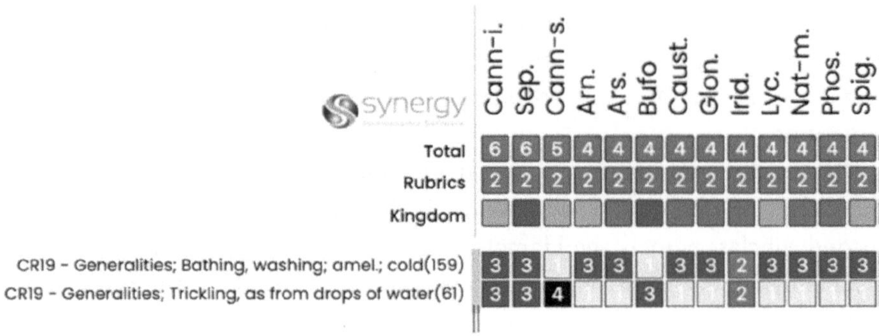

We can also then look for the other symptoms in this case and confirm our remedy selection —

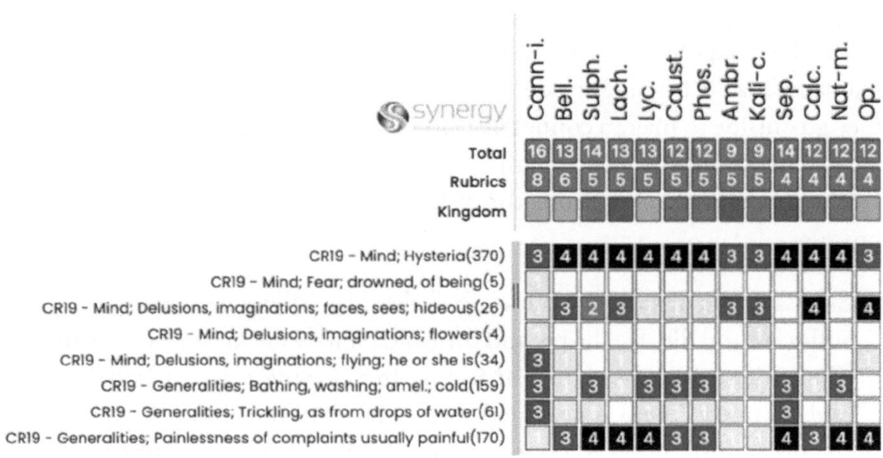

To summarize our analysis of this case here is the information —

Superclass	2
Kingdom	Plant
Subclass	Hamamelidae
Order	Urticales
Family	Cannabaceae
Remedy	Cannabis Indica 1M

The patient responded very well to the remedy and we can see this in her 8 month follow up —

- Constipation is 70 - 80 % better. Attacks of violence, suicidal thoughts much better. No attacks of cutting or scratching herself at all. Not a single episode in last 3 months. Smoking, alcohol not consumed. Remains very positive most times of the days.
- Her mother hears her conversation with her friends – it is mostly very much positive. Tends to smile, share her feelings with family members. She is becoming open to grandparents.
- Cold shower at night stopped.
- Dreams of rape, brutality also stopped.
- All Allopathic anti-depressants, anti-psychotic medicines stopped.

Case 5

This is the case of a 44 year old female who is suffering from Sjogren's syndrome. Let us review this case so as to understand the themes of the second Superclass further.

The patient begins by narrating several of her complaints —

> She has a severe back pain which has been diagnosed as a prolapsed intervertebral disc. She has swelling of her cervical lymph glands. Dryness of her eyes, very low appetite and fatigue. There is also swelling on the left side of her neck. There is a swelling in her ankle which has been diagnosed as Rheumatoid arthritis after several tests. And an overall diagnosis of Sjogren's syndrome which we can see from the collection of her symptoms. She also mentions that she is taking many allopathic medications.

We ask how all of this started —

> *Ok, it started way back in 2007 when I left my full-time job. Then I was not very active, and I had no regimen, exercise regimen at all before that. But then in 2008 I started doing a lot of kickboxing and did the half marathon with minimal training, may be the training was not adequate, not the correct thing, maybe that led to the back problem. Also, there was a big change in the whole outlook of life, I was working full time and now I had to start working on my own. I wanted to do something, continue with professional life, it was little different and difficult to manage this transition.*

This is an interesting way of expressing it, that there was a 'transition'. We ask her to describe this 'transition' in more detail —

> *I was working in a bank and that includes going at a regular time, having a routine schedule, reporting to someone, getting a monthly income. Everything works as per schedule as per process, now when you are on your own, things are different. So, you have flexible time which is one of the reasons I gave up the job also, as it was difficult to get adjusted to because I had worked for 17 years and then suddenly, I didn't have a specific routine, so maybe that change was a bit disorienting.*

We ask her to describe this further —

> *It takes a little while to get adjusted to the change, in the sense that now you are looking to different aspects, maybe you tend to look into, automatically you tend to look into more what is happening in the house, what are the maids doing, what are the in-laws doing, and what are the children doing, and you know those kind of issues come and occupy your mind more. And you feel you need to make some contribution here now, because you have a lot more time. And maybe you do feel that you are imposing on them, and they are all set with their normal life, and you are the new entrant in their life, so to speak you know. In everybody else life at home, at times I felt like I was imposing on them, now I was making them maybe eat at regular time and eat proper food. When I was not at home and they came home from school, they would just eat whatever they wanted. They would just laze around and do whatever they wanted. And now I was putting them in some kind off, I thought it was a routine kind of schedule for them also, in the sense that making them eat on time, or making them do their homework, making them clear their room, things like that.*

At this point we can understand that this change in her life has had a big effect on her, but we still do not know what the experience is for her, so we stick with this and ask her what it was like for her to be in this situation —

> *Systematic. You feel comfortable, you know everything is going in a predictable way, like you catch a particular train, and you know that there is a bus waiting for you. In the sense nothing uncertain nothing untoward is going to happen. Things move as per schedule, as you planned it, you planned to leave at a particular time, you planned to reach at a particular time, that nothing will harm you, nothing will go wrong suddenly.*

Asking further about this comfortable and safe she describes a protected space along with a hand gesture, so we ask her to just describe this gesture –

> *Maybe a cocoon kind of thing, it's the same thing I think, you are ok, you are taken care of. You are self-contained kind of, you have everything that you need within that place, and we are ok. You are independent, your needs are fulfilled within that place and your just satisfied.*

Two elements of the case have started to become clear. There is comfortable, protected space where nothing can harm you. And there is the issue with something uncertain suddenly happening. It is important at this point not to jump to any conclusion. We could hear the words 'comfortable' and 'protected space'. This could make us think of the first Superclass. A sudden uncertain thing happening could make us think of the 4th Superclass, with its need for stability. However, we need to make sure that we have understood the entire dynamic. To do this we ask her why she gave up the routine and comfort if she was happy with it. —

> *I wanted to do something more different, not moving much in the corporate ladder. So, again that was also because I could not when you have a family and try to have a career it becomes very difficult to divide yourself equally, it just doesn't happen like that. And then I felt yes that I wanted to be more with kids and home, rather than here because this was not moving in the direction I wanted it to go anyway.*

We ask her to describe not moving —

> *Not moving as in stagnant, I was doing what I like to do. But I did not want to do it forever. I was not doing anything different. I was not having any value, stuck in my place, not enjoyable, not challenging. Nothing different. Same thing over and over again, then it becomes useless. It becomes dead. Just repeating, lifeless, no energy, nothing to keep you excited. No fun, something that you enjoy doing, something that you like to do that would be exciting, you feel energised, you feel alive, you feel that you are doing something meaningful.*

This dynamic is starting to become clearer to us. If something uncertain happens she wants to be able to feel comfortable and safe. After a while this comfortable and safe routine can become stagnating for her. She feels lifeless and dead. There is no fun. We can begin to see this is the 2nd superclass.

To be certain of this we need to examine the case from other aspects. We ask the patient to describe a stressful incident in her life —

> *I was supposed to take my daughter for a sports meet. And that was on a Monday so I had prepared everything on Sunday and its quite a tedious thing and you have to think of lunch and dinner and what time you'll leave and what time you'll get there and what she will do there and everything. So, I had done all that, I knew Monday, Tuesday Wednesday I had to keep myself completely free. Because I would be with her, so we planned everything and ready to almost leave at 8 in the morning on Monday and suddenly my husband says I'll take her, so I was at loose end you know. I had cancelled everything that I had planned for the next 2-3 days and suddenly I am out of the picture and now I have nothing to do. And I am wondering my full mind frame is now shifted, now I have to suddenly think of now what do I do.*

This is a very interesting example as it clearly shows the sudden unexpected change which interrupts her routine. So, we ask her to describe the experience to be in this situation –

> *I was very angry and irritated, helpless. Even now instantly tears will come out of my eyes, choked in the throat. it's like a big lump (and she points to her throat), just like somebody is squeezing your throat and not allowing the words to come out or the anger to come out. You feel like some rope is tied on your throat, it's like you can't swallow and there's like a hollow pain inside the throat. You almost can't breathe, try to take a couple of deep breaths, and calm down. You just want to scream but it doesn't come out actually. You just feel I want to take a couple of deeper longer breaths, just to get rid of the tightness in your throat.*

We have the dynamic of wanting a safe comfortable space especially when something sudden unexpected happens. This space can be lifeless and repetitive. We also have this sensation of constriction and difficulty to breathe. There is the desire for a deep breath.

Having a clearer understanding of this aspect of the case it is time to investigate a different area of the case, so we ask the patient what fears she has —

> *I am afraid of being dependent on anyone or anything. To not to be able to live without that person or that thing, it could be a something like you*

> *know asking if I don't have a regular income then I must ask for something. I would not be able to function as i want to function, or I want to live if I did not have that, it could be a person it could be a medicine, it could be anything. It feels helpless, it's like weak and useless, like a vegetable or something, a potato. It is a useless lump.*

This is very interesting as we can see the features of the kingdom here; we can see the issue has to do with capability. She doesn't want to be dependent on anyone as she may not be capable if they are not there to help you. However, there is still more information to be gained here, so we ask the patient what the exact opposite of this feeling like a 'potato' is —

> *Something fun, maybe like an egg. You hatch and become into a chicken. An egg has life in it and it will change into something dramatically different. There would some process going on in the egg to change into a different being, sprouting and getting into life. There must be some major process going that the egg turns into a chicken.to an innocent like child or something. It would be fascinating to see and egg suddenly changing into a chicken, it's exciting. Chicken must be flabbergasted in suddenly being a chicken. Surprised, stunned maybe he must be feeling little scared also. Suddenly changed into a different environment and he has to get used to so many new things now. But I guess he will learn automatically.*

This is a fascinating part of the case. We see all the discrete elements of the case come together. We can see the dynamic of the 2nd superclass. They want to go inside to a safe comfortable space when there is any sudden expected danger. Once inside this can be boring. We also have seen the kingdom features, namely the Mineral kingdom. The mineral kingdom group in the 2nd Superclass are the Carbons.

We know that it must be a carbon remedy. We also know that the 2nd row of the periodic table to which Carbon belongs has everything to do with the birthing process. Carbon represents the stage where the baby is still in the womb but it is time to leave it. They have a doubt whether they have the capability to have an independent existence. We have also seen the sensation of choking and needing to take deep breath. This is common to the Carbon remedies.

At this point we know enough to prescribe a remedy for the patient. Yet, in order to be certain, it is worth seeing some more features of her case.

She mentions that she and her husband are very different to each other. We ask her to describe this —

> *I am an introvert, quiet, shy. mostly, till I get used to a person, and make friends, get comfortable, and he is completely different always surrounded by people. Loves to socialise meet friends, party. And I like that because it's fun, exciting to meet new people, go to new places. Opposite is sitting at home, reading a book listening to music. I like that more, but I realise I can't do that all the time because then that would get terribly boring at some point of time, being blank and not knowing what to do with yourself. The potato comes to mind. You just being in one position, and not knowing what to do with yourself and not knowing how to keep yourself occupied, happy really.*

When we look at the rubrics of the case, we get our confirmation.

	Carb-v.	Calc.	Acon.	Chin.	Nat-c.	Merc.	Sil.	Ars.	Caust.	Bar-c.	Sep.	Thuj.	Alum.
Total	25	36	35	34	34	33	33	32	32	31	30	28	27
Rubrics	11	10	10	10	10	10	10	10	10	10	10	10	10
Kingdom													
CR19 - Throat; Choking, constricting(430)	4	4	4	3	2	4	3	3	4	4	3	3	3
CR19 - Throat; Lump sensation(317)	2	4	3	3	3	4	3	2	4	4	4	3	3
CR19 - Throat; Swallowing; difficult(423)	3	3	4	4	3	4	3	3	3	4	3	3	3
CR19 - Generalities; Warmth; amel.(515)	4	4	3	3	4	4	4	4	4	4	4	3	4
CR19 - Stomach; Thirst; often, frequent(95)	1		3	3				4			1		
CR19 - Mind; Timidity; bashful(81)	1	3		3	3	3	3		1	3		1	1
CR19 - Mind; Anxiety; palpitations; with(207)	1	4	4	4	4	3	2	4	3	1	3	3	2
CR19 - Mind; Anxiety; perspiration; with(121)	3	4	3	4	4	3	3	4	3	3	4	4	3
CR19 - Mind; Sensitive, oversensitive(527)	1	3	3	3	3	1	4	3	3	2	3	3	3
CR19 - Mind; Weeping, tearful mood(610)	4	4	4	4	4	4	4	4	4	3	4	4	4
CR19 - Mind; Starting, startled; noise, from(118)	1	3	4		4	3	4	1	3	3	1	1	1

The remedy we prescribed was Carbo veg 200 for two days followed by one dose of LM 6 daily. A year later:

- No complaints at all
- HCQS – had taken for 6 months – tapered & stopped
- No allopathic medicines now

- State of mind – more patient and tolerant
- Doesn't get upset easily
- Able to control to a big extent
- 90-95% - better

Quantitatively the patients ESR and CRP all came back to normal levels.

Superclass	2
Kingdom	Mineral
Subclass	2nd row
Remedy	Carbo vegetabilis

Case 6

This is a case of a 52-year-old male who has been diagnosed with irritable bowel syndrome. Using our previous analogy of the Atlas we will go through this case step by step, classifying the information according to its relevant category. This case is an excellent demonstration of the characteristics of the 2nd Superclass.

The patient began by listing the complaints which he has come with —

> *I am a known case of hypertension as well as having high cholesterol levels. I also have a G6PD, this doesn't hamper me in any way it is just that I am restricted to certain medications. I just avoid certain foods. Along with this I have been having problems with my rotator cuff on the right-hand side for the last 10 years. The pain goes down from the shoulder to the elbow and it extends backwards to the scapula.*

The patient then lists some modalities —

- <swinging the arms when running
- <raising the arm at 90 degrees
- >cold fomentation
- <exertion
- >massage

The patient now comes to the main complaint —

> *My main issue is irritable bowel syndrome. If I take any supplements, they have an impact on my stomach. There is a lot of gurgling in the stomach,*

> *gas building up in the stomach. I have a problem of constipation for 10 years. Sometimes I pass motions 3 times, normal motions these are not loose. There is bloating in the abdomen. I feel why am I going to pass motions so often? I have cramping pain in the abdomen which happens 2 hours after eating. I feel better for passing flatus and motions. I want to maintain my good health. I don't want to age faster than that. My elder brother has blood cancer. So, psychologically I feel what if it is in the family. My sexual drive hasn't been great. I don't feel much urge and there is a problem with erections. It is not as stiff or as hard as it was earlier. This is ever since I started the cholesterol and BP medicine. There is no real pressure on me as such, I don't understand why this is happening… in this lockdown, there has been stress on my mind.*

At this point we ask the patient to tell us about the stress —

> *I have been working in the stock market. This caused a lot of pressure. The clients would be screaming and shouting. By the time I would get home, I would still be thinking about work. There was a lot of pressure. If anything occurred that day like any mistake or error, I would take it to heart. I am a sentimental and soft guy. I am quite emotional. I don't cry but I do take it to heart. I keep the frustrations within me. I don't vent it out. I have never even shouted at my team. I am patient that way. I will teach my team in a soft way. Even with helpers, the drivers I never shouted. Even if anyone shouts it affects me. I feel bad, I feel what right does this person have to shout at somebody else? That person is also human. If it was me at the receiving end of the shouting, I don't cry and I'm not aggressive. I just let it pass. Aggressive meaning, I don't shout back or hit or attack back.*

What have we gathered about this patient already? He doesn't argue, doesn't fight; he goes inside himself. It sounds a bit like the Ranunculaceae. There is the inability to fight back, a softness, everything hurts and injures as if he doesn't have a skin

He is not fighting, there is no violence or escaping or bursting out. Everything is sensitive, vulnerable, soft. We don't come to any conclusions but just note these things.

We ask the patient to give us an example —

> *If my wife shouts at the driver or talks rudely to him, I feel bad and tell her not to talk to him like that. What if I am him? What if I would be shouted*

at like that? It is a horrible, demotivated feeling. In life bosses have shouted at me. They have raised their voice. I don't react immediately. I will first say I am sorry. I feel it is best not to argue. I will accept the blame immediately. I hate arguing back. I hate arguments. I don't stop thinking then, I am very sensitive. For example, if something goes wrong in the office and the boss says to me this is right or this is wrong, then I would hate to defend myself and argue. I will feel sad internally, but I will never express. I will go into a shell. I will introspect at that point. I will become very quiet. I will disconnect from the rest of the discussion. I will switch off for the next few minutes. When I have gone into my shell there are no real physical attributes that happen like palpitations or perspiration. What happens when I go in is I become very quiet. My mind is switched off from the flow of things. It is completely switched off but just for some time – like a snail for example, it will go into the shell for 2 minutes when there is danger and then come back again. (Here the patient gives a hand gesture bringing both hands together)

We ask about the hand gesture and the patient describes it —

Protect me. To be safe and no harm.

The snail is protecting itself by going into the shell and becoming smaller. Similarly, I become small. I wish I am not here. I become invisible. I become small and invisible because I don't want further harm.

I go into a shell- I become very quiet – I withdraw, I go inside, I introspect, I become quiet and switch off… this is his response, going in, disconnecting – it sounds close to the first superclass. This information is very clearly signifying the patient's superclass as it is his basic reaction. Similar to our initial experiment , where we looked at our basic reaction to a situation, he describes what his basic reaction is at a very deep level.

The patient continues —

See like a boxer – he will bow down on knees and protect himself (HG), go into my shell. To be in a shell. To prevent any further harm. I am becoming as small as possible.

We ask him to describe the HG a bit more —

The image of a snail comes to mind. It will be getting small, invisible. Shell is protecting the whole body. Just like a snail, a whole soft part of the body goes inside the shell. Protecting themselves from harm. The soft part does not have self-protection. So, you need other parts like the shell to protect the soft parts of the body. Your guard is up, now I am safe. Now my soft part is not exposed. I feel no further harm can happen to me. Now my harder part is going to protect the rest. The hard part is like a big cement block. A pillar. Protecting the rest of the body. Protecting the soft part. I have created this wall by my own self. It is the size that fits and the durability that protects. My own cement wall which I have built myself. If somebody argues or punches immediately the cement wall will come up. Nobody can break this cement wall and hit me on my soft parts. It is similar to what a snail does when you touch it, it goes inside the shell, the shell is protecting the entire soft part of the body. This shell is created by itself. Similarly, I would bring out the cement wall which is created by myself. Then I am safe. Then when I feel safe, I will put down the cement wall down and then I am back out again.

'Becoming smaller' sounds like the third Superclass word 'shrinking', but you can see the idea here of becoming 'small' is to become invisible – so that one is not harmed. One goes into a shell, to prevent any harm. His hand-gesture of making a fist – is like a snail, become small and invisible. The whole soft part of the body goes inside the shell. Soft part doesn't have protection

What differentiates the kingdoms? When he says 'My harder part will protect my softer part. It's me for myself – my harder part will protect my softer part. To be dependent on someone else, would be more mineral. But here you see a survival strategy.

We ask the patient describe the word safe —

That no other harm can happen to me. I can do anything inside that wall and nobody can harm me further. By having this self-created cement wall, I am 100% protected. If I don't put down the cement wall it feels horrible.

But living within a cement wall is not always good. Then you are cut off from rest of the world. Living in four walls 24/7. You will not allow yourself any exposure or growth. It feels claustrophobic. Not able to breathe fresh air. Boring.

Claustrophobic feeling - I had done an MRI once and I will never do it.

I don't feel claustrophobic in car or airplane. Sitting up in room all the time for long. I can't do that. I need to see around, what's happening? I need to breathe fresh air.

> *Within a cement wall – I am scared. It is like sitting in a jail with 4 cement walls and locked up in that little cubical. That would be the worst point of my life. Being alone, not really seeing any daylight. I am not in favour of darkness. I don't prefer much darkness. I prefer mornings to the night. I feel scared if it's dark lonely place. Jail like feeling, dark and dingy. Fear of uncertainty ahead.*

This is the 2nd Superclass. When safe you can open the gate. Opening and shutting; in and out, this differentiates the 1st from the 2nd Superclass. 'Boring' also comes in as a feature of the 1st . In the pepper family (Piperaceae), Ennui (boredom) is relieved by entertainment. She stays in, reads a book, or watches a movie. The difference between the 1st and 2nd Superclasses is that in the 1st they remain inside. In Superclass 2, they come out to get sensory stimulation. 'Claustrophobia' in the 2nd Superclass is about being bored inside, and wanting to go out, unlike in the 5th Superclass where one feels stuck in there and wanting to burst out.

> *When I am a free bird, I can choose my path. I can go and fly where I want to. Floating. Now last 6 months I have left my job. Last 25 years I felt like a slave, being dictated. I felt like I am in a jail. Like a bonded labourer. You are tied. Your legs and hands are tied. You are being told what to do. No independence. Same way you are sitting in a jail is not independence.*

We have to further differentiate between the 2nd and 5th Superclasses. In Superclass 5, there is claustrophobia, and need to break free. There can be similar expressions in Superclass 2. It can be confusing! What is the difference?

In Superclass 1&2 being enclosed and inside gives feeling of safety and security. On the one side it is safe and secure inside. Yet, dark and limiting so you need to come out. However, when you come out, you see that the world is harsh and cruel, and you need to go in again. In and out, this the 2nd superclass. There is this alternation.

To find being inside suffocating and need to break out, this would be the 5th superclass. There is no alternating between in and out.

The patient continues —

> *Being in jail is like being tied within those 4 walls. I will be sweating; I will be angry. I would want to kill myself. I would try to break those walls.*

I would feel like vomiting and claustrophobic. Fear of the unknown. What if I am stuck in machine or the jail forever? Then I will have to break the jail wall to escape and come out.

If you are stuck, not able to move – then would panic, how do I move? If I don't try and move now, maybe I will be stuck deeper. If I don't jump out, then I might go deeper in the wall. If I am in a hole and I don't jump out, I will go more deeper in the hole. The hole becomes deeper and it will be more difficult to come out. Deeper hole – like a swimming pool. I hate swimming pool. I only go when my feet touch down. In any deeper end I hate it. If I go deeper, then I can never come out. If I keep going down, there is no end inside to going down.

Hole – dark, dingy, lonely, breathless. Is there enough oxygen for me to survive? Then I will break the wall or jump out the hole as soon as possible. If I am not capable of doing it on my own then I would want someone to help me.

Jump out – break the walls of the jail, break the walls and the chain. Then it would feel relaxing, calm. I feel very independent.

Opposite – being in jail, being tied, being stuck. MRI machine. There was no way to come out of that MRI machine. Come out – Is coming back to normal. Freedom. Relaxed feeling. Like floating in thin air. No worries and no tension. It feels light in the head. No gravity. Nobody is pulling you down.

At this point when we are classifying our information we are sure it is the second Superclass. So far, we have had some soft hints that the kingdom is animal but we need to take it further and confirm. We direct the case to some new areas —

What dreams do you get? —

In childhood I would dream that I was there with my mother going to a doctor. It was difficult to park the car. There were small streets and hawkers. Feeling helpless. Limitations of not being able to help. I feel little cold and sad.

What are your fears? —

Fear of dark, alone. I feel somebody else is in the room and he will come and kill me. May be with a gun or knife. If it's in dark I will not be able to see also. I usually come down from terrace in the dark. Fear that somebody is there and I cannot see. He might harm me. They can harm me in the dark. Hit me or kill me. Hit me with knife or gun. Fear of being in a jail. Alone in the dark jail. Fear of swimming in deep. But I don't get scared when I drive a car very fast. I get an adrenaline rush. Charged up. Energetic. I feel young. I feel I am not old.

Old – is more related to not able to do things that young people do. But I accept it. I don't get frustrated.

Here we can see the idea is that something will come and kill him. The issue is one of victim and aggressor. People control her, tie him up. Now we can clearly see that we need an animal remedy from the 2nd superclass. This approach of classifying the information is very helpful. We can be confident in our remedy selection .

From this point on the rest of the case becomes very easy. We are so close to the remedy. We just need to find the particulars and get our final confirmations.

We ask about the patient's childhood —

I am born and brought up in Mumbai. I was the youngest of 3 children. When I was young, I had little bit of asthma and it recovered with homoeopathy. When I was 26 years old, I developed fistula in rectum and I had first surgery of my life. Another surgery I had of blocked nasal passage and DNS. It was done in 2012. Since then, it's been very smooth. I am married and I have one son who is 22-years-old.

What are you sensitive to? —

I am sensitive about shouting or yelling. If somebody is making judgement about somebody else.

What are your interests and hobbies? —

I hate movies. I cannot sit through movies. I feel frustration. I feel fidgety. Claustrophobic. You are sitting on that one chair. Stuck, locked in one thing. I want to move around. I would rather prefer watching movie at home because in theatre I feel locked up in the chair. I cannot move my body. Like going in a flight. If you are sitting in economy class and in the middle seat is the worst experience. You are stuck in that seat. I like to walk around. I feel more alert at certain times of danger. Alert means to be on guard. I can quickly react to whatever that's happening. I am very methodical. My cupboard is always neat and clean. I am systematic. Medicines are properly kept.

Physical generals? —

- Appetite - good
- Thirst - thirstless
- Desires - spicy++, extra salt, chilli powder, green vegetables. Meat ++ chicken and fish
- Aversion - too much mustardy
- Sleep- I sleep well. I keep pillow on head like a protection. And I sleep with cuddling the pillow.
- Position on left side
- Urine- ok
- Motions- ok
- Sweat- profuse
- Thermals- feels more hot but fan hitting me on the head gives me headache

Past History —

Dryness on one side of the face. It comes intermittently even now. Even body has dryness.

When I was 21 years of age, I had alopecia on the beard and took 2 years to recover. Now there is no issue.

Chicken pox Typhoid, malaria

Family History —

Mother- Diabetes mellitus, had breast cancer

— End of Case —

Let us look at the classification of this information.

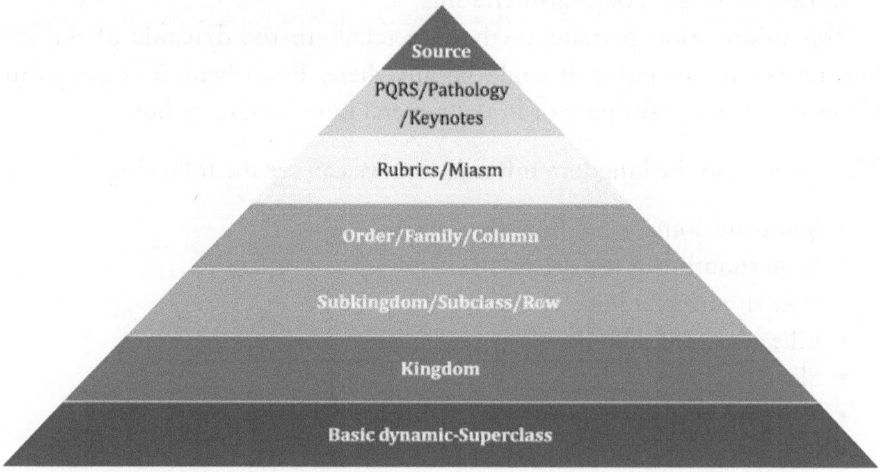

Let us go through this information in this case —

Firstly, what is the basic dynamic? We can see that for him, his basic dynamic is 'in and out'. When in, he wants out, and when out he wants in, and he alternates between the two. So, this is Superclass 2.

Then we see victim/aggressor which is animal kingdom.

The main animals in the 2nd Superclass are the gastropods (snails). Superclass 1 includes bivalves and Superclass 5 has cephalopods including Sepia. It is the gastropods that are in and out. The snail goes in and puts up the cement-like wall; then when there is no danger, it comes out.

Once you are sure of Superclass and kingdom, you can zero in on a specific group of remedies. Once you get there, then you could use any information which indicates the order, family or the row or column of the periodic table, or peculiarities or miasm, pathology or source quality. All this will help you come to a specific remedy in that shortlisted group.

This kind of classification and hierarchy of information is very important. You must know which information in the case belongs to which category. If you put one in the other, it doesn't work.

Let us, once again, go over some of the Superclass features we see in this case.

He is very sensitive, small things affect him.

When he goes in and disconnects, and he finds it boring!

There is no light, it's dark and dingy. Outside is not boring, but inside is dark and boring, like being in a jail, locked in and alone.

Outside you have light, the adrenalin rush, you are charged up and young!

In/out; dark/light; boring/interesting.

This information pertains to the Superclass, to the dynamic of the 2nd Superclass. At this point, it could go anywhere. From here, it could go to Cannabis or to a gastropod; or in the mineral kingdom, to carbon.

Now coming to the kingdom information, we can see the following –

- Someone doing something to someone else
- Wife shouting at the driver
- Boss shouting at him
- Like a bonded labourer
- Slave
- Tied and told what to do
- Aggression, hit and kill
- Someone will come and kill me with a gun
- Someone is there and he might harm me
- Pulling you down

Always someone is doing something to me or to someone else. So, we can see that the issue is that of animal kingdom.

Then within the animal kingdom we can see all the features of the Mollusca —

- Soft
- Shell
- Safe
- Guard up
- Exposed
- Alert
- Danger
- Harm
- React quickly
- Protection
- Restricted

Within the Mollusca we can see the features of the Gastropoda —

- In and out
- Like a snail - Goes into the shell for a few mins when there is danger and then comes back out again

- It protects itself by going into the shell and becoming smaller. I become invisible
- Shell protects the soft part from harm- soft part does not have self-protection
- Created the hard cement block, wall by my own self
- Size that fits and durability that protects
- Nobody can break this wall-100% protected
- Similarly, I would bring out the cement wall which is created by myself and then I am safe
- When I feel safe, I put down the cement wall and then I am back out again
- Can't be inside 24/7 feels claustrophobic, no growth

Then we can look at the rubrics of the case —

	Nat-m.	Cypra-e.	Ars.	Phos.	Stram.	Ign.	Calc.	Plut-n.	Puls.	Lyc.	Acon.	Sep.	Rhus-t.
Total	37	13	37	35	35	35	33	14	34	34	32	32	32
Rubrics	13	13	12	12	12	12	12	12	11	11	11	11	11
Kingdom													
CR19 - Mind; Delusions, imaginations; floating; air, in(122)	3	1		1	1		2	1			3	1	
CR19 - Mind; Fear; panic attacks, overpowering(124)	1	1	2	3	3	1	1	1	1		4		4
CR19 - Mind; Helplessness(128)	3	1	1	1	3	3	1	2	1	4		3	3
CR19 - Mind; Hide; oneself, desire to(90)	1	1	3		4	3		1	3	1	1		1
CR19 - Mind; Mildness(135)	4	1	4	3	3	4	3	2	4	4	3	4	4
CR19 - Mind; Sensitive, oversensitive(527)	3	1	3	4	3	4	3	1	3	3	3	3	1
CR19 - Mind; Sympathetic, compassionate, too(179)	3	1	3	4	1	3	1	1	4	1	2	2	
CR19 - Mind; Timidity(248)	3	1	4	4	4	3	4	1	4	4	3	4	3
CR19 - Abdomen; Pain; cramping, gripping(727)	4	1	4	4	4	4	4	1	4	4	4	4	4
CR19 - Abdomen; Pain(1195)	3	1	4	4	2	4	4	1	4	3	4	4	4
CR19 - Extremities; Shoulders; right(282)	3	1	1	1		3	3	1		3		1	1
CR19 - Skin; Dryness(397)	3	1	4	4	4	1	4	1	3	4	3	3	3
CR19 - Face; Dryness(350)	3	1	4	2	3	2	3		3	3	2	3	4

It is a good time to use the repertory when you know what Superclass and what kingdom or subkingdom you are in. Then the differentiation features can either be rubrics, keynotes, pathology, peculiarity, source. Any, or all of this.

When you see the rubrics, you see Cypraea Eglantina.

We can filter our repertory search to only show us remedies from the animal Kingdom. We will notice that the top remedies all come from the mollusc group —

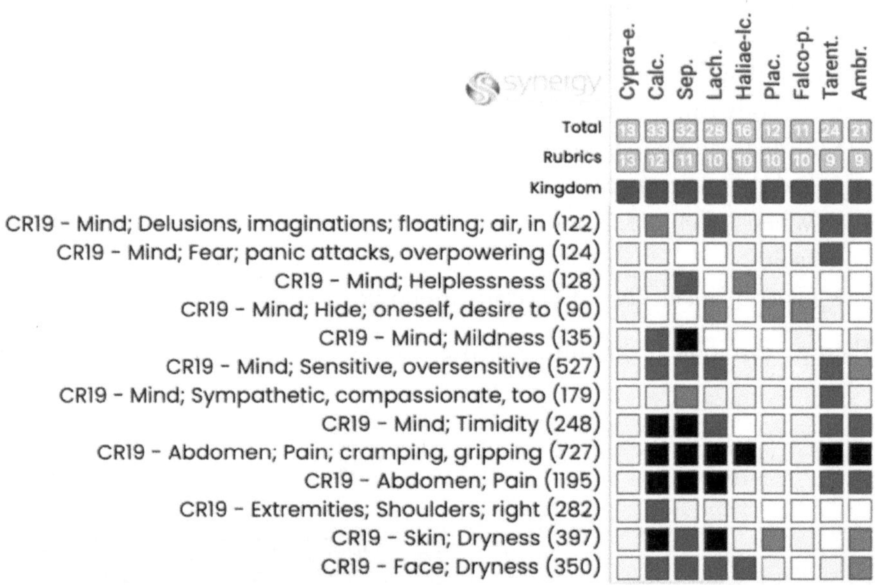

During the case taking, he gives one peculiar characteristic symptom. “I am flying or floating in the air, like there is no gravity”. This he mentions several times.

Anne Schadde’s book “Listening to Stone, Wood and Shell” has the proving of Cyprea Eglantina (the Cowrie Snail).

Listening to Stone, Wood and Shell ×

DELUSIONS, imaginations; floating in air (71)
DELUSIONS, imaginations; floating in air; Bett/bed (6)

43 Sensation as if not living in the ordinary world; sensation as if floating. (19-06 + 19-27)
44 Everything appears to be unreal, irrelevant, strange; I feel limitless, not grounded, as if floating (19-34)

Listening to Stone, Wood and Shell ×

73 I am lying in bed and have the feeling as if I were floating above the ground (9-17)

The prescription must be looked at from all angles. Not only kingdom, sensation, Superclass. The patient kept saying I feel like a snail. This is useful after you have clearly seen the rest of the case. Otherwise, jumping to a remedy just from that would be very risky.

There are some other features… and it is important to know how to understand these in context of the case —

- Stuck, cannot move
- Panic
- If I don't try and move, difficult to come out
- Hole is dark and dingy. Feel lonely and it is breathless
- Is there enough oxygen for me to survive?
- Need help, what if am not capable of doing it on my own?
- What if I am stuck forever?
- In or out
- I want to break the wall or jump out of the hole as soon as possible
- Want to break the walls
- There is no end inside to going down

You cannot ignore or neglect such graphic images: air hunger, stuck, can't move, feeling lonely. It seems similar to carbon which is also Superclass 2. There are many themes that remind us of the birth process such as "I need to come down, and get out, I need to move, can I survive without oxygen", "If I don't get out it will be difficult, no oxygen, I need to break the wall, come down, go down."

Every remedy will have some quality of all the remedies which are in the same Superclass. This is the beauty of it! But one aspect will be very prominent, which belongs to that one remedy which is the remedy for the case.

In one remedy of a particular Superclass, one element could be very intense. In another, it will be there, but subdued. The idea of the Superclass helps you to understand the totality of the case. Otherwise, you might think it looks like Carbon. Yes, it is close. You could also think of Cannabis indica with the floating and flying sensation, seeking excitement and thrill. You will find common elements between the remedies in a given Superclass.

To complete our classification of information —

Superclass	2
Kingdom	Animal
Phylum	Mollusca
Class	Gastropoda
Remedy	Cypraea eglantina

The patient was given Cypraea Eglantina 1M twice a day for two days and repeated every month.

This was the patients follow up information after 1 year and 5 months;

- I am doing very well.
- IBS has improved a lot.
- No bloating, pain, or cramping
- Frequency of motions has reduced
- Pain in the shoulder has completely gone off
- Mentally I feel so calm, there is no anxiety now.
- Got a dream: – someone is coming to attack. Feels closed up. I curled myself inside to become invisible. Feel safe but tight.

The dream indicates that he still requires the remedy which he takes once per month.

Case 7

To explain the features of the 3rd superclass more clearly, we will discuss a case. This is the case of 58-Year-old female who comes with the main complaints of Psoriasis and eczema.

We start by asking this patient what the problem is, and she narrates her complaint of the psoriasis –

> *I was learning pottery four years back, got eruptions and patches of dry skin on my fingers. It started becoming worse. I stopped pottery and went to a homeopath, they said it was psoriasis, I took their remedy for about 8 months, and it went away. Then I developed eczema on the feet. She told me I was stressed, and that the psoriasis would come back when I was stressed. I tried meditation and things were alright for a bit. Two years back I had jaundice. Then something like chikungunya began. Knees were so bad I couldn't stand up. Started ayurvedic treatment and began strict control over diet. Things were not working out. Then I got fever. Joint pains became less after 3-4 days. Then infection and face puffed up like a ball. Then I went to Kerala. Had massage with hot oil, after this got huge blister on feet. As if top skin was parting from bottom skin. Would just cut it away. This gradually developed into bad psoriasis. My confidence was shaken.*

The patient has described her main complaints quite generally and we can't see any peculiar symptoms.

She continues —

> *My hands have started erupting. Feet are getting better, but hands are getting worse. I have been a healthy person. I have an enthusiasm for learning new things. My dad passed away four years ago; things have been going downhill since then. He used to love all aspects of life. He was a very obedient father of four daughters. He was in a coma; we heaved a sigh of relief. His passing away was very comfortable, he was always surrounded by love. At least two people were always around. I had always given him as much love as I could. I don't remember feeling traumatized or shocked. He went very suddenly, the evening before he had been fine. It felt as though someone up there had blessed him. Subsequently two of my sisters had a big falling out. That just broke! The feeling that nothing could separate us. That has traumatized me. That has shaken the core of my being.*

Still the patient tells us quite general information. These are all common situations and reactions and nothing peculiar comes up, so we take the patient to a different area and ask about her dreams —

> *I am Whatsapping my best friend that my mom has died peacefully.*

We want to try and understand this dream a bit better, so we ask what she means by dying peacefully —

> *To go to sleep and never wake up. To look at death coming to you and to smile.*

We still haven't understood this in the context of the patient, so we ask what the opposite of dying peacefully would be —

> *To die in an emotionally or physically traumatized way. To die in a physical violence, like sticking a knife in you. I don't know If I had the strength. Not like slicing through a cabbage.*

This is where the case starts to become interesting. We go from peaceful death to violence and then slicing a cabbage. This doesn't make sense. All we need to do is stay with this until we can see how it fits in the case, so, we ask the patient to describe slicing a cabbage —

> *Cabbage is a very easy vegetable to cut. The knife doesn't slip. It has layers and layers. It cuts easily. It cuts smoothly. It provides enough resistance; in*

contrast you are more likely to cut your fingers when cutting an onion. The surface of an onion is slippery.

Now logically this still doesn't make sense. How can you go from violence to comparing cutting a cabbage to cutting an onion. This is the beauty of homeopathy. That which is peculiar is interesting and important to us, so we then ask to describe what it is like to cut your fingers —

> *Ouch! I did it again. A sharp pain. It is like a very sharp cutting pain. Its sudden, it has gone a little deep. The knife has gone a little deeper. When a little bit of skin comes off you don't experience pain. When it goes deeper it touches your nerves and you feel the pain. You must wash your hands. It's like a point. Something which is only at that particular place. It's like your muscles are hurting it's a big area that has a pain. When you cut your finger, it is just one narrowed down point where you have the pain.*

This is the peculiarity of the case. We now have our first particular symptom, we will need a remedy in this case which has cutting pain in the fingers. There is still so much information which will need to collect before we can get to the remedy. For now, we store this information and continue with the patient. Since we have been successful with a dream, we now ask the patient to tell us another one she can recall —

> *The most joyful dream I have ever had. I was on a seaside, I was tied by rope on the back of a jeep. The jeep took off really fast and I took off in the air, I took many minutes in the air, just dancing and swirling and swooping in the air. Not bound by gravity, light enough to stay afloat in the air. So much joy within you. It makes you light*

This is also an interesting dream, so we ask the patient to describe 'light' —

> *Feels like you are not there, not bound by a physical body. Not limited by a physical body (HG). Something that ties you down.*

All we need to do is guide the patient. It is important not to distract or divert the patient. Keep asking them to describe what they are talking about, and the experience of it in the body —

> *As if tied to a chair. Scary, frustrating. Like my heart beating really hard. Be really tense. Trying to break those bonds. Using all my strength to loosen the bonds. Gritting my teeth. My stomach would not feel very good.*

From this second dream we have started getting some hints at the Superclass. We can see theme of 'being limited'. But we need to confirm this, so we ask patient to tell us another dream —

It was the movie 'nightmare on elm street'. The guy comes back to people in their dreams and manages to kill them. The procedure of killing is extremely violent and bloody. He tears them open with his nails. Saw it in the first year of my marriage. I dreamt that I got a call from this guy, I put the phone down. I thought it was real, there was no division between dream and reality. I couldn't believe it was a dream at all.

The dream she starts narrating is a nightmare. It sounds quite terrifying, but we shouldn't allow this to sway and misdirect us. Nightmares can be very common as well as all sorts of horrific situations. We shouldn't immediately jump to a group such as the Solanaceae every time someone tells us a nightmare. What is important is what is the deepest experience within the dream. This is more important than just the subject or the situation in the dream, so we clarify this further –

Terrifying, so scary. I think heart had stopped. Was ready to burst into tears.

Again, terrifying isn't enough, we need to understand the experience of terrifying, so we ask further —

As if your heart is going to stop or burst. Tense or so tense inside (HG two fists clenched)

The patient now shows us a hand gesture, this is the where the energy is, so we need to concentrate on and this and ask them to describe what they are showing —

Opposite is light and free. This is scrunched. Something has become really tight.

This is starting to confirm our earlier observations of the 3rd superclass. She spoke of being limited. We need to stay with it and be absolutely sure, so we ask the patient to describe the word "tight" —

Shrunk into the smallest possible thing. Like a ball of iron vs a ball of rubber. Rubber will bounce it is happy. Iron is like "tak." It is dense, feel like it will create a dent. The iron would be like heavy and dark and not capable of expanding or bouncing.

From the nightmare we have come back to the 3rd superclass themes. There is the idea shrinking in order to fit within a limit. The opposite is expanding beyond the limit and no longer feeling limited. At this point we are sure that it is the 3rd superclass. We ask a confirmatory question just to test our hypothesis, so we ask the patient how it would feel to be limited —

It feels sad, it feels as if you had been tied down. Very frustrating, very scary. I can imagine continually resisting. Trying really hard to break the bonds. Slump back again, gather all my energies. To get out of that space. A physical space. A closed room. It would be dark. No windows. Small, closed dark room. But enough light to see what I am doing. My heart being really tense. (HG - clenched fist.) As if there is a weight on my heart. As if my heart is feeling constricted. Not able to beat at its normal. Shrunk. To become smaller.

Our confirmatory question has paid off. We can see how it all comes back again to the themes of the third Superclass. Even the original hand gesture has come back so we can see that the patient is only talking from her state. This is so well represented by this hand gesture. The patient explains it in terms of constricting, shrinking, and becoming smaller. This again highlights the dynamic of the 3rd Superclass for us.

By now we are sure that this is the 3rd superclass. We should always go to different areas of the case. We ask the patient about her interests and hobbies. The patient says she likes to sing and dance so we ask her to describe this further —

When dancing I feel like I am not thinking. Totally absorbed in the music. Graceful. Parts of my body are following my instructions. I feel strong, light. A dance is a flow, it's not static or heavy. Like water or a bird. They flow. I feel very happy. As if I am part of, or at one.

The patient has taken us into a new area. We need to try and see how this will link back into what we already understand of the patient. So we ask her to describe what the experience of being at one would be like for them —

As if I'm not there. There is no physical limiting body. A body is tied down by gravity. It's limited by its own construction.

And very beautifully the patient brings us back to our anchor which is the idea of ' limit' of the 3rd Superclass. So, at this point we can try and classify the information which has been given. We already know the Superclass, but what is the kingdom?

For this we need to see what the patient experiences in various situations, dreams, fears, etc. Does the patient experience a sensation and its opposite, or is the experience one of lack within oneself, or is it an experience of one versus the other. In this case, in every situation the patient has the experience of being limited, constricted, tied up and shrinking. The opposite is the feeling of wanting to expand and become bigger, going beyond the limitations of the physical body. This points us to the Plant Kingdom.

We know 3rd subclass of the dicotyledons (Caryophyllidae) belong to the third Superclass. We can reflect back on the characteristic features of the 3rd Subclass from Section Two. We are able to see them reflected in this case.

We can also see some of the other themes of this Superclass such as the idea of doing good deeds. This comes through when we see in her nature that she has a strong desire to connect with others and to help them. This patient does a lot of social work and since the last 10 years been working with girls from a rescue home. She also says that she likes to do anything which helps other people otherwise she feels selfish. This symptom (desire to do good deeds) is an important feature of another remedy from the same subclass namely *Cereus bonplandii.* However, this may not be the remedy of the patient, since this quality of helping others can be found in most of the remedies of this Superclass, even if it is not specifically mentioned in the rubric.

Having understood that the remedy we need is from the 3rd subclass how do we find the remedy we need? By taking the specific symptoms we elicited from the dream. The patient describes cutting a cabbage. From this we realise we need a remedy from the 3rd subclass which has the specific cutting pain in the fingers. So, if we look in the repertory, we will find what we are looking for;

- Extremities; Pain; cutting; fingers – peti
- Extremities; Pain; cutting; fingers, first, thumb – peti

There is only one remedy from the Caryophyllidae in these two rubrics. That is *Petivaria tetranda.* But we can't leave it at that, we must always confirm the other rubrics of the case (by using the reverse repertory or by limiting the repertory search to rubrics of that remedy), as seen below —

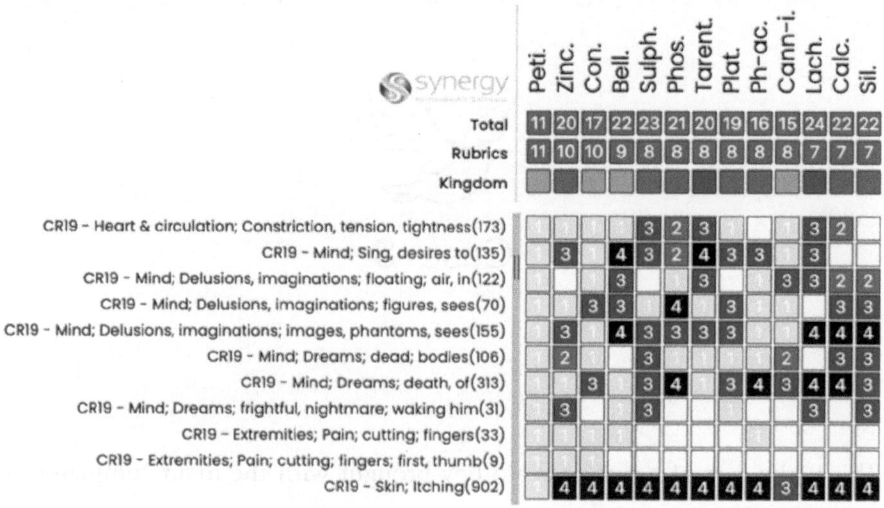

Based on all this, the patient received *Petivaria tetranda* 200, and this was her follow up after one year of treatment —

> *Physically my skin is much better. The spots have gone, and the patches have reduced in size. There is no itching and also no pain in my back. I am feeling extremely energetic now, no longer tired like earlier. Even if I exert myself physically, I feel energetic and enthusiastic. I am also feeling much calmer and more relaxed. Not stressed or worried like before. My irritability has reduced. I feel like I am going through the best phase of my life. Not having scary dreams like before, I hardly recollect them. There is no impact of the dreams on me now.*

Superclass	**3**
Kingdom	Plant
Subclass	Caryophyllidae
Order	Caryophyllales
Family	Portulacaceae
Remedy	Petivaria tetranda

Case 8

This is the case of a two-year-old boy brought with the main complaint of recurrent styes.

The patient's parents narrate the main complaint —

Eye-allergy and styes

Started a year back, parents are not sure, but he was playing and by mistake must have put some sand/mud in his eye; though parents cleaned it up immediately, they didn't see any particle but after 2-3 weeks redness of eye and since then his stye keeps coming often. Stye is in different position and can be on upper or lower eye lid. Presently stye is coming only in right eye. Sometimes entire eye lid is swollen. Earlier left eye lid was swollen for a month. Presently his upper eyelid is swollen, eye is pinkish-red and watery. Whenever his eye is affected, he will be lethargic, he avoids anything bright, he likes dark and cold environment.

When he is not well, then parents will take him out for a ride in the car with air-conditioning on, at night and he will feel better. He will try to keep his eye closed or cover it with his hand. Cold water seems to help. He will be cranky, wants to cling to mother.

His basic nature is also to cling to mother and paternal grandmother, but when he is sick, he will cling more. When not sick, he will go to other family member for some time, but then he wants to go back to mother or grandmother.

He is a Covid baby - was born in May 2020 and he has been inside the home as parents were scared of taking him out from the fear of getting Covid. When eye symptoms are severe, he will also get running nose and eye complaints will also increase.

Nose discharge will be on the same side of affected eyes. Discharge will be thick or thin, sometimes white, sometimes watery clear, sometimes yellowish. He keeps touching his eyes and keeps saying that it itches. He tries to rub it with his hand especially outer canthi. He listens to parents that he should not itch, and he understands when parents tell him to control. Earlier he had discharge coming from the affected eye—yellowish discharge, thick. Eye lids will stick together.

Appetite —

Okay, 4 meals in a day. When hungry, he will be irritated and stop playing. Parents will understand that he is hungry, he will ask for milk at times. If he is irritated and cranky, parents hit him and he will ask for milk. When sick his appetite is poor.

Thirst —

He likes water and drinks enough during the day. Small quantity often.

Cravings —

Ghee, salt, chapati (bread), bhindi (okra). He likes cold stuff, even when he is sick, he wants cold milk. If cold milk is given, he will drink more quantity as compared to warm milk, he doesn't like warm water. He likes milk+++ and fruits, sweet lime juice, dry fruits- almond, cashew nuts, pistachios, banana chips. Cheese+++, sweet also he likes. He likes noodles, Maggi (noodles) – and can eat even after eating.

Agg —

Cashews affect eye redness

Bowels —

regular

Sweat —

Not much, if he sweats it will be on back, he will sweat in sleep at times. Even his head and pillow are little wet, he cannot tolerate heat.

Sleep —

On abdomen, on right side. Mouth is open – during sleep when sick, like if his nose is blocked. He needs touch of mother while sleeping, he is okay if he can feel the touch of someone. His toes are pressed to bed and parents have to loosen it up, parents feels that his feet are stiff/tensed when he sleeps. He will cry with eyes closed in sleep (recent development for 2-3 weeks). He will keep crying for some time, it is inconsolable, and he won't open his eyes, they will carry him and move around, try to pat him. They are trying to wean him off breast feeding and possibly weeping is related to it.

Thermally —

Hot, after cyclonic rains when the weather is little cooler for a week, his eyes seem better and when it starts to be warm then his eye symptoms worsen.

Past history of febrile convulsions twice - June 2021 and Dec or Jan 2022 – now parents are careful and don't let his fevers go above 102.

Family history: Paternal Grandmother - allergic cough from smell, Father - allergic cough from dust

Milestones —

All on time or before time.

Vaccinations —

All given as per the government

The parents are asked to describe his nature —

He had desire to eat chalk and mud earlier, when examined his haemoglobin was a little low. When mother told not to eat then he would cry. He has a little OCD – he wants bathroom to be either completely dried or completely wet, but if only a wet patch is there in the bathroom he doesn't like. He will ask to wipe it properly. He will keep cards/toys in its box. He will keep things in place. If something falls down, he will want it to be put in place. He will do it also, though not very neat as he is just 2, but wants it to be put properly in place or its box. He is shy, takes a long time to mix with people. If some guest comes to their house, he will not go to them, if they stay for 30-40mins, he will go but maintain a distance from them, if they stay for 4-5 days then he will mix up. He would want to be in his comfort zone (his room). He is curious to know about them and what they are doing, but he will keep distance from them. If someone tries to hold him – he won't cry immediately but when they leave him, he will go to mother crying.

His memory is sharp. He can name the eye drops. He knows the alphabet well. If parents tell V for Vicky, then he will say V is for Violet (how it is taught). His memory is good.

If he will ask for cold milk and if mother takes the milk and put it in microwave thinking that he won't understand but he knows that microwave is for heating and would throw a tantrum. Once doctor told him not to eat mud and he remembered it and told mother that doctor told not to eat mud as it is not good. He likes to play with pebbles/stones of any size. If he goes out, he will bring some stone with him. He will hold one of the stone in his hand.

He is talkative with family and people whom he is comfortable with. For e.g., with maid he will talk, though he will keep distance from her. He is verbose, he will say "Vicky is eating corn" or "Mother is coming". He will weep on small matters, get emotional especially when mother says no to him. He will cry as if he is complaining that mother said no to him, if father says no, he is ok. Generally, he will show his tantrum towards mother. He is not very demanding for toys and is not stubborn. He has anger, he will be emotional when something unfair happens to him. Like his elder brother takes something, then he will be angry and tries to take it back or complain to mother. When mother won't listen to him then he will be angry and start to cry. If he asks and he is given something, then he will cry. At times while playing he will hit others even without reason.

He gets detached easily/he doesn't get attached easily. For e.g., if some animal is rescued and brought home and then when they heal the parents will let go the animal, he won't be emotional. His elder brother will miss and cry.

He is independent- does quite a lot of things by himself. Like if he is given a glass of water/milk, then he will drink it himself. He shares with everyone in the family- be it a chocolate or some snack. He is very precocious.

He is systematic and won't break or let things fall from his hand. He knows that if he will put his hand in the door it will hurt. For him parents never had to put any table corners, his walking and running is quite stable, and he would not fall much. When he started to learn to walk, if he is about to fall down he will sit.

What makes him happy —

Likes listening to music and even hums along.

Likes watching cartoons

Fears —

Of dark - he won't go into a pitch-dark room. He will get up and look for someone, he will be teary. he doesn't like house fly, though he is not scared of it

Sensitivity —

If his stone is taken away, he will be upset.

He is clear about what he wants to wear or watch on TV. He dislikes to wear tight clothes. He won't wear socks, wants half sleeves shirt/t-shirt. Won't wear sandals for long.

For adventure rides he will sit in any ride and won't be scared, same way in play zone, elder son won't go for it, but this fellow would go quickly. He likes oil massage on head and likes to comb hair. He doesn't like to apply anything on his body even if he is hurt, he won't allow to apply any antiseptic cream.

Mothers' history during pregnancy —

Planned pregnancy C section—as first child's delivery was also C section. No medication during whole pregnancy. Allergic cough during last month of pregnancy for 10-15 days (took Homeopathic remedies)—suddenly developed cough especially in the night after sleeping and suddenly woke up coughing, had to sit up and it will go on and on and she was not able to lie on back. She had to lie on recliner sofa and as soon as she would lie down on bed then it would start again. Sometimes it will stop and if she would lie down then it would start again. Had to recline on some sofa but could not lie down completely [During covid times—she was using a lot of sanitisers could be the cause of it] throat irritation, dry cough. No phlegm. Dryness of throat – desire to drink something to wet the throat.

Once her BP was very low and it was not measured on digital BP machine—but after resting it was better.

Cravings —

Chinese, spicy food.

Aversion —

Jeera (cumin) the smell of it.

We ask the mother about her mood during the pregnancy —

Stressed due to covid- worried that elder son should not get covid. Father-in-law was on dialysis and elder son was close to him, so I was constantly stressed about family getting infected.

There was no house help. Mother-in-law was there but everything had to be done by us such as cleaning utensils, vegetables. I had elder kid also to take care of. Until I delivered, I was stressed. Both physically and mentally. Elder child's school was online, father-in-law had to go for dialysis and husband had to take him every week. Child was born in May 2020, and there were lots of restrictions in hospital. Only husband could visit and there was no mental support after delivery. I suffered from postpartum depression, even my parents could not visit. All responsibility was on me—elder son, newborn, house chores etc… I felt bad as elder son was neglected as I had to take care of newborn and house chores. Post-delivery I had fever within 7 days. It was not covid but still it was there for 10 days, and I was very depressed. Elder son was used to sleep with me since his birth and I couldn't sleep with him during pregnancy as he kicks hard in sleep. So, I had to keep him away from me. As living with in-laws—I felt I didn't get full attention of husband and complained that he was not giving time. I felt no one cared. I wanted to go to my mother's place but couldn't go and felt that support system was missing.

We ask her about a support system —

I was alone, no one to share my feelings with, husband was busy with job, taking care of his father, felt that if she could have been with mother then I could have shared my feelings, which I couldn't share to mother-in-law. With own mother I could express myself. I don't want to do certain work now and I can do later etc. Which is difficult to mention to mother-in-law. I am very introverted and cannot share feelings with anyone. My younger child (the patient) is more like his father, certain traits of OCD is from me. I have tendency to suppress anger and not express it, especially after children were born. I keep things to myself and don't express it to anyone, not even to my mother. I feel that since we are trying to wean the child off from breast feeding, the child feels that I am going to abandon him. When child is crying and if I call him, he won't go to me. He wants me to go to him and he will cry with his eyes closed. He wants me to breast feed him quickly. He listens to father but not to me. If I ask him to have a glass of milk he won't, if father or brother gives, he will have it. With me he shows his tantrums but with father he is little obedient/disciplined.

— End of Case —

How do we analyse a case like this? There are different options or ways of approaching it. We could go via the symptomatic approach as there are some interesting symptoms in the child related to the stye. This can be a good way to do but there is some risk involved when we only observe one aspect of the case.

So along with the symptoms there are two other aspects we can include in our analysis –

1. Genius
2. System

Together, the symptom, the genius and the system we call the synergy approach. When we use these aspects of the case synergistically, we can be sure of the remedy we prescribe. In this book we mainly deal with the system part, as the Superclass falls under this umbrella. However, when you go through our cases you will be sure to see these other elements included in every case. If you wish to learn more about using these different aspects as part of the synergy approach I would refer the reader to my book, "*The Synergy in Homeopathy*".

What is the Genius part of this case. We need to look at what we are dealing with. The main problem we are dealing with in this case is allergy. The mother had allergy during the pregnancy. We also see the history of allergy in the family with the paternal grandmother and the father and we also see the allergy in the child. Based on this we require a remedy where allergy is one of the main ideas.

Another aspect of the Genius in this case is the manifestation of the physical complaint. It is in the eye and it has manifested in only one part. So, this idea too must form a central core of the remedy.

Now we can take a look at the System aspect of this case. We can start with the description of the patient by the father. He says the patient is independent but only with familiar people. Only in the home. He can show curiosity with new people but there is some discomfort. There is a kind of limitation. The child is comfortable only in a limited space. This is a quality of the 3rd Superclass – Limitation and expansion.

The child is very organised. He wants everything in its proper place. The child is also quite cautious as well as fastidious, he is very clean. These are soft clues towards the mineral kingdom.

We know that the group from the 3rd Superclass in the mineral kingdom is the 3rd row of the Periodic table.

We can see that the child is dependent on the mother. There is attachment and clinging to the mother. Yet, he is very clear that he wants to be independent of the mother. He wants to make his own choices. He wants care and nourishment from the mother but he wants to be independent about the clothes he wears etc.

These are the qualities of the 3rd row of the Periodic table (care, nourishment, identity and choice). This confirms our understanding and correlation of the 3rd superclass and the mineral kingdom.

He is dependent and independent. Shy but curious. So, he must fall in the middle of the 3rd row.

This is the information of the system which points us at Silicea.

We need to look at the main characteristics of Silicea. These are;

- Allergies
- Ailments from foreign bodies

From this we can see there is a hyper reaction to foreign bodies in Silicea. This is what an allergy is. This directly corroborates what we were looking for in the Genius aspect of the case.

Silicea is the main remedy for allergy and also suppuration. We can see the greenish discharge from the eye. It also covers the characteristic allergic cough of the mother.

The second aspect of the genius which we mentioned was the manifestation in single parts. When we read Silicea from "*Soul of Remedies*" we see the following —

> *The pathology in Silicea also often exhibits the qualities of fixity and obstinacy - chronic suppurative processes, keloids, fistulas, etc. They tend to develop problems in single parts like glands, sinus, headache, keloid, and*

often Silicea has only one problem. It is as if all their effort is concentrated in filling up that one weak spot in themselves.

We can see this same idea represented by the rubric - CR19 - Mind; Monomania.

Silicea is one of the main remedies in this rubric.

So far we have shown how the system and the genius come together at the remedy Silicea, but we need to confirm the 3rd aspect: The symptoms. So, we can show the following Repertorial analysis —

synergy	Sil.	Puls.	Sulph.	Calc.	Nux-v.	Phos.	Thuj.	Lyc.	Nat-m.
Total	23	43	27	25	25	25	17	25	22
Rubrics	15	14	11	10	10	10	10	9	9
Kingdom									
CR19 - Generalities; Food and drinks; lime, slate pencils, clay etc., desires(29)	1	3	1	3	3		1		3
CR19 - Generalities; Applications; cold; amel.(177)	1	4	4	3	1	4	1	3	3
CR19 - Eyes; Sties, styes; recurrent(17)	3	3	4					1	
CR19 - Mind; Clinging; mother, to(16)	1	3							
CR19 - Generalities; Food and drinks; warm; drinks; aversion(28)	1	4				4			1
CR19 - Mind; Weeping, tearful mood; sleep; during(112)	3	4	3	3	4	3	3	3	4
CR19 - Mind; Fastidious(115)	1	4	3		3	1	3	4	3
CR19 - Mind; Timidity; bashful(81)	3	4	3	3	2	1	1	4	1
CR19 - Mind; Cautious(55)	1	4	1	3	3		1	4	1
CR19 - Cough; Sit up, must(73)	1	4	3	1	1	4	1		
CR19 - Cough; Lying; agg.; down; head touches pillow, as soon as(10)	1	3							
CR19 - Back; Perspiration; sleep, during(16)	3		1	4		3			
CR19 - Generalities; Convulsions, spasms; heat; during(67)	1	1	3	1	4	1	2	1	3
CR19 - Mind; Strangers, in presence of; agg.(68)	1	1		1	3	1	3	2	3
CR19 - Mind; Precocity(67)	1	1	1	3	1	3	1	3	

The symptoms confirm the choice of Silicea which we can prescribe with confidence which comes from a strong synergistic approach.

In this case the Superclass aspect was a little subtle as compared to some other cases. However, we can see the features of the nature of the patient as well as the mother's history during pregnancy. There is the strong correlation with the 3rd row of the periodic table which also overlaps somewhat with the Superclass features giving us a deeper understanding of the basic nature of the person from the 3rd Superclass. This case is also a great example of circumspection. We have to see every aspect of the case and analyse all the information and see how things fall into place. The synergy approach is an amazing tool in case analysis and we can see in the follow up the true success of the approach.

The patient received Silicea 200 twice a day for two days which was followed by LM6 daily. After 3 months of taking the remedy, the eyes were completely fine. Only once during this period was there a little discharge. This too cleared up completely. He is very cheerful and active and is starting to express himself more. He will even get a little angry and express himself. Earlier he wouldn't let his emotions out but would shut them in.

Case 9

This is the case of a 26-Year-old female suffering from depression and emotional problems.

The patient begins narrating her complaints –

> *Irritable from ovulation day onwards till 28th day. I cry, throw huge tantrums, and talk about divorce. I say things that are very rude. Now, I am very short tempered. I react to smallest of things I have low self-esteem. I have lot of complaints about the way I was raised. As a child had abusive father who was esp. abusive towards my mother.*

Here we can see that there are mood changes related to her hormones. Along with this you have the feeling of low self-esteem. These are some soft clues towards the 3rd superclass.

The patient goes straight into her emotional state –

> *Last April I got married. It was arranged marriage. Towards wedding I was indecisive. The boy's family hasn't accepted me too well. There was stress in marriage too. He is very controlling. He puts me in box. Restricted, confined, stuck, caught up, constricted and suffocated. (HG) This is a cage. My future will be controlled. I will be something which I don't want to be. Dead. Over. Run. Get out of here. I want to get out of that box. Free space. Open and blue. Free air and water. Carefree. Dancing. Laughing. Twirling. Spinning. Running around beach. frock flying in the air. Me twirling. No concerns.*

Happy. Move more. Spinning, lot of space there. Free flowing. Open blue, calm see. Breeze. Blue water. - It is like that picture (points to the HMP logo which can be also seen in this book) My hands up in the air HG, singing, ballet dancing, free. Space where I can be myself. Here I am HG hands coming together, tied, controlled. Restricted. There is something that is controlling me. Here all is closed up, tight, suffocating. I feel that there is a rope and I am tied by rope, moreover in the upper body. Tough and strong rope. I am struggling to free myself. Helpless and finished. It's over and I will die like that. Choking sensation in chest. I have a bad cough while I cry. Girl without all these concerns, without these pressures. Social standards which I need to cross. Someone sets up a level. Doesn't have all these people. I took up the exam after marriage, to prove myself to my in-laws. Prove my worth to them. I feel ashamed now. I feel like a failure, lost. Fear of being alone, rejected. Again, not being accepted. I feel performance in every phase of life. If I can't perform, it is death. Everything is finished. I am asking for divorce. Finished. I am out of that one box, one cage. Divorce, is something that my mother didn't do.

Now my biggest worry is what will my mother do? I try to mother her now. Protect her. Sacrifice. Give your all to that person. You be very compassionate.

Let us see the main expressions in this narrative. We see that she is indecisive. Restricted. Confined. Like in a cage. And she wants to get out of the box into a free space. At this point it could be as much a feature of the 3rd superclass as it is of the 5th. What is the difference? The difference is that in the 3rd superclass, staying within the restriction is somewhat self-imposed. The feeling is that, "I need to stay within boundaries in order that I am accepted, cared, nourished." The feeling is, "I need to be worthy of being accepted." These expressions in the above narration indicate the 3rd superclass rather than the 5th.

The patient tells us her dreams —

A rowdy football player, touching me. I tried calling husband but he didn't come. Disgusted and disappointed. Perversion expressed on me. Touching my body. Helplessness.

Her fantasy?

Desire to be top notch doctor. Very popular. Well accepted by everybody. People will want to come and see me. People would like me. In-laws would be proud. I would defeat my husband. You lose and I win. Powerful. I have everything in control.

Now I can control. I am higher [HG] level, I am above everybody else below. Content. Over. Fulfilled. One aspect is that I am controlled and other is that I have achieved. Once I achieve it there is same free feeling that I told you. You have everything with you.

You see her emphasis on doing things where she will be accepted. Along with this now we see the themes of the kingdoms. You see the theme of comparison, control by another person, the question of who is higher? who is lower? etc. So, this way, we need to differentiate between superclass features and kingdom features. Here you see features of superclass 3 (constriction/expansion, need to accepted, etc) and kingdom features (higher/lower, controlled/controlling, etc) So, we need to look for an animal remedy within the 3rd superclass.

Her fears? —

I will end up a housewife. I will be controlled like that. Fear of lizards, rats. I live in land where there are no lizards. I feel very safe. I come out bathroom and I feel someone is there. I feel angry or rage towards in-laws, they are cheap. Not cultured. Aimless. No goals. Like my father. He was reckless person with respect to money. Loud and arrogant person.

You see here again feeling of one vs the other (I feel rage towards the in-laws) You see comparison(they are cheap)

The patient shares the following generals —

Appetite – ok. Diminished before menses
Thirst – thirsty esp. before menses
Craving – chicken, spicy. I feel fire should come out and then soothe it with my coffee, ghee, butter.
Stools – normal. Prolapsed haemorrhoids only during stools
Perspiration – profuse on palms and feet always esp. when I am nervous.
Nervous about exams. Performance pressure.
Thermal – hot pt. vertigo with warmth
Menses – regular

Pain in vertex on fasting. Pain extends from vertex till jaw

At this point we did the WISE process with the patient and showed her the picture of Woman 1 —

> *Trying to be defensive that something coming to her. I can see her inner body through it. Other end there is a man abusing her. Strong force which she is trying to repel. Powerful tall, hefty man coming against her abuse. She is slave. Helpless cry. Dark shady room. Dim light. Closed. Pushed against the wall. One man in the room. She doesn't look shocked. Only helpless. Her hands are very dirty. Dragged on the floor. She is screaming but no one hears her. Place is aloof, isolated. No people around. One corner. Miles together nobody is going to hear here. Outside is beautiful, lot of land, empty roads, no cars, good amount of green, dry grass, no noise. She wants to go there. She feels caged inside. As if she has been locked in, someone has locked her inside. She wants to escape but she can't. As if tied down. Constricted. I am trapped. I feel like I am bonded. You are not free. Free means you are free, like a free spirit. No one can hold you. No one can control you. You can move. You can move very fast. It is rapid. Experience is of thrill, (HG) like this, very good experience. Released.*

Explanation- You can see the themes of animal kingdom of one abusing the other. You see the themes of being caged, locked in, constricted. These themes are similar to what we have seen earlier. By doing the WISE process we confirm that these are the central experiences in her case.

We show the patient Woman 2 and repeat the process —

> *She is looking at the direction where there is dining table with lot of people. sitting. They have mocked her. She is lifting herself up. Voicing opinion. Destroying her as a person. She wants to be something but because of this comment she is not able to perform. She has been left out. Treated not right. Lonely. Empty. Unwanted. Rejected. Hated. Not accepted. Secluded. Room by yourself. Alone and crying. Failure.*

Here again you see the theme of one vs the other. You see the theme of being rejected, not accepted. You see the theme that in order to be accepted you have to perform. The animal remedies in superclass 3 are the birds. The patient gives many words evocative of birds such as caged, freedom, space etc. She also gives themes of speed, movement. Then she gives specific themes of "being like a slave" or" being controlled by a powerful figure who abuses her". During the WISE process, she gives graphic images of being in a dark, shady room, dim light and being totally isolated. This image is quite similar to what happens to the falcon. The falcon is caught, trapped by the falconer and kept isolated in a dark room for many days. And even after it is let out, it is under the total control of the falconer. It needs to perform for him in order that he receives food. It is not able to break free from his control even though physically he is not tied to him. When we examine the rubrics of Falco Peregrinus by using the repertory, we see the following —

- *Abuse ailments from*
- *Appreciation desires*
- *Delusion, he is dominated*
- *Delusion she is a prisoner*
- *Delusion expansion of space*
- *Delusion under superhuman control*
- *Delusion trapped he is*
- *Delusion he is worthless*
- *Forsaken feeling, isolation sensation of*
- *Freedom desire for*
- *Opinion longing for the good opinion of others*

After taking treatment for a year the patient shares the effect the medicines have had on her —

> *Much better emotionally. Moods remain calmer with the medicines. I feel free. Now the chest constriction and restriction are completely gone. Now I am bolder. I feel stronger. 10 months back I felt that my life is doomed. But now I feel very free. Free means no restriction. No judgements.*

We can see the hierarchy of information as follows;

Superclass	**3rd**
Kingdom	Animal
Family	Aves
Remedy	Falco peregrinus

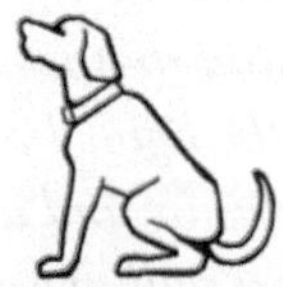

Case 10

This is a case of a 57-year-old male, who came with post-operative rectal cancer and complaints of headache and insomnia.

This patient was diagnosed with adenocarcinoma of the rectum, he proceeded to have it surgically removed, where there were post-operative complications and he ended up in ICCU, the recovery took 4 months. The patient has completed chemo and radiation therapy. He has a colostomy bag with an ileostomy having been performed. The post-operative complications were the failure of the wound to heal with the formation of a fistula, accompanied by continuous discharge of pus, which is yellowish, greenish, greyish. The patient also must pass a bowel motion around 10 times a day, and whenever there is food intake. He is also losing weight. At the beginning of the consultation the patient states his main reason for treatment is to avoid a relapse.

The patient narrates his symptoms prior to the diagnosis as follows —

> *Used to get frequent motions before 4-5 years of the diagnosis. This would happen 5-6 times in a day and 3 times in the morning. There wasn't much quantity but the urge was very strong, where I had to rush, I could control it but it was very urgent. The consistency and colour were normal and occasionally there was a strong odour. The report also showed there is a large simple cyst in left kidney, but the doctor has said its nothing to worry about.*

The patient then goes on to describe the frequent headaches —

> *The headache is worse in the sun and when I'm hungry. While hungry I also get eructations. There is a throbbing pain which starts from the neck, occiput and whole head esp. the right-hand side. In any area that pains if I press, I used to burp and that would make it feel better. During headache I want to switch off the light. I also want to rest. The headache also feels better when I apply pressure and when I vomit. Sometimes I will even induce vomiting, the vomit will appear yellow and has a sour taste. When I get the headache I want it to go away as soon as possible. And I would prefer to be alone, I will become irritated and angry if someone comes and tries to talk to me.*

Next, he describes the complaint of insomnia —

> *I am taking a sleeping pill, Zolfresh 10 mg at night since the surgery, even before that sleep was not sound. At a stretch I cannot sleep more than 5 hours. I get up after 3 hours of sleep. Usually, I wake up at about 1-2 am. Then can't sleep again for half an hour, or an hour, sometimes all night.*

These are his physical complaints. We know that his cancer was an expression of a deeper state in the body. We need to understand him at a deeper level. This is so we can treat the state which has brought about the cancer. This will also help prevent the relapse. We begin with asking him what was bothering him the most in his life. We ask him whether there was any stress which he thinks could be related to the cause of the cancer. His answer was very interesting —

> *My daughter brought a pet in our house, a dog. My wife and daughter were fond of him. But I didn't want him in the house because of uncleanliness. Sometimes he sits on floor and wets it with his saliva and stains would be there. I got irritated because of him. I didn't want him here, wanted them to arrange someplace else for him. There was his smell, I was just not comfortable. I didn't feel at peace. I just wanted him to be taken away. It should not be in front of me. Now since 6 months, he is given to wife's friends. I said, I don't want him, anyhow arrange for him to be shifted there. Send him anywhere but not here. I was very uncomfortable in his presence. I used to get irritated due to uncleanliness and hair fall, even though it was cleaned immediately by the staff. I feel uncomfortable restless in an unclean place. Concentration goes to that point only, what is not correct. Can't do*

anything else until that is corrected. Why my wife and daughter are not listening to me? I didn't like the sight of him. I felt helpless. I understood we could not just throw him out. He should go to a good house but not here. I used to shout at the dog. At times I used to drag him out. We had arguments and fights in the house because of him. This stomach problem and cancer is may be due to him (the dog), because I used to shout at him, drag him. I had a guilty feeling. I thought I am getting these health problems because I am very negative with him. Used to tell my family this. Guilt was that he is an inexpressive animal, so we should not do anything wrong and I thought I was doing wrong. He should be removed to avoid what wrong was being done with him.

Now this is very unique; how many patients have told such a story before? We can understand that this is a peculiarity. As we go further in the case that pattern that will further emerge. We will see it in every aspect of the case, but for now we can make a note of it and see what comes up. So, we ask him what other stressful incidents were there in his life –

Changing our house. I have wanted to change house since last 6-7 years. Wanted to move to a better place but it hasn't worked out. I have been dreaming of this new house. There, I will be able to enjoy my life, have friends. Here we don't socialize much. I think, if we move we can socialize. Currently where we live it is a congested area, where we want to move is an open area.

Inside the house we are comfortable. We don't feel congested in the house, but when going out, we have to go through heavy traffic. That is irritating and very inconvenient. People avoid to come to our place because it is difficult to come, no parking available.

In a traffic jam it takes more time. You leave assuming it will take 15 mins, but then it would take more time like 25 mins. It is a feeling of irritation, should get out. Sitting idle in the car waiting for the traffic to move. You feel mentally restless. - I tell the driver to shout at some other driver and tell him to move aside.

Here there is congestion, everything is mingling. It takes time for vehicles or people to come to this place where we stay. It gets unorganised. It's like they are moving in the wrong direction. They get stuck. They get held. There is hindrance, obstacle. You are not allowing person to pass because of wrong direction. If I am moving in a direction and someone comes in front of me, he blocks my way, or I come in his direction. Blocking (HG).

There is also a mental block. We have a way of thinking. We stick to it and don't listen to anyone else. Block, obstacle, barrier. You are being stopped, blocked. If there is any obstacle and circumstances that are such that you can't move further because of block or barrier.

We are now able to put together some important elements of the case. The first issue is of the dog, where he feels uncomfortable with it in his house. Then in another stressful incident for him he talks about the feeling of comfort. When we try understanding what is 'discomfort' he begins to speak of a block, obstacle and barrier. These elements are becoming clearer for us. We are starting to see the Superclass. We need to clarify further, so we ask what the opposite of this block feeling would be —

Smooth, free, no hindrance. Moving as it should move, the flow is proper. Everything is flowing properly. Life is comfortable.

And again, the idea of comfort comes up… so we ask him to describe a comfortable life –

A life where you are organised, happy family, organised family, organised business, socially active and happy. You are able to do whatever you wish to do. Able to do whatever you want, need in your lifestyle. Lifestyle means – living properly, good house, good education for children, good house, car. All doing exercise, routine, eating properly, good fun, family, good house, car, good children.

We can now see the themes of the 4th Superclass. We can see the idea of comfort vs discomfort. What is comfortable for him? His description of a comfortable life is maintaining the status quo. We can go further in this case and see more features of the 4th superclass. We continue and he tells us of another stressful incident in his life —

Main stress is my daughters marriage. She is 31 and not yet married, we are searching for a groom since 5 years. I think that normally she should have married by 26-27 years, we are 3-4 years late and after my diagnosis, I want my responsibility to be taken care of as soon as possible. We couldn't find the right match, something or other. What we required we couldn't get. There is worry, stress, helplessness.

How should I move further? Which door to knock? How should I get proper direction? How should I get the way out, proper channel, proper direction – move further? Right direction. How to go ahead, you can't when there is some obstacle, some problem. Obstacle is when things not working properly to make your way. Obstacle is barrier, that stops, something stopping you. Moving further, move in progressive way, whatever you are doing with target, but situations not favourable those are obstacles, barriers.

Here the patient again comes to the idea of the obstacle or block or barrier. We then ask the patient to tell us what his fears are –

Will everything work out or not, finances, house, business, daughter's marriage. Will it be completed smoothly or not? I have the resources but the things have to be right in their place. When I need finances, property should be sold and property in the right place. Sometimes life is like a jigsaw, there are blocks, have to be organized. I have all the blocks, I have to organise that because it is unorganized, and then everything is affected. Like every aspect of life is affected, family, business. If it is organized, all will be fine, smooth and happy. Happiness, content, completeness is there, Life is settled. Everything going smoothly. Everything working how you want.

The patient tells us that when things are going well everything goes smoothly. This word 'smoothly' is important in the context of what he has told us earlier about the blocks and barriers. We can see this is exact opposite. We are also able to understand the kingdom of his case and how it fits into this dynamic. When there is a situation the patient either feels comfort or discomfort. This is determined by whether things go "smoothly" for him or not. If he is feeling discomfort, then there is some obstacle or barrier to his comfort. From all this we can understand this his experience is in the realm of sensitivity and reactivity (plant kingdom) . This dynamic of his desiring to find a comfort zone belongs to the 4th superclass. The dicotyledon subclass which belongs to the 4th superclass is the Dilleniidae.

We now ask the patient what dreams he gets –

I had repeated dreams in my childhood that either my father or grandfather, in red clothes running holding my hand. Felt good, happy safe and very comfortable. Because with your elder and holding his hands there are no worries. Felt in safe hands, happy , safe from the world. No one can harm me because my father is holding my hand. It felt comfortable, easy. Like how it feels when surroundings are normal, without unfavourable atmosphere. As it should be. When everything is as it should be, then it is normal.

We can see the features of the 4th subclass coming up again in the dream. The idea of comfort and maintaining the status quo; there shouldn't be any discomfort. And also we see that the family is the source of the comfort.

At this point in the case we ask the patients wife to tell us about him —

> *He is a perfectionist. Keeps things in order, very methodical. Wants to know everything. Very curious, if children and me are talking he wants to know what we are saying. Gets angry very fast, if we don't listen to him. He feels what he says is right. If children ask if they can go out he says why? (They are 31 years and 23 years) He needs to know every detail of it. He scolds when he is angry and then just keeps quiet. Fond of mobile, 24x 7 he is on WhatsApp, if asked anything he says please don't interrupt. you don't know what I am doing.*
>
> *If we have a discussion like daughter's marriage, if he is talking to his brother, he often says, don't talk in the middle, don't interrupt. You don't know anything. These days very irritated for no reason. Very caring - if he has yelled at me and I do not talk to him, he comes and consoles. Stress – related to financial problem, he thinks he has not reached the level he wants to. He is an introvert, limited sets of friends, that too from school but close ones. Best friend expired last year – he was affected, didn't share much.*
>
> *He is too God fearing and religious. Wants to follow rituals. Says, if we flourish more in business if we do this. Disciplined – everything should be according to him. Children should come on time for meals and sit with us. Likes company of sister, wants everyone esp. the family to come home. He has 7 sisters, wants to go out with them. Loves giving. Very generous. Never stops us from spending.*
>
> *His cupboard is never cluttered, he cleans It himself. If I keep one paper somewhere else, he yells, why did you touch it? So, I stopped cleaning his things. Can't make up his mind very fast. If we decide to go for a night show, he says he will go, he books tickets then says is it ok if he does not come, he wants to be home. When asked about God he says I fear God, if I do something wrong God is looking. Wrong means – cheating someone, hurting intentionally, in business can harm anyone and be the reason of loss.*

This description from his wife is very useful and tells us a lot about him. When we analyse it we can see all the 4th subclass features. The first thing she tells us is how fastidious and perfectionist he is. He doesn't want anything out of its place. He takes comfort in this and any change to his routine disturbs and irritates him. We can also see this routine in his religious beliefs. He has to follow all the rituals and do it in the right way or he will experience discomfort. This can also be seen in the irritability when he is interrupted. When can see how irritated he gets from any change in the flow of or in his flow of thoughts. We note the importance of the family for him and how they give him comfort. He, therefore, wants them around all the time. We can see the features of the 4th subclass in every aspect of this patient. We can see that it is even confirmed by those around him. We have all this information but it is never a bad idea to confirm our thoughts. We decide to do a WISE process with the patient.

We show him the first picture of the WISE woman and ask him to describe what is happening —

> *She is afraid and emotional. Saying go away leave me alone kind of expression. She is scared and emotional. May be some warriors may be attacking her or her family and she is asking that they leave her. Maybe she has seen her side of people being slaughtered. Great shock and sorrow. She is seeing her people dead or attacked, with weapons, or hitting her family, children or husband.*
>
> *Seeing the damage to the family or close ones. If some close family member is being attacked, it comes as a shock or sorrow. She is saying go away from me, leave me alone. Please leave me. She is crying. What damage has been done to family, she was not spared. She must have been attacked.*

From the WISE process we can again see the theme of the family coming through. Later on in our analysis we will see how to further apply the WISE to confirm our remedy.

In our analysis thus far we have already located the Superclass, the kingdom and the subclass. Now, how do we find the remedy? We shouldn't forget why the patient has come to us. He came stating that he wanted to avoid relapse of the cancer. So, we need to focus on the site of affection.

We need a remedy which has some effect in cancer of the rectum as well as on fistula. Using the search function on Synergy Homeopathic Software we look for all remedies in Homeopathic literature that have cancer within 3 words of rectum and in the same remedy as fistula. We limit our search to remedies from the Dilleniidae —

This gives us a clue, but we still need to confirm further so we check the other rubrics —

synergy	Paeon.	Puls.	Sep.	Calc.	Lach.	Ars.	Carb-v.	Graph.	Kali-c.	Nit-ac.	Phos.	Sulph.	Caust.	Lyc.	Merc.	Nux-v.	Thuj.
Total	13	26	26	25	25	24	24	24	24	24	24	24	23	23	22	21	21
Rubrics	9	8	8	8	8	8	8	8	8	8	8	8	8	8	8	8	8
Kingdom																	
CR19 - Rectum; Urging, desire(596)	3	4	4	4	4	4	4	4	4	4	4	4	4	4	4	4	4
CR19 - Rectum; Cancer(85)	1	1	3	1	1	3	1	3	3	3	1	1	1	1	1	1	1
CR19 - Rectum; Abscesses, suppurations; perineum(8)	1												3		3		
CR19 - Generalities; Fistulae(147)	3	4	4	4	4	1	4	3	4	4	4	4	4	4	4	1	3
CR19 - Stool; Frequent, too(326)	1	4	3	4	3	4	3	4	3	4	4	4	3	3	4	4	3
CR19 - Head; Pain, headache; right(559)	1	3	4	4	3	4	4	3	3	3	3	1	3	3	2	3	4
CR19 - Head; Internal; sunlight; agg.(283)	1	3	1	1	3	3	1	1	1	1	3	3	1	1	1	1	1
CR19 - Head; Forehead; eyes; above(578)	1	4	4	4	4	4	3	3	4	3	4	4	4	4	3	4	4
CR19 - Generalities; Pain; eructation amel.(126)	1	3	3	3	3	1	4	3	2	2	1	3		3		3	1

We can even repertorize the information we got from the WISE process; this should also be in the remedy —

synergy	Paeon.	Haliae-lc.	Cast.	Chin.	Stront-c.	Plut-n.	Lsd	Bros-g.	Culx-p.	Fic.	Plac.	Alumn.	Med.	Mur-ac.	Plat.	Aran-ix.	Coli.
Total	6	6	4	4	4	4	4	4	4	4	4	3	3	3	3	3	3
Rubrics	4	4	4	4	4	4	4	4	4	3	3	3	3	3	3	3	3
Kingdom																	
CR19 - Mind; Dreams; death, of; family, in(41)	1	1	1	1	1	1	1	1	1	1	1	1	1	1	1	1	1
CR19 - Mind; Dreams; death, of; relatives(57)	3	1	1	1	1	1	1	1	1	1	2	1	1	1	1	1	1
CR19 - Mind; Dreams; death, of; family, in; parents, of(20)	1	1	1	1	1	1	1	1	1	2	1	1	1	1			1
CR19 - Mind; Dreams; quarrels, strife(142)	1	3	1	1	1	1	1	1	1						1	1	

We still have other areas which we can get further confirmations for the remedy. We can consider his childhood dream namely of his father/grandfather holding his hand. We can find the following rubrics in Paeonia —

- Mind; Dreams; family, own
- Mind; Dreams; parents, of

A very important general symptom is his sleep. He says he wakes up after a few hours of sleep at around 1-2 am and then can't go back to sleep. We find the following rubrics of Paeonia –

- Sleep; Sleeplessness
- Sleep; Waking, night
- Sleep; Waking, midnight, after

Now we can be sure. This remedy Paeonia is known best for rectal complaints, and we see that it also has his specific delusions/dreams and characteristic generals .

The patient received Paeonia 200. Later it was changed to 1M. After 1 year of treatment he gave this follow up:

> *The headaches have reduced considerably. Not got a single episode in past 2 months. Only occasionally if I have indigestion, I get the pain. The sleeplessness was much better actually. I was able to sleep through the night. Since the past few months, sleep bit disturbed again, after daughter's engagement broke off. However, have stopped the sleeping pill. Can remain active throughout the day, not exhausted or sleepy even on the days of having disturbed sleep. My energy levels are very good, not tired at all.*
>
> *Mentally I can* **see** *changes in myself. Feeling more stable not taking stress as I used to take before. Worries are always there but I don't keep it in my mind. My stress levels have definitely reduced compared to before. I have a normal routine now. I had a dream where I was attending some function with my father, there was a good feeling a happy moment.*

The patient also had his PET scan take prior to treatment —

Comments:
Treated case of carcinoma rectum; as compared to previously PET/CT scan dated 01.04.19: present follow up PET/CT study shows:

1. **Thick walled serous collection in left side of lower anterior abdominal wall abutting bowel loops as described demonstrating persistent high grade metabolic activity likely suggesting localized infective aetiology. Further evaluation may be considered.**
2. **No new FDG avid lesions noted elsewhere on present whole body survey.**

And repeated the PET scan after 10 months of treatment with Paeonia —

IMPRESSION:

In a Known Case of carcinoma rectum. Underwent colostomy surgery on **20-11-17. Post** chemotherapy, post radiotherapy on follow up, present PET-CT scan reveals:

ABR and colostomy status noted.

- Metabolically active disease is present in left side of lower anterior wall as described above, likely infective etiology. As compare to previous FDG PET/CT scan it is **reduced in size and metabolically activity**.
- Renal cyst is seen is noted in left kidney and single calculi is seen in right kidney.
- No evidence of FDG avid any other lymphnodal or any distant metastasis in present scan.

Clinical / histopathological / other investigational correlation & followup is suggested as needed.

This case is a good illustration of the features of the 4th subclass and the 4th Superclass. It also shows how we need to approach cases synergistically. We need to cover all the aspects of the case. The system, the symptoms, and the genius, the pathology. Then we can be much more confident about the result. We checked every area of the patient's life. We made sure it was covered by both our system and the symptoms as seen by the rubrics.

Superclass	4
Kingdom	Plant
Subclass	Dilleniidae
Order	Dilleniales
Family	Paeoniaceae
Remedy	Paeonia

Case 11

This is a female patient of 28 years old who is suffering from hypoplastic anaemia.

Before appearing for the consult, the patient had the following investigations —

Haemoglobin: 10.8
Platelets: 59000
Large platelets on smear
WBC- 4800

The patient begins narrating her complaints —

It started with fever & low platelets. I was advised proper diet and was on B12 injection, the haemoglobin increased. Then again in April it decreased. I had gone to learn Jainism and was fasting for a month. I became very breathless & tired while climbing stairs. When haemoglobin was checked it was 4.3 & platelets were low. Then Bone marrow test was done. Then started treatment and was diagnosed with Myelodysplastic syndrome.

Then a year later I fell pregnant but at 6 weeks I had to abort due to the low counts. My menses have been irregular with heavy bleeding for the last two cycles. Otherwise, I have no other symptoms.

We ask the patient to describe her nature —

> *I am reserved with strangers; it takes time to mix with them. I think they will come and talk to me, or that they should approach me. What if they don't like me? Our nature might be different. They might not like my nature. I am sensitive and emotional, if someone says something, I believe them easily, trust easily, I am naïve, I can't even imagine that they can fool me.*
>
> *I can get angry at times, I have to control or think, in spite of explaining still if they don't understand, I have to keep control, I keep thinking in mind to leave it… or a fight will happen, the relationship will break, the affection between us will decrease. We won't talk to each other. Generally, if you get angry with people you love, you can express it to them.*

What do you like to do? –

> *Talking to friends, I like sharing with best friends, now after marriage I can't share, it feels better after sharing. Listening to songs. Watching movies, my favourite are suspense and action movies.*

What are your fears? —

> *I am afraid of dogs, I will hide behind someone if it comes near, they could bite me, and I would have to take an injection. Also, I am afraid of cows, I heard that many people died when hit by cow and I have fear of death. Also fear of speed is there, when in car if speeding there is the fear of an accident, I will chant or tell them not to speed. Cockroaches too! I dislike them I had a bad incident with them. I am not afraid of darkness or ghost. I can startle from noise.*

This is quite strange, I have never heard of anyone being killed by a cow. They are very peaceful quiet animals they generally don't hurt anyone. So, this is a very extreme fear, so we should make a note of this and not let this fear out of our analysis at a later point.

What do you not like to see on TV? —

> *Anything with pain, like cutting throat with blade, that would be very painful.*

Here too we can see the fear of pain and suffering… so we are beginning to form a centre of the case.

What dreams do you get? —

> *Of lions & tigers, there are lions coming in the house, they might kill someone, I am thinking how to save myself, I went to another house where there were no lions, I felt safe there. I had been in a room, the lion was moving around in the balcony, I was thinking how to get out. It can kill me, it would grab my neck with his teeth, it would kill me, it would be painful.*

This is a very subtle case in terms of the Superclass. We need to be observant to pick it up. When we take into consideration all the information, we can begin to create a bigger picture. In this dream we can again see the fear of pain and suffering.

However, what is the main response in the dream? It is to find a place of safety. We probe deeper and ask her what safety means to her. Pay attention to her answer —

> *Secured, no fear of pain or of dying. There is a protective layer or wall around. There is no fear inside, you are inside, and a layer is covering you. Its transparent layer, soft.*

At this point it could be very easy to think of the first Superclass : to go inside and shut oneself off from the outer world. This is where we must be careful with how we sort the information.

This is not the Superclass dynamic. This is the sensation of the remedy as we can see the experience and its opposite. The experience of the dream is of pain and suffering. The opposite of this experience is to be secure, safe, and protected. So, when we classify this, it would come under the remedy information not the superclass.

What are you interested in? —

> *Want to start own business, I have done Pharmacy graduation. The main purpose is to earn, because of my illness there are lots of expenses, I feel bad that lots of money is wasted after me.*

What happens to you when afraid? —

> *If there is some sudden news or tension or before exams or I get fear before going for blood check-up, then I will pass motions.*

Tell us about your drawing… what is the feeling there? – (The patient had drawn a spiral)

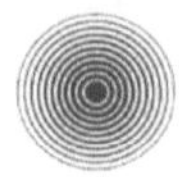

> *Feel confusion, not able to come out of it, how to get out? I feel fear. It is like an island; you are not able to get off it as its surrounded by water. There is no food or water. You are not able to contact anyone. It would be a difficult death; you don't have any water. You could have a headache. How would you tolerate hunger or thirst. Someone should come to help. Or get some phone. You have no energy, you can't walk, you will die.*

An important theme in the 4th Superclass is that of the comfort zone. And what is a comfort zone? It is an area in life where you are totally free from any disturbance. You are completely comfortable and stable nothing can shake your foundations. The problem one has in the 4th Superclass is when you leave this comfort zone. This is exactly what the patient is describing from the doodle. She is describing the exact experience of leaving her comfort zone. Where she would feel like she is deserted on an island. What is important to her, to have food and water. These are very important things without them one would not be able to be comfortable. And for her the experience of being out of the comfort zone is one of pain, suffering and death. You can see how beautifully the Superclass and the sensation interact. Her basic dynamic is to try and find her comfort zone. When out of her comfort zone she will experience it as pain and suffering – the sensation of her remedy.

We can also see very clearly from this experience on the island that in this case there is an issue of capability. She will not be able to manage on her own. This same feeling pervades throughout the entire case. We can also see it through the fear of relationships breaking. If that other person goes away, she will suffer. One of the central issues is also an inability to manage on her own. This is the central issue of the Mineral Kingdom. Now we know we need a remedy from the 4th superclass, the mineral kingdom and with the fear of pain and suffering.

The patient mentions —

> *I like eating bricks and the smell of mud. I would chew on pencil and slate pen.*

She also mentions –

> *I have a childish nature, I am mature enough, but I like to watch cartoons, I like to play games with my brother's son. We do puzzle solving, reading small children's story things like that. I like the cartoons Tom & Jerry, Oggy and cockroaches, Scooby doo etc… I like cartoons which teach you something. I like to solve puzzles, as you are using your brain. I like mathematics a lot.*

This is all just information which can be used to help build up our remedy picture. We already know that it must be a remedy from the 4th superclass with the fear of pain and suffering. Now we can see that there must be something slightly childish in the remedy as well.

The patient has the following generals —

> Cravings: spicy++, salty snack, sweets+++
> Perspiration: armpits, odour
> Menses: Abdominal pain for 3-4 hours
> Sleep: Increased, likes to sleep, there is a problem waking up, have a headache after nap
> Positions: I like to sleep on abdomen. People say it's not good to sleep on abdomen so I have started sleeping on sides
> Thermal: chilly++ feet & hands gets cold easily, I can't tolerate cold
> Have cracks in soles, mainly the heels

The patient also is complaining of lower back pain —

> Lower back pains are worse when lying on back. It is the lumbosacral region; the pain is on lying. And there is stiffness which is worse after movement.

— End of case —

Going through all the data we have collected, we understand the basic dynamic to be that of the 4th superclass. The need for stability and wanting to be in a comfort zone. This is expressed in mineral kingdom features. When one is out of their comfort zone, they lack the capability to manage on their own. They fear that they would experience pain and suffering. We can then do a sectorial analysis with our repertory to see each of the different areas expressed in the case —

The patient's nature —

	Calc.	Bell.	Carc.	Nat-m.	Lach.	Puls.	Phos.	Nit-ac.	Caust.	Kali-c.	Med.	Lyc.	Plut-n.	Sulph.	Ars.	Acon.
Total	25	22	14	18	17	15	14	12	17	15	15	14	12	10	9	14
Rubrics	9	8	8	7	7	7	7	7	6	6	6	6	6	6	6	5
Kingdom																
CR19 - Mind; Weeping, tearful mood; admonition, from(18)	3	1	1	1		1		1		3		3				
CR19 - Mind; Weeping, tearful mood; reproaches, from(20)	1	1	2	1				1		1			2			
CR19 - Mind; Fear; animals, of(134)	4	4	4	3	3	3	3	1	3	2	4	1	2	2	1	3
CR19 - Mind; Fear; dogs, of(51)	3	4	1	3	1	3	1	1	3		1		2	1		
CR19 - Mind; Fear; accidents, of(73)	2	3	3		2	2	1		3				2		1	2
CR19 - Mind; Fear; death, of(279)	4	4	1	3	4	4	4	4	4	4	3	3	2	2	4	4
CR19 - Mind; Starting, startled; noise, from(118)	3	4	1	4	3	1	3	1	3	4	3	3		1	1	4
CR19 - Mind; Fear; pain, of(37)	1	1			3		1				1	1		1	1	
CR19 - Mind; News; ailments from, agg.; bad(74)	4		1	3	1	1	1	3	1	1	3	3	2	3	1	1

Dreams and fears —

	Calc.	Verat.	Merc.	Tax.	Phos.	Cimic.	Hyos.	Lach.	Op.	Med.
Total	10	8	5	4	9	7	7	7	7	6
Rubrics	5	4	4	4	3	3	3	3	3	3
Kingdom										
CR19 - Mind; Dreams; animals, of; biting him(35)	1	1	1	1	3					1
CR19 - Mind; Dreams; dogs; bitten by, of being(15)	1	2	2	1						1
CR19 - Mind; Fear; animals, of(134)	4	4	1	1	3	3	3	3	1	4
CR19 - Mind; Home; go, desire to(76)	3	1	1	1		1	3	3	3	
CR19 - Mind; Fear; murdered, of being(38)	1				3	3	1	1	3	

General characteristics —

	Calc.	Caust.	Sulph.	Sep.	Nit-ac.	Calc-p.	Con.	Lach.	Tax.	Nat-m.	Phos.	Merc.	Sil.	Graph.	Carb-v.	Kali-c.	Puls.
Total	27	22	32	29	27	23	22	22	10	25	24	21	18	24	23	23	22
Rubrics	10	10	9	9	9	9	9	9	9	8	8	8	8	7	7	7	7
Kingdom																	
CR19 - Generalities; Food and drinks; salt or salty food; desires(158)	3	3	3	3	4	4	3	1	1	4	4	1	1	2	4		1
CR19 - Generalities; Food and drinks; sweets; desires(295)	3	1	4	3	3	1	1	1	1	2	3	3	1	4	3	4	3
CR19 - Chest; Perspiration; offensive; axillae(55)	3	1	4	3	4		1	3	1		2	3	4		1	3	
CR19 - Sleep; Waking; difficult; morning(48)	3	1			2	4			2								
CR19 - Generalities; Sleep; after; afternoon sleep(90)	1	3	3	1	1	1	4	3	1	3	2	1	1	3	3	1	3
CR19 - Sleep; Position; abdomen, on(55)	2	1	3	3		3	1	1	1	1	1						3
CR19 - Generalities; Cold; agg.(768)	4	4	4	4	4	4	4	4	1	4	4	4	4	4	4	4	4
CR19 - Extremities; Coldness, chilliness; hands(375)	3	3	4	4	4	4	3	4	1	4	4	4	2	4	4	4	4
CR19 - Extremities; Coldness, chilliness; feet(466)	4	4	4	4	4	1	4	4	1	4	4	4	4	4	4	4	4
CR19 - Extremities; Cracks, fissures; feet; heels(45)	1	1	3	4	1	1	1	1		3		1	1	3		3	

The experience in the Doodle —

	Calc.	Bry.	Sep.	All-c.	Fl-ac.
Total	3	4	3	3	3
Rubrics	3	2	1	1	1
Kingdom					
CR19 - Mind; Fear; death, of; hunger, fasting, from(1)	1				
CR19 - Mind; Fear; starvation, of(11)	1	3	3		
CR19 - Mind; Fear; suffering, of(29)	1	1		3	3

The patient's other complaints —

	Calc.	Lyc.	Kali-c.	Nat-s.	Vib.	Agar.	Carc.
Total	7	7	5	5	5	3	3
Rubrics	3	3	3	3	3	3	3
Kingdom							
CR19 - Back; Pain; lumbar region, lumbago; lying; agg.(59)	3	3	1	1	1	1	1
CR19 - Back; Pain; lumbar region, lumbago; motion; amel.(75)	1	1	1	3	1	1	1
CR19 - Back; Pain; lumbosacral articulation(112)	3	3	3	1	3	1	1

From all these different areas the same remedy is appearing : Calcarea carbonica, a remedy from the 4th row of the periodic table. This is the corresponding row in the mineral kingdom to the 4th Superclass.

It is interesting to see in the repertorisation of the doodle we can also see Bryonia. This is one of the main plant remedies in the 4th Superclass.

This extract from *The Soul of Remedies* highlights the essence of Calc carb as seen in this case;

> *Thus, the main theme of Calcarea carbonica is a need for protection. But in order to get this protection the person does not need to make any effort - all he has to do is show a vital reaction. There is a feeling of being too weak to face the cruelty and roughness of the world.*
>
> —
>
> *Calcarea carbonica tries to build a protective wall of defence around himself. This will ensure that he is safe, secure, and covered like a developing embryo within an egg.*

Further to understanding the 4th Superclass with Calc Carb I also wrote in "*The Soul of Remedies*" —

> *The main feeling of Calcarea is the need for stability and security.*

This is the exact dynamic of the 4th Superclass. To try and reach a place of stability and security. This is why we so often see the image of a house in this Superclass as it symbolizes all these features.

The patient was prescribed Calc carb 1M followed by LM8 daily. She reported the following after 1 year of treatment —

- *More confident, more relaxed, and stronger*
- *I don't hesitate to say things to strangers or new people*
- *Dreams of lions have completely gone*
- *Menses are regular now*
- *Back pain is better*
- *Craving for slate pencil is better*
- *Fears have reduced*

We can also see the changes in the Blood analysis –

DATE	13.9.19	22.10.19	24.12.19	30.7.2020
HB	10.4	10.8	11.4	12.1
RBC	2.36	2.92	3.16	3.90
PLATELET	59000	88000	96000	106000
WBC	4800	58000	6100	6800

Superclass	**4**
Kingdom	Mineral
Row	4
Remedy	Calcarea carbonica

Case 12

This is the case of a 27-year-old female who is suffering from Polycystic ovarian disease.

She begins by describing the main complaint –

When the periods start then there is spotting, and the spotting doesn't stop without taking the tablet regestron. There is no cycle for one year, no fixed pattern. Periods are not very painful now, earlier they used to be heavy and painful. Was on treatment with another homeopath and had got 3 cycles which were good with heavy flow. Before and during periods I get numbness in the palms. I don't like my periods because there was a lot of pain earlier and I would have to be at home for 2 days and I would have to take injections for it. There is heaviness of the breasts before menses.

I am also suffering from allergies for the last 4-5 years every summer. Had developed itching on the body and swelling on face and lips. The scratching was unbearable. Then would get red eruptions like mosquito bites. It is aggravated by dust and better when taking a bath or applying ice. Happened more behind the knees and on the face. Two weeks back I had very high fever then the allergy went. I used to take cetirizine every second day.

Another complaint I have are these skin eruptions. They started 6-7 months back. A friend had it and maybe I got it from her. Big annular lesion brownish. With severe itching especially at night in sleep. On the right forearm, on the abdomen, on the thigh.

The patient is asked to tell us a little bit about herself —

I get irritated very easily. I am very attached to my mother my grandmother and my husband. For the others I really don't care. Earlier I was very short tempered, but now I am not. if I did not like something I would shout and get angry. Whenever I get angry, I start crying, I won't be able to form a sentence. I mix up words that time. If things don't go according to my wish, I get angry. I don't like to be told what to do and what not to do. I like going out on holidays. I am married for 1.5 years, we used to go every month initially but of late we don't, and I don't like it, and I don't like it. Feels I am losing the best period of my life. I am not an organized person. I don't like keeping things in place. I don't realize also if the things are not in place. I am not liking his mother and I complain about it, and he does not like it, so I fear that I won't have that bond that we had. I am very confused, sometimes I feel I want to go back home. I feel something is wrong with me (weeps). She does a lot for me, makes my dabba in the morning, keeps no work for me when I come home but still, I don't know, I don't like it. I am not accepting the things the way they are. I am not letting things go. I remember grievances all the time and I take it out on my husband.

What are your fears? —

Water, I don't go to swimming pools, I am scared of drowning.

Scared of talking to people. I feel they will start judging me. I am reserved, I don't like talking to people much. There are two sides, on one side I will go on talking, talking, talking and on the other side I can be very quiet. I am scared of losing my mother or my grandmother. I am very close to them.

What dreams do you get? —

Dreams of flying I feel I am doing something new and good, flying and hopping without touching the ground. It felt good. I always wanted to do that, hop, and not touch the ground. I am happy. I am climbing invisible steps. Dreams of what I have to do the next day. Dream of teeth falling out. I feel I will have to go to the dentist, and I don't like going to the dentist. Dream of being naked, I wasn't ashamed as no one was actually looking at me. I felt exposed that time, I felt vulnerable that time, somebody would come and touch me. Normally in a crowd if someone tries to touch me my first instinct is to push him aside, hold the collar and push him. I generally feel dirty if someone stares at me also. I feel dirty and disgusted

> *when I hear of things in the news. At that time, I feel strong. Strong means physically strong. After 2-3 minutes I will be shaken, and I would want to cry, I will not know what to do next. I won't let anything happen to me or anyone around me. This topic is very sensitive for me, if someone is touching my breast. Even when I hear of rape, I feel a lot of anger and my head starts paining. If anyone is saying anything to my mom, I won't allow that.*

Here we can see some features of the Kingdom and the sub-kingdom. She has the fear of talking to people as they will judge her. This same feeling comes in the dream. She dreams of being naked and feels people are looking at her and she feels shame. There is the feeling that someone will do something to her.

This is the animal kingdom along with the common feeling of dirtiness and shame. She is very sensitive to rape, which is the act of someone doing something to you, another key theme in the animal kingdom. Along with the animal themes we can see the Sub-Kingdom themes of the Mammal group. She has a very strong attachment with her family and one of her fears is that of losing them. This feeling of dirtiness and shame is also very common in the mammal group. We can see these themes in remedies like Lac fel, Ambr and Lac can. At this point we have also gotten a hint of the miasm. The feeling that everyone is watching her could indicate the sycotic miasm. This is a strong indication for the sycotic miasm this feeling of being observed. It came out strongly in the proving of Aq marina a very sycotic remedy.

The patient continues —

> *Leaving my home was the most difficult thing. Everything in my house was fixed, my bed, my room, my cupboard everything was scheduled for 26 years. I did not like the change. If I get used to one thing I can't change it, I don't give away my old stuff also. I am not happy with my job, and I want to change the job, but I don't like change, so I don't want to shift a job. Feels what if I am not able to adjust, what if I am not able to mix with the new people. I feel comfortable in old environment. I don't feel like adjusting in new things. I remember on my first day of school or college I would always like to skip the first day. One day I will prepare my mind. No, no tomorrow you have to go and then I would manage to go.*

Here we can see the features of the 4th Superclass, this aversion to change. They don't want any change to their routine. Any change will affect their stability.

We could see this earlier as well when she spoke about being newly married and living with her in-laws. She could not give a reason why she doesn't like them. She says they do everything for her and are good to her. When we recognise her Superclass, we can understand how this big change in her life affects her so much. We understand why she feels so uncomfortable with it.

We ask the patient about her nature as a child —

> *I was very shy, didn't talk to anyone, I didn't have friends. I had a constant fear that my parents didn't like me, I was very average. I was very attached to my granddad and grand ma. I played with them full day; I usually didn't go out.*

What was the main fear as a child? —

> *I was not able to get good marks, fear that dad will not like me because of that. He will not be proud of me, they would neglect me. I felt anger, I would want to hurt myself by suicide or something.*

Why would you get that feeling? —

> *Because they shout at me when I didn't get good marks, that means they didn't like me. I would get lot of headaches at that time, every second day. I would get calf muscle pain. I was an athlete that time. Usually in the afternoon at 12.30, I would tie a handkerchief tight around the head.*

We confirm the patients' general symptoms —

Appetite: occasionally more occasionally not hungry at all
Thirst: sometimes very thirsty and sometimes not thirsty at all.
Stool/Urine: No changes
Thermal: I don't like cold weather, I feel colder, I tolerate the heat better. Don't like the fan much. Covers and sleeps.
Perspiration: not much
Desires: pav bhaji (spicy mashed vegetable dish), Maggi (noodles), I like the taste of tomatoes +++ - raw or cooked. I like biryani (spicy rice dish) - again it's the tomato puree in it is what I like.
Aversion: ladyfingers (okras) , lentils, raw onions
Sleep: not satisfied with my sleep, don't feel like getting up in the morning, sleeps sound.

— End of case —

This is quite a short case, and the analysis should be quite simple. As we discussed during the case, we could see the features of the 4th Superclass. This sensitivity to being disturbed and losing stability. And the aversion to change. Along with this we can see the Kingdom themes quite clearly. This is the animal kingdom and the subgroup of Mammals. The Mammal group themes are quite clear. In the Mammals there is a strong dependency on the group. There is a very strong connection with one's immediate family. There is the constant fear that they will be thrown out of the group. In this case we can see that is her main fear as a child. If she doesn't live up to the expectations of the family they will cast her out.

We can also see how this ties in with her Superclass dynamic of the basic need for stability. She requires the family for stability and if she is thrown out of the group she will lose her stability. This is why she felt so much pressure to get good marks. Within the Mammals we will also often see the conflict of the individual vs the group. We can see this with the issues between her and the in-laws. She cannot complain too much to her husband otherwise she fears she will be thrown out. Losing her stability in the form of the family unit.

By this point we realise we are looking for a remedy from the 4th superclass. It must be an animal kingdom remedy from the Mammal group. We could also see some of the features of the sycotic miasm. If we take some of the rubrics of the case, we can also see which remedies come in the analysis —

synergy	Lac-c.	Nat-m.	Sep.	Puls.	Phos.	Lach.	Lyc.	Thuj.
Total	26	20	15	21	14	13	12	11
Rubrics	9	7	7	6	6	6	6	6
Kingdom								
CR19 - Vertigo; Walking; gliding in the air, sensation of, as if feet did not touch the ground, while(25)	4							3
CR19 - Mind; Delusions, imaginations; despised, is(46)						3		
CR19 - Mind; Forsaken feeling(299)	3	3		4		3		2
CR19 - Mind; Sadness; menses; before(81)	3	4	3	4			4	
CR19 - Mind; Sadness; menses; during(60)	3	3	3	3				
CR19 - Mind; Delusions, imaginations; dirt, dirty; he is, she is(28)	3							
CR19 - Female; Menses; late, too(303)	3	4	4	4	4	4	4	3
CR19 - Chest; Pain; mammae; menses; before(75)	3	2	2	3	3			
CR19 - Generalities; Food and drinks; spices, condiments, piquant, highly seasoned food; desires(123)	3	3		3	4			

The top remedy is Lac caninum, a mammal remedy which falls in the 4th superclass. We can read the description of the remedy from "*The Soul of Remedies* and see its main issue". We can see how it belongs to the 4th superclass;

> *This remedy has in it the nature of the dog, an animal that has been totally controlled and civilized so that it has to suppress its basic animal nature and can only express its controlled, civilized side. It is dependent on its master for food and so it is out to please him. Its survival depends upon keeping its master happy by its performance, its affection, etc. It has to perform, or it won't be wanted anymore, and its master will kick it out. This need to please is the animal side of Lac caninum, but the dog knows that no matter how much it tries to please, it will never be equal to the human. It feels inferior, knows that it is at the bottom of the hierarchy. The animal side is also malicious (if you pull a dog's tail, it will bite you).*

From this description we can understand the dog's basic need for stability and its reliance to humans for this stability. This description is also a very good analysis of the patient's behaviour itself and we can see how she is living this type of pattern.

Superclass	4
Kingdom	Animal
Sub-kingdom	Mammal
Order	Canidae
Miasm	Sycotic
Remedy	Lac caninum

The follow up of this patient taken after 1 year shows great improvement;

- The patient is now 4 months pregnant!
- Skin and allergic complains have been good for one year
- Health wise is much better
- The recurrent headache is not there now
- Mentally much better, anxiety also better
- The restlessness and stress have reduced
- Anger, irritability, and snappishness has completely settled down
- *I am in a much calmer state of mind*
- Sleep has gotten much better because the stress is better
- Nausea of pregnancy has stopped completely and has good energy level

Case 13

This is the case of a 52-year-old male who was suffering with Gastro-oesophageal reflux disorder, fibromyalgia and hypertension.

His chief complaints are as follows;

Body pain —

- *Especially pain in the shoulder and tightness*
- *Stiffness of muscles, feels like a ball is there.*
- *It feels as if the whole left side of the body is not properly joined or aligned with right side and as if it is not in a unit with the right side.*
- *Also feel fatigue, dead tired by evening. As if all my energy is drained.*
- << *stress*
- >> *movement*

Back pain —

- *Severe excruciating pain*
- *MRI showed stenosis of the lumbar and cervical vertebrae.*
- *The doctor said that even though I am 50 years old, my spine is that of an 85 year old.*
- *Pain is worse if I cycle more than 50 kms. I am a physical guy , I like these things . You can even say I am an overly active person.*
- *Feels like my back is collapsing and can't hold itself up.*
- *I need to lie down at that time.*
- *Pain is in the tail bone, dull pain. It feels like roots of a tree are collapsing.*
- *Feels like my back can't keep up with the weight of my body.*

Gastro-esophageal reflux disease –

- *Lot of acidity*
- *Feeling of swelling and bloating in the abdomen*
- *Pain as if something hard in abdomen*
- *Pain if I eat, even with 2 Rotis (flat bread) – I get lot of pain*
- *Like a cricket ball is stuck inside. It is under the heart, above the naval.*
- *Leads to anxiety*
- *Belching is a lot*
- *>> by walking*
- *<< with tea, coffee and alcohol*

Hypertension —

- *Since many years*
- *Used to feel uneasiness when the pressure was high. Taking allopathic medicines for it so it is in control now.*
- *Have been making lifestyle changes, like stopping alcohol and have restricted my food.*

Having collected all the information about the complaints we then ask the patient how this all began —

> *It started 3 years back when I had just moved to Mumbai. My brother died the very same month. He was super fit, all his medical reports were fine. This was a shock for me. I have become so anxious and insecure after that. Even if I feel a slight pull in my chest, I feel I am going to have a heart attack and the pains increase as my anxiety increases. Everything gives me a feeling that I will be wiped out and dead. Life can be snuffed out in one second. I can die. I may be there next week or I may not be there. When I read of people dying I feel very sad and so very anxious. I keep thinking this can happen to me anytime. Unseen fear has gripped me. I feel Oh, God!! Is it the end? Is it the end? This anxiety comes on anytime while travelling, walking or even just sitting. It's a constant 24 hour restlessness. All this has come after my brother's death.*

This is a very interesting response and we can see that we are entering the level of delusion. So, we need to probe this situation and we will come to the sensation of the case. So, we ask the patient to tell us some more —

> *Earlier I used to feel that being fit is an insurance for health and that it would protect from disease. Now since my brother was super fit, he could*

> *walk 100 km and still died, I have realised that it is not an insurance against anything. In 15 mins he just died! Whatever you do, at the end of the day you are exposed to all the harmful elements of uncertainty and death. Since then I feel vulnerable and shaken. Even my mother's death shattered me. She was my pillar of strength. She managed my house. I have lost all my family, literally all I grew up with. Anything can strike at any time. I feel as if things are uncertain.*

Having seen the previous cases of the 4th superclass we can begin to recognise the characteristic features. We can see the idea that a sudden change in the status quo aggravates. He had been having a steady life and then suddenly something happened to disturb it. Now he is not so sure of his security or stability – his health.

He says he felt vulnerable and shaken, and then shattered. His mother was his pillar of strength. Anything can strike at any time. While we can place this in context of the 4th superclass, yet there are some very peculiar and individual words he is using. We can also see some of the features of the plant kingdom. He shows a great sensitivity to an event it is experienced as a sensation. Therefore he is likely to need a plant remedy.

Looking at the 4th subclass these words of 'shatter', 'pillar of strength and 'suddenly strike' don't seem to fit into any of the families of the dicotyledons. So, we need to start considering what other groups of the plant kingdom we find in the 4th Superclass.

The patient continues with the narration of his case —

> *After my brother's death I jumped back to work in 4 days. I kept pushing it back and not thinking of it. Suddenly it hit me and I got numbness and shooting pain in my left side, like a rocket. I went to the hospital and the doctor gave me many restrictions. I came back thinking now the game is over! I have the fear that anything may strike anytime like a heart attack or a stroke. I get scared if I see an ambulance. With my mother I knew that she was going to die because she was in the ICU for 10 days before. With my brother there was no inkling , just a call that he has gone. It shook my faith in life. Brought to fore the extra fragility of life. You can drop dead any time.*

We ask the patient what does 'fragility' mean? —

> *Anything can break at the drop of a hat. It can be shattered any time without any warning. Like a glass shattering, you hurl a stone at glass and it just shatters and is completely destroyed.*

There is a polarity in this case which is emerging. We can see the two sides as follows —

Pillar of strength	Weak
Not affected by any kind of crisis	Fragile
Physically fit	Shaken
strong	Shattering
	Falling
	Broken

This polarity is the main theme of the Gymnosperms. The most well-known remedy from the Gymnosperms is Thuja. In Thuja (and Conifers as a whole) we know the sensation key words are:

- *Breakable, brittle, easily broken, delicate, flimsy, fragile, frail, defenseless, weak, vulnerable, unprotected, unguarded.*
- *Connect, together, cut off, disconnect, fragment, break away, break up, break, cracked, cut off, unconnected, shattered, fall apart, fall to pieces*

Considering the theme of polarity in the Gymnosperms we have understood the following —

- On one hand brittle, fragile, easily broken, can be split from the slightest things, any fall or vaccination can aggravate.
- On the other hand, I can stand strong, invincible, cannot be destroyed by any kind of disaster/crisis – fire, earthquake, flood, storms, or decay.
- Resilient – I can stand firm, nothing can shatter/break/shake/destroy me
- Sensitivity to things which can break me down, split me and make me fall down
- (Oh! I have a scratch, this can kill me, this can give me a stroke.)

In the Gymnosperms some trees are tolerant of extremes of weather, temperature, snow, fire, wind, rigid, strong, firm and some are fragile, brittle, slight weather or temperature changes can have a major effect on them.

In the Gymnosperms we can also see a polarity between solidity and hollowness which is also present in our case —

- If I am hollow, I can be broken, if I am solid, I can stand firm.
- Solid like a trunk of a big tree - nothing can break. (Mother was a pillar of strength I was strong.)

There are some more important themes in the Gymnosperms —

1. exposed vs being covered —
    - GYMNOS (NAKED, not covered) and SPERMS (SEED)
    - Something inside is very delicate, very fragile, so needs to be covered with something hard – Cones (Conifers)
    - They need hard cones to cover
2. Needles and stitching pains —
    - Pains of these remedies are needle like
    - Conifers – have sharp needle like leaves
3. Old age —
    - They always refer to old age.
    - Patient: "My spine is 85 years old, age is catching up, now anything can happen"
    - In old age we feel fragile, will break easily
    - From something solid, you have become brittle
    - Bones can break
    - Gingko biloba is the remedy for premature old age
    - Teeth can break, bones can break
    - Immunity to cold weather, wind, storm becomes less (physical influence that can damage the system)
    - You want to be covered and not exposed
    - So, there is cautiousness, carefulness
    - I cannot eat that/touch that – this or that can destroy me
4. Anticipation - something will happen —
    - Dreams: Fire, Storm, Disaster
    - There is anticipation of:
      Crisis, Misfortune, Disaster, Ordeal, Storm
    - All these mean the same thing.
    - The main idea is whether one will be able to deal with crisis, storms in one's life and yet be standing upright and not be broken into two or many pieces and fall down.
    - One is anticipating a crisis all the time.

The question here is —

- Can I take more storms?
- Can I withstand it?
- Will I be standing after this crisis?
- Any crisis, that can break you in all possible ways, uproot you, make you fall down.
- Do I have the resilience to stand after such a storm?

They are concerned with crisis in —

- Reputation
- Finances
- Political crisis
- Social crisis

It is interesting to us that the Gingko tree was the one that survived the blast at Hiroshima.

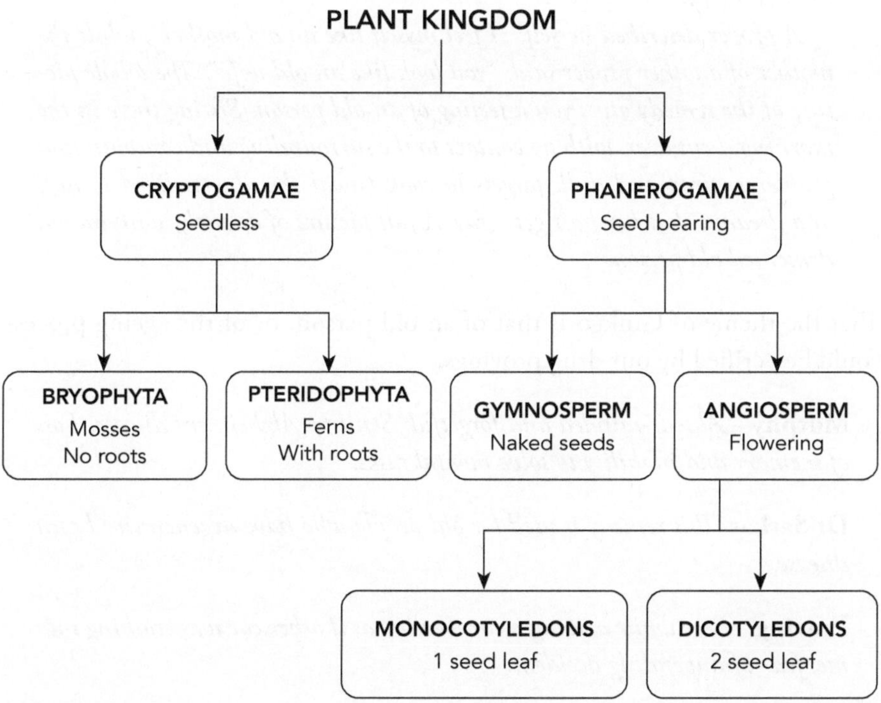

The Gymnosperms are a group of seed-producing plants. All Gymnosperms are found in four major divisions —

Ginkophyta

1. Ginkgo biloba, also known as the maidenhair tree, is the only living species in the division Ginkophyta, all others being extinct. We can understand Gingko further from the following;

   Homeopathic Links 1992- *Dreams of water, flooding, and a characteristic fearful waking from dreams. Dreams of robbers and fights. Another dreamt of falling down and breaking her head in 3 parts. They were all fearful dreams wherein the prover woke with a fright and felt unrefreshed in the morning. Dreams of bomb explosions, of escaping and death in the family, of graveyards, of misfortune. Dreams of millions of ants, of corpses and of being dissected. Most of the dreams confirmed by the provers were of water, ships, worms, battles, and war and that their bodies were opened. Always fearful.*

   A prover described herself: "I feel myself like an old mother", while the mother of another prover said: "you look like an old wife". The whole picture of the remedy gives you a feeling of an old person. Sitting there in the morning, bent over, with no contact to the surrounding and concentration problems, tired and dull, forgets to cook (what she always liked to do), and dreams, that her hair gets gray. A full picture of a lonely, withdrawn, demented old person.

That the theme of Ginkgo is that of an old person, or of the ageing process could be verified by our drug provings.

Murphy - *Absent-minded and forgetful. Senility. Alzheimer's disease. Loss of memory and inability to solve mental tasks.*

Dr Sarkar-*This remedy is used for old people who have degenerative brain disease.*

Proving - *Fear while driving a car. Feeling as if other car was crashing into me; fear of impending accident.*

I am standing with 5 others under a group of trees. The wind picked up; one can hear rustling in the trees. Suddenly there is a loud cracking noise, we all look up. I saw a brittle, broken branch hanging down. All of a sudden, a young man was hit on the back of his head with a piece of wood that came down extremely fast. He collapses bleeding. Apprehensiveness was in the air. The wound looked as if the piece went right through his head... Then I see an old man (a shaman, I am wondering?) helping his apprentice to carry a sack with the same pieces of wood...

Desert, catastrophe, we have shovels to dig a big whole for a mass grave; we start to dig a hole in the middle of the desert. It is war time, many people die.

About earthquakes, numbing noises, ground drops into an abyss in front of my eyes; encounter with a woman; it is as if we stood on top of a volcano.

About a cosmic catastrophe, a huge explosion; strong nuclear and electromagnetic powers are influencing me; complete darkness, just a pulsating tone; I wasn't able to realize whether I was moving with a gigantic speed or stayed in complete calm.

Feeling: around me is hell, but I am still in heaven

The high tide washes away our tent and everything we brought with us for our vacation. I get into a panic, feeling of a threatened existence.

Cycadophyta —

1. Macrozamia spiralis
2. Stangeria eriopus
    - mind; DREAMS; accidents, of (119) *
    - mind; DREAMS; accidents, of; crash of airplane (14) *
    - mind; STRENGTH; increased, mental (58) *
    - mind; THOUGHTS; clearness of (157) **
    - mind; TRANQUILLITY, serenity, calmness (304) *
    - mind; TRUTH; tells the plain (35) *
    - mirilli's themes; FRAGILE (141) *
    - mind; PROTECTED, feels (5) *

Gnetophyta —

1. Ephedra vulgaris
    - Plantae; Spermatophyta, Gymnospermae; Cycadopsida; Gnetatae; Gnetaceae
    - mind; DREAMS; body, body parts; amputated and sown on again (1) *
    - mind; DREAMS; body, body parts; cut off (25) *

- mind; DREAMS; falling (149) *
- mind; DREAMS; head, heads; cut off (9) *
- mind; DREAMS; head, heads; new put on (1) *
- mind; DREAMS; teeth; breaking off (12) *
- mind; DREAMS; teeth; falling out (26) *
- mind; TRANQUILLITY, serenity, calmness (304) *
- mind; TRUTH; tells the plain (35) *
- mirilli's themes; FALL (366) *
- mirilli's themes; EMPTY (270) *

Mirilli Isolation –

Delusions: division between himself and others
Delusions: separated, world, from the, that he is

Ephedra proving –

> *In spite of the very threatening event, I was not at all excited, no fear, no panic. Normally this kind of experience would have wracked my nerves. I remained absolutely calm and relaxed."*
> *"I am sitting on a camp-bed with three other persons and hovering in the air (to me apparently nothing extraordinary at all) and we are carried up very high. Then we plunge down vertically towards the sea, and we say to ourselves: That will hurt. At the same time, I realize that I want to remember this dream. That is why I miss the moment we hit the water. Anyhow the fear is not in due relation to the danger."*
>
> *"While ascending in an elevator the lift runs out of control. It does not go up anymore but dashes downwards very rapidly. I am amazed rather than terrified, there is no panic at all. I am absolutely convinced that nothing will happen to me." Again, the dreamers are lacking the due feeling of danger and menace although they are dashing down and have to be aware of a deadly impact any moment.*

Coniferophyta —

In the remedy Thuja —

- mind; DREAMS; accidents, of (117)
- mind; DREAMS; accusations; crime, of wrongful (22)
- mind; DREAMS; battles (28)
- mind; DREAMS; danger (192)

- mind; DREAMS; misfortune, of (74)
- mind; FEAR; misfortune, of (108)
- mind; FEAR; ordeal, of an (9)
- mind; FEAR; wind, storm, of (17)

These show anticipation of—

1. Crisis
2. Misfortune
3. Disaster
4. Ordeal
5. Storm

All these mean the same thing. Hence, we can say that the main idea is whether one will be able to deal with crises, storms in ones' life and yet be standing upright and not be broken into two or many pieces and fall down. One is anticipating a crisis all the time, and this is a big crisis.

In summary we can say the feeling in Gymnosperms is —

> *my roots are not able to withstand a crisis. They will break. I have to stand firm.*

Gymnosperms	
• *Ginkophyta* • *Cycadophyta* • *Gnetophyta* • *Coniferophyta*	
Brittle Fragile Easily broken Fall Fractures	Strong Invincible Can stand any kind of disaster: wind, fire, flood, earthquake, storm, crisis Decay
Exposed Naked Sensitive	Covered Hard Warts, tumours, keloids
Needles Stitching	
Old age Old people Premature old age Fragility in old age	

If we continue on with our case, we will see these themes quite clearly and will also look for the individualising symptoms of our remedy. We ask the patient to tell us his fears —

> *Fear of darkness in childhood . Fear that something will come out from the dark , like some wild animal. This was especially in any new place. Fear of death and disease. Even if there is a slightest scratch, I imagine that something big will happen. I have to be fit and strong in case there is any physical or mental emergency. I am reaching an age where I can drop dead anytime. Anything can happen that can decapitate me or make me bedridden. I have always tried to protect myself. Since childhood I wanted to protect myself and so I built my physical body. So that if 5 people come then I can fight them and manage. In Delhi, I never had the feeling of being protected by someone. I was the one who had to protect others. And so I made myself fit physically.*

We ask the patient to tell us about his childhood —

> *When I was young, I was the go to person. I was immune to all these fears. I would always be the calm one and take control of the situation. My father was not fit. I have had to take him to the hospital may be 300 times or more. My brother was in the Navy so I was the only person at home. I had to be calm and collected. I would take control over such situations. All this has completely shaken now.*

Again, we can see all the features of the Gymnosperms coming through as discussed. It is also interesting to see them in the light of the 4th superclass. We can clearly see that this fragility of the Gymnosperms is closely linked to a loss of stability. We know that Gymnosperms commonly have very shallow roots and will fall easily. This is beautifully correlated with us placing this group in the 4th Superclass. We then ask the patient to tell us more about this shaken feeling —

> *Lost that ability. It's like a tree that was standing strong and now suddenly has become uprooted. It has a 5-8 foot diameter trunk, massive tree, having huge branches creating shade. Now the roots have got termites and it has deteriorated completely. It cannot carry its own weight. It is stuck at the root and tilting to one side. If it is not treated it will fall.*

Even the patients physical generals highlight this theme of fragility –

- Desires- sweets, oranges, eggplant, mango
- Used to like alcohol but have given up. Careful about what I eat.
- Tea agg
- Coffee agg
- Alcohol agg
- Used to smoke but gave up because mother had Interstitial Lung disease and it could have affected her.

Now having gone through the case we have seen the various information which we have sorted through leading us to the Gymnosperms. But which remedy do we choose? This is where we can use the physical complaints to individualise and point us to the correct remedy. When we look at the main complaint it important to note that 1000's of patients have acidity, yet very few will say that they have a sensation of a cricket ball in-between the chest and navel. Our remedy has to be a Gymnosperm remedy which has this symptom.

So when we look at the materia medica we see the following;

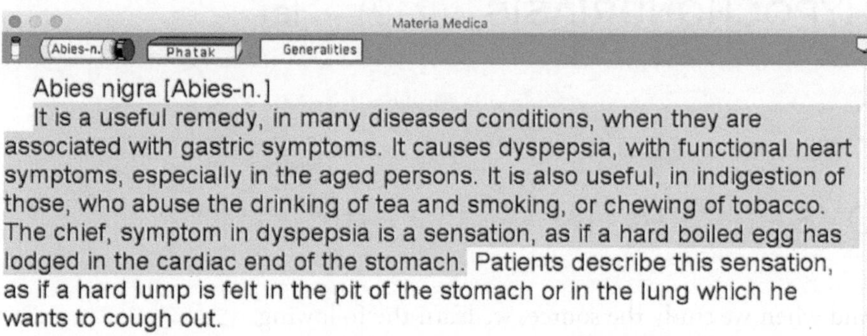

Abies nigra [Abies-n.]

It is a useful remedy, in many diseased conditions, when they are associated with gastric symptoms. It causes dyspepsia, with functional heart symptoms, especially in the aged persons. It is also useful, in indigestion of those, who abuse the drinking of tea and smoking, or chewing of tobacco. The chief, symptom in dyspepsia is a sensation, as if a hard boiled egg has lodged in the cardiac end of the stomach. Patients describe this sensation, as if a hard lump is felt in the pit of the stomach or in the lung which he wants to cough out.

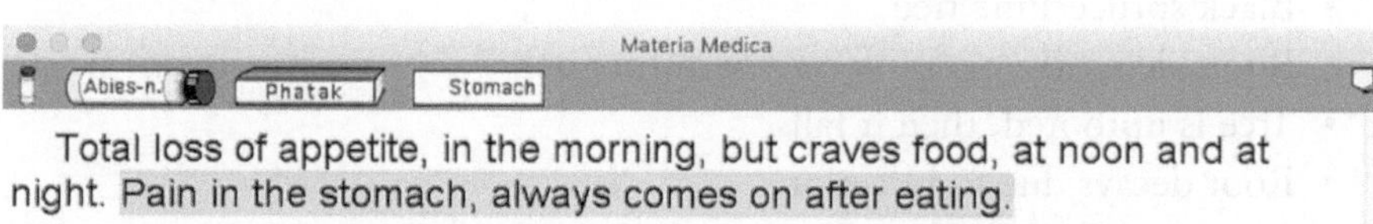

Total loss of appetite, in the morning, but craves food, at noon and at night. Pain in the stomach, always comes on after eating.

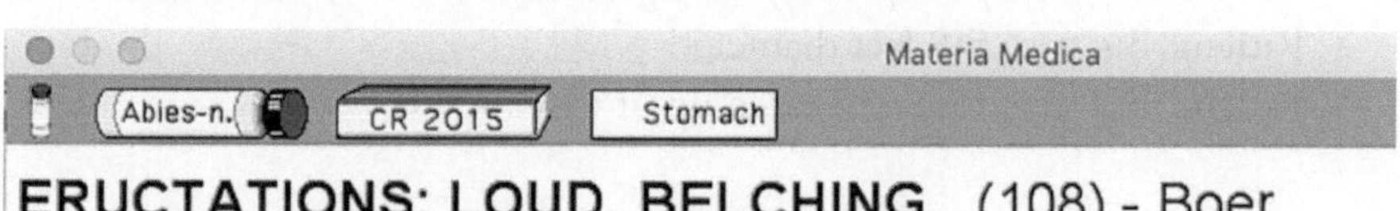

ERUCTATIONS: LOUD, BELCHING. (108) - Boer

Materia Medica

Abies-n. | CR 2015 | Stomach

LUMP SENSATION. (89) - Alle
LUMP SENSATION: EATING, AFTER. (14) - Alle
LUMP SENSATION: CARDIAC ORIFICE. (8) - Alle
Lump Sensation: Pit Of Stomach. (10)
LUMP SENSATION: EGG AT THE CARDIAC ORIFICE, AS IF A HARD BOILED, AFTER EATING. (2) - Alle
LUMP SENSATION: HARD. (12) - Alle

STONE SENSATION. (137) - Farr
Stone sensation: eating: agg. (21) - Ken
STONE SENSATION: PIT OF STOMACH. (17) - Farr

Tea: agg. (33) - Boer

Materia Medica

Abies-n. | CR 2015 | Mind

HYPOCHONDRIASIS. (219) - Her

Materia Medica

Abies-n. | CR 2015 | Mind

DYSPEPSIA, IN. (31) - Farr

And when we study the source, we learn the following.

- Black spruce/Pine tree
- Roots decay they get infected with fungus
- Tree is uprooted, then it falls.
- Root decays due to infection.
- Roots are not very deep in Gymnosperm
- Patient: Big tree: 5-8 feet diameter
- Patient: Big tree, roots get eaten up, it tilts and decays

We also understand a bit better what he means when he says —

Decapitate ⟶ You get cut off

Superclass	**4**
Kingdom	Plant
Classification	Gymnosperm
Order	Coniferophytes
Family	Conifers
Remedy	Abies Nigra

The patient was prescribed Abies nigra 200 and he gave us the following report after 1 year 6 months of taking treatment –

- *No pain in the back, shoulder, or body.*
- *No lethargy, feeling of fatigue or tiredness- >100%*
- *Acidity, feeling of hardness as if something stuck is gone 100%*
- *There is no physical problem at all now*
- *Mentally much better. Not feeling anxious like before*
- *In between felt anxious once because many old people died suddenly so I was worried about that, but it's not like it was earlier.*
- *Have reduced all allopathic medicines.*

Case 14

This is the case of a 4-year-old girl who was brought with complaints of Recurrent urinary tract infection, epilepsy, gastritis, asthma, and autism.

The patient had been born at 30 weeks of gestation with several congenital malformations. She was hospitalised for 2 years after birth and has undergone 14 surgeries up till now on her pancreas, stomach, duodenum, bladder, and kidney. The mother narrates —

She has a very low immunity and has frequent vomiting because of severe esophagitis with reflux, due to malformation of the stomach. The vomiting is worse when crying or laughing. She has to be fed through a gastric tube. We have to frequently admit her to hospital for severe urinary tract infections (UTI) which are recurrent which require antibiotics frequently.

She also suffers from epilepsy. Just the other day she was admitted in the hospital for 1 week as she had two seizures, one after the other. Nothing out of the ordinary occurs before the seizures. The seizures always occur during sleep. Her left side of the face, eyes and mouth are pulled back. Her left arm was stretched out and left arm and left leg were shaking. Occasionally this occurs on the right side.

When she was younger the duration of the seizures would be 10-20 seconds.

Now the duration is longer. The last one lasted for 10 minutes. It is Tonic-Clonic type seizure. When one thing goes out of control like if she gets a seizure, she ends up with a UTI or an asthma attack and has to be taken to several doctors at one time.

The Asthma attacks are frequent, they are worse from strong smells, dust and cold temperatures. It starts with a dry allergic cough, which becomes productive later.

Many paroxysms of cough one after the other and she vomits with it. It is worse lying down and at night, around 9-10pm and also worse around 5am. And better when propped up. She becomes more restless during the asthma and there is blue discoloration around the mouth. If not able to control it at home we have to go to the hospital.

She is also diagnosed with Autism. There is no speech yet. She bites her clothes. After her surgery, one year ago she began to pull out her hair when angry. Because of this she has started developing bald patches. They had to cut her hair very short. She still does this. She is also sensitive to sound.

Currently the patient is taking the following medications —

- Nitrazepam (Sonebon) ¼ (5 mg) 3x/day
- Depakene (Valproic acid) 2.5 ml 2x/day
- Levetiracetam (Keppra) 2.5ml 2x/day
- Trileptal 5.5 ml 2x/day
- Doxazosin 1ml 1x/day
- Oxybutynin (Retemic) 3ml 2x/day
- Enalapril 2 ml 2x/day
- Esomeprazole 20 mg 1x/day
- Azithromycin 3.5 ml 1x/day
- Salbutamol spray

The patient developmental milestones occurred as follows —

- Teething : 7months
- Sitting : 9 months
- Standing : 2 and half years
- Walking with support : 2 and half years
- Walking without support : 3 years
- No speech
- No urine control

The patient is also allergic to latex, milk and milk products and will suffer anaphylaxis with exposure to them. We also managed to get the following physical generals of the child –

- Appetite : Normal, eats well
- Thirst : very less
- Desires : Salty food, Eggs, Tea, Fruits
- Aversion : Meat, Fish, Fried food
- Stools: Normal
- Perspiration : Back, Neck
- Sleep : Normal, on back or left side

Having received this information we ask the mother to tell us about the child's nature —

> *She is calm. She is not hard working but she does what she is supposed to do. Plays at the time of playing, eats when called for food. She has no problem with others. If I need to go out and leave her, she is fine as long as she has something to play with. She is a very tranquil girl not an agitated child. She is affectionate and likes to hug and she likes to go skating. Her teacher says she remains isolated at school.*

By now we had made the following observations of the patient —

> Constant movement. For a major part of the case she was playing by herself.
>
> Did not trouble the mother much. Listened when told something.

An essential part of case taking in paediatrics is to ask the mothers history during pregnancy so now we ask her if she had any observations —

> *My pregnancy was difficult. I had Diabetes and Hypertension so there were many food restrictions. I felt many times that I won't be able to carry it to term, that the baby would have some problem. I had many ultrasonography's done but nothing showed up.*
>
> *I had bleeding all the time. I was always on alert. I had nausea but not much vomiting.*
>
> *It was a very, very difficult pregnancy. I felt like I was sick throughout, not as if I was pregnant. I had no appetite and I lost 12 kgs.*
>
> *The worst part of the pregnancy was that there was so much pain in the bones and the body. Pain in my hips, I could not sleep because the pain*

was maximum and unbearable on lying down. I couldn't move or turn and could not even get up on my own. I needed someone to help me all the time.

It was too much pain. A strong continuous pain. I had to keep on moving and walking to feel better. I used to constantly walk a bit, sit and then walk again. There was like an impatience in me. I had to get up all the time.

We then ask the mother to describe her mental state in this period —

Stress was high especially as my husband started smoking and drinking at home while I was pregnant. It really bothered me and I used to get high blood pressure and bleeding due to the stress. I don't like anyone smoking close to me. I don't like the smell of alcohol. This is because it reminds me of my step father who was an alcoholic.

It was very disturbing. It is a part of my life that I don't like to remember much.

I get nervous and feel uncontrolled. My mom married my step father when I was 1 year old. He used to drink. He molested me all the time. My mother took me to live with other relatives because of this. He is the model of the worst man that can be on earth. I felt disgust, anger, sadness and it brought me panic!!! When I was in the bathroom, he would spy on me. On lying down at night, I could never have a good sleep because he was always around my bed room. My bed room didn't have a lock because he would remove my lock so that he could get in. When I was 17, I decided to get out of my house. I was lonely. My mother gave me no assistance. She saw what was happening but she didn't help me. She said it was our secret and that I couldn't tell anyone. I didn't know what to do. I was in a conflict. I didn't have anyone to help me. I had to go and live with this sick, highly jealous fellow. He tried to kill me. He even brought a revolver to kill me.

He did it because he was jealous that another man may like me or that I may like another man.

The mother is describing an intense situation but it is important to remember that it is the experience of the situation which is of most importance to us, not the situation itself, so here we ask the mother to tell us what her inner experience was in this situation —

I was disgusted about myself. I didn't want anyone to see me. If I could become invisible, I would have done that. I started to have black out episodes. I would have fainting spells from the age of 12 until 17. I fainted because my pressure would go up.

He always said that it was not serious enough to take me to the doctor. He was jealous and always there besides me. One day I got a severe pain in my stomach. It was sudden.

I was fine doing something and suddenly I got this big pain and I fainted, lost my senses.

We now ask the mother to tell us some of the dreams she would get —

Dreams that my mother died. I was scared of losing her. It was my biggest fear and constant dream. I wanted to die each day. I couldn't sleep. I didn't like to see him.

I normally have dreams that always mean something. I sometimes dream that animals are talking to me. I know then it may have something to do with the health of my children or my own health.

We ask the mother what dreams she got during the pregnancy –

My most disturbing dream, it was in another dimension. I was with my husband and we left this plane and went to a different place. I dreamt about the devil. A battle with the devil. It was very dark, very black and there were some flashes of light. It was when those flashes of light came that I saw the devil. They looked like a goat but also a man. They had the horns and face of a goat but on a man's body. They didn't have hands, they had knives instead. They were blowing (phoooo) and when they did this it was as if I lost sense of everything. I nearly lost balance. I felt dizzy and I let go of my father's hand and we got lost from each other. We re-met each other in the darkness and we would hold hands again. But then the devil would come and do the same thing again. They would blow and I was not scared but it was a bad sensation. I felt dizzy, I fell over, I lost a sense of things. When I woke up, I knew immediately that this spiritual battle was connected to my daughter.

We ask her to tell us more about this spiritual battle –

I was fighting with the devil in another dimension. I wanted to win the spiritual battle.

I didn't have the strength to win that. I was very, very tired when I woke up, it was as if I really experienced that. I knew it was connected to my daughter.

We ask to be told more about the flashes of light and being in another dimension –

> *It was a desperate situation. It was desperate!!! I wanted to get out of that situation.*
>
> *But I was weak and I was not able to get out of it.*

When trying to understand the Superclass of a patient it is very important to focus on the basic reaction. What is the most basic response in stressful situations. Here the mother says her response is to get out. While we do not jump straightway to the conclusion of the superclass this is a very good hint and gives reason for us explore this a bit more. So, we can ask about 'get out'.

> *To wake up from that and go to a light place. To not see the situation anymore.*

It is important to stop the patient from using their rational and logical mind. It is very helpful to ask them to describe something unrelated to anything that has been said previously. This forces them to use their imagination and allows us to step into the unconscious mind. So, we ask her to describe the expression 'get out' unrelated to the dream –

> *Liberate self, free self, to get out means to leave behind something and to start something new. To change places. To come to a new phase. I felt privileged because God showed me what was happening. He showed me that there was a battle.*

We want to understand a bit more. We now ask the patient to describe 'a battle' in general. We try help them to use their imagination by asking it generally —

> *A spiritual battle in which I tried with all my strength to resolve the situation of the dream. I couldn't manage alone. In my head I knew that there was God, who would help me to win this. This feeling was so much so that when I woke up, I prayed and asked God to help me. I am a person who has a lot of faith in God and I know that my life is ruled by God and God made me see the battle that was taking place. There was really a battle happening with my daughter. When I woke up I prayed to God because this battle that was happening was out of my hands. I couldn't manage to resolve it. My strength was not much but God's strength was not little. I prayed for her*

life. They wanted to take my daughter's life away. I got this dream one week before I went into labour.

We have been receiving good information up till now. We still need to try and put it into context with everything else we have heard. So now we try a different tactic, we ask the mother to describe her step father's nature. This is not because his nature is relevant to the child. It is often easier for people to project their own issues onto others than it is for them to tell about themselves. When we ask the mother to describe her stepfather what we will actually hear is what she is sensitive to. This will give us an insight into her state and will also be a part of the remedy–

He is a bad person. He is evil, very evil. Revengeful. Person with a bad character. He cannot be trusted. He is a retired police officer. He made us watch him beat up people in prison. He threatened us with his gun or knife. He always had to have the last word.

He was very, very authoritative. Everything had to be done how he wanted it to be done.

My mother suffered a lot with him. He didn't respect anybody. He thought that he was above the law. He thought that he was above everybody. He killed people with no justification whatsoever. He beat people up with no need for it. Things had to be under his domain. He was a model of a horrible man whom I had in my life. He molested me.

We have gotten some good information from this question but now we need to separate the experience from the situation, so, we ask the mother to describe her inner experience -

I felt dirty and ashamed of myself. Angry with myself. I didn't want him to see me.

I felt almost as if it was my fault. Later in life I had contacts with other women who were abused and molested and it is a feeling that we normally have. We are guilty for existing and we don't want to be seen. Want to be invisible. Wanted to be invisible so that they don't see us in the world. Today I am better in this aspect. I have tried to resolve it. It is difficult to resolve but I am better in self.

I wanted to kill him. When I was 17, I used to sleep with a knife under my pillow and I was sure that I was going to kill him. If I had not left the house when I did, it would have become a big tragedy. He didn't dare to come into my bedroom when I was sleeping with a knife. I had difficulty in life because of this. If a man looked at me and saw me as a woman, I would see my stepfather's face.

This was the information from the case taking. We need to look at those features in the case which are repeated and striking and that which represents the dynamic. This is where we can see the Superclass.

Firstly, we have our observation that the child is constantly moving. Then we hear the mother's story where she tells us how her home was not a happy place. There was a lot of violence and her feeling was that she had to get out. This is the most basic reaction of hers as we also see it in her dream. She describes how she wants get out, and also to free herself.

It is also very interesting how the symptoms she manifested during the pregnancy are physical pains. These force her to move all the time and don't allow her to lie down.

When we see all these in conjunction with each other it becomes very clear that this is the 5th superclass.

The aspect of the case we can look at is the kingdom. In this case we can see that there is a sensitivity to a situation and then a reaction. This points us to the plant kingdom. From her reactions to her husband and her step-father it might seem to be an experience of victim-aggressor and therefore pointing to the animal kingdom. Persons and remedies from the 5th and Superclasses have many animal like features, though they may be from the plant or mineral kingdom or even a nosode. The difference can be quite subtle. Here the mother says she felt abused by her step-father and even wanted to kill him. This seems so animal-like. Similarly, many remedies in the sixth Superclass such as Mercurius and Hyoscyamus have the desire to kill, though they are mineral and plant remedies. Here we have to see that the animal quality is one of me vs the other. Who is stronger, who is weaker. In the above case, the desire to kill in the mother is a reaction to the situation. However, feeling I want to get out, to move, to change, etc is far more her basic reaction than wanting to harm her step-father. It is more a sensation than a comparison. This points to the plant kingdom. I can understand that this can be confusing and it did take me some time to know the difference.

Having seen that the common thread in the case is the need to get out, the mental feeling of stiffness and stuck and also in the physical symptoms and the constant need to move, we need to investigate the Rosidae group of the dicotyledons. This is the 5th subclass and correlates with the 5th superclass.

The main sensations we will find in this subclass are

- Holding and releasing.
- Tight, squeezed, stuck, rigid, stiff, can't move, can't breathe, claustrophobia, can't bear tight clothes
- Movement ameliorates, change desires, travel ameliorates, need to get out

When we look at the orders from the 5th Subclass and some of their key features (Section Two). We can understand that in this case we have seen the features of the Sapindales. The main focus in the case was, "I want to get out, I have to move."

This is also validated by the observation of the child's continuous movement. We see this in the mother too , esp. in relation to her pain which forced her to move and the dream where she wanted to get out. The stressful situation in her home also gave her the feeling "I just wanted to get out". From this we can understand how we saw the 5th superclass through the qualities of the Sapindales. In the Sapindales there is a family which we know very well, the Anacardiacaeae. They have the exact sensation we are looking for in this case. The stiff, stuck caught sensation with the reaction of always being on the move.

Now we start narrowing the search for the remedy. We must know that in each case there is something which is unique and specific. This will distinguish remedy out from the other remedies in the same family or group. In this case what was most clear was the Miasm along with a few PQRS symptoms and mental characteristics.

The PQRS symptom that we see in this case is in the situation with the stepfather. The mother says that she was in a conflict. This idea of an internal conflict is also seen in the dream of the battle with the devil. A spiritual battle where we see the Devil and God. This conflict with self is a very characteristic symptom of *Anacardium.* It is typically represented by the symptom feels one has 'the devil on one shoulder and an angel on the other'.

The Miasm which we can see in the case is a mix of Cancer and Leprosy miasm. In the child we see the Cancer miasm clearly though the child's very obedient behaviour. The mother uses the word tranquil to describe her. We can also see elements of the Cancer miasm in the mother when she talks about her childhood. She speaks of feeling nervous and uncontrolled. The dream for her was a very desperate situation, where she tries with all her strength to resolve it. She prayed to God as what was happening was out of her hands (she is not in control). Then we can also see the Leprous miasm in her feelings of disgust, dirty, ashamed, angry with self, guilt for existing, don't want to be seen, want to be invisible and wanting to kill him.

There is a plethora of information, and it can help to use the 8-box method to ensure that we have investigated every aspect of the case.

Pathology Organ Affected	Local Symtpoms Lsmc Pqrs	Phyiscal Generals	Mental Symptoms
• Recurrent UTI • Epilepsy • Gastritis • Asthma • Autism	• Vomiting <crying, laugh, coughing • Seizures: left sided, During sleep • Cough <lying, night, 5 am >propped up • Restlessness	• Thirst less • Desire: Salt, Egg, Tea, Fruits • Aversion: Meat, Fish, Fried food • Perspiration: Back, Neck • Agg: Milk, Latex	• Constant movement • No speech • Bites clothes • Pulls hair • Calm • Obedient • Sensitive to sound • Affectionate
Dreams	**Physical Symptoms In Pregnancy**	**Mind: Mother**	**Kingdom**
• Mother-death • Talking-animals • Battle with devils • God helping me	• Bleeding • Pain in hips • <lying down, turning • >motion • Restless	• All the time alert, nervous, uncontrolled • Disgust • Invisible • In conflict **Nature of Stepfather** • Jealous, evil • Wanted to kill • Authoritative	• Plant: • Sensitivity and reactivity **Subclass** • 5th **Sensation** • Have to get out, has to move **Miasm** • Leprosy, Cancer

We have now sorted out all the information into the 8 boxes and it is important to find a remedy which covers all the boxes. We will also use the repertory to confirm all our selection. It is very helpful to limit our repertory search to remedies from the 5th subclass only.

The symptoms of the child

	Anac.	Carb-v.	Sep.	Nux-v.	Bry.	Con.	Nit-ac.	Sil.	Calc.	Nat-m.	Carb-an.	Tub.	Sulph.	Dros.	Hep.	Hyos.	Rhus-t.
Total	19	29	29	28	26	26	25	25	24	24	17	15	27	26	25	24	2
Rubrics	9	8	8	8	8	8	8	8	8	8	8	8	7	7	7	7	7
Kingdom																	
CR19 - Mind; Affectionate; children kiss and caress(17)	1	1		1							1						
CR19 - Cough; Violent(226)	4	4	4	4	4	4	3	3	3	3	1	1	4	4	4	4	4
CR19 - Cough; Cold; taking a(53)	1	4	4	4	3	1	3	4	1	3	1	3		3	4	1	3
CR19 - Cough; Lying; agg.; bed, in(91)	1		4	3	3	4	1	3	3	1	1	1	4	3	1	4	3
CR19 - Cough; Suffocative(239)	1	4	3	4	3	3	3	4	3	3	3	3	4	4	4	4	3
CR19 - Cough; Convulsive, spasmodic(320)	3	4	4	4	4	4	4	3	3	4	3	1	4	4	4	4	3
CR19 - Stomach; Vomiting; cough; during(149)	3	4	3	4	4	3	3	3	4	3	3	1	4	4	4	3	4
CR19 - Cough; Night; agg.(355)	4	4	4	4	4	4	4	4	4	3	4	2	4	4	4	4	4
CR19 - Generalities; Food and drinks; salt or salty food; desires(158)	1	4	3		1	3	4	1	3	4		3	3				

The symptoms of the mother's history during pregnancy

	Rhus-t.	Anac.	Rhus-a	Mangi.	Rhus-g	Rhus-v.
Total	13	2	3	3	1	1
Rubrics	4	2	1	1	1	1
Kingdom						
CR19 - Female; Hemorrhage, uterine, metrorrhagia(387)	4	1	3	3	1	1
CR19 - Extremities; Pain; hips; lying; agg.(43)	4					
CR19 - Extremities; Pain; hips; walking; amel.; while(23)	3					
CR19 - Generalities; Turning; bed, in(136)	2	1				

The symptoms of the mother's mental state and dreams

synergy

	Anac.	Puls.	Nux-v.	Op.	Stram.	Lach.
Total	15	14	12	11	9	8
Rubrics	9	6	6	5	5	5
Kingdom						
CR19 - Mind; Delusions, imaginations; attacked, is going to be(36)	1		1			
CR19 - Mind; Delusions, imaginations; bed; someone; in, with him, her(18)	1	3	1	3	1	1
CR19 - Mind; Delusions, imaginations; devil, devils(46)	3	3		3	3	1
CR19 - Mind; Delusions, imaginations; persecuted, that he is(79)	3	1	1	1	1	3
CR19 - Mind; Delusions, imaginations; religious; redemption and devil, about(2)	3					
CR19 - Mind; Delusions, imaginations; trapped, he is(47)	1					
CR19 - Mind; Dreams; vexatious; disgusting(12)	1	3	3			
CR19 - Mind; Reproaches; oneself(98)	1	3	2	3	1	1
CR19 - Mind; Kill, desire to(100)	1	1	4	1	3	2

We shouldn't forget the nature of the stepfather either as this was the sensitivity of the mother –

synergy

	Anac.	Nux-v.	Hyos.	Plat.	Lach.	Sulph.	Lyc.	Phos.
Total	24	36	33	33	30	26	31	27
Rubrics	12	11	11	11	11	11	10	10
Kingdom								
CR19 - Mind; Love; perversity; sadomasochistic(5)	1							
CR19 - Mind; Love; perversity(28)	1	1	2	3	1	3		1
CR19 - Mind; Lewdness, obscene(51)	1	3	3	3	3	1	1	3
CR19 - Mind; Dictatorial(99)	1	3	1	3	3	3	4	3
CR19 - Mind; Kill, desire to(100)	1	4	4	4	2	1	4	3
CR19 - Mind; Unfeeling, hard-hearted(108)	4	1	1	3	3	3	1	1
CR19 - Mind; Abusive, insulting(113)	3	4	3	3	1	3	4	
CR19 - Mind; Jealousy(133)	3	4	4	4	4	1	3	3
CR19 - Mind; Striking(143)	1	4	4	2	1	1	4	3
CR19 - Mind; Lasciviousness(159)	1	4	4	4	4	3	3	4
CR19 - Mind; Malicious, vindictive(167)	4	4	4	3	4	3	4	3
CR19 - Mind; Alcoholism, dipsomania(181)	3	4	3	1	4	4	3	3

When we put all the information together, we get to the remedy *Anacardium orientale* and as we have shown not a single piece of information that was provided was ignored or left out of the analysis, every area has been covered. We can summarize the classification of information as follows —

Superclass	5th Superclass
Kingdom	Plant kingdom
Class	Dicotyledons
Subclass	5th Rosidae
Order	Sapindales
Family	Anacardiacaeae
Miasm	Leprosy/Cancer
Remedy	*Anacardium orientale*

Anacardium 10M followed by LM 10 was prescribed to the patient and after one year of treatment the patients mother shared the patients progress —

> *She is doing much better. No seizures in the past 5 months. (Used to have 3 per week).*
>
> *Last UTI was in august, since then she has not had an episode. No asthma or cough episodes. No recurrent infections and hospitalizations (Used to get hospitalized weekly acutes).*
>
> *She has been off antibiotics since 5 months.*
>
> *She has become more aware. Speech is slow but she has started interacting.*
>
> *She has started connecting to people. She used to be very inactive, now has become very active.*
>
> *She has started becoming very mischievous now like children of her age. Laughs and runs away when she knows she has done something wrong. She was unable to do things properly now she can pull a chair, open the door, she even flushed my cell phone in the toilet!!! Threw all the detergent powder into the laundry when I was not attentive. Starts shouting when not given candy.*
>
> *The change with the medication has been dramatic.*

Before treatment	After treatment
Nitrazepam (Sonebon) ¼ (5 mg) 3x/day	Nitrazepam (Sonebon) (1 mg) 3x/day
Depakene (Valproic acid) 2.5 ml 2x/day	Depakene (Valproic acid) 2.5 ml 2x/day
Levetiracetam (Keppra) 2.5ml 2x/day	Levetiracetam 2.5ml 2x/day
Trileptal 5.5 ml 2x/day	Doxazosin 1ml 1x/day
Doxazosin 1ml 1x/day	
Oxybutynin (Retemic) 3ml 2x/day	
Enalapril 2 ml 2x/day	
Esomeprazole 20 mg 1x/day	
Azithromycin 3.5 ml 1x/day	
Salbutamol spray	

— End of Case —

Case 15

This is the case of a 22-year-old Male who was suffering from Psoriasis. He begins the case narrating his complaints.

I have Psoriasis, it is on my scalp. Occasionally eyebrows and beard.

On allopathic cream – elocon topical cream (steroid). Since a year it started with dryness of skin. There is no itching as such. There is flaking in dry skin. White flakes come up. No other problem

We ask the patient what the effect of the complaint on him is —

It has been a bit annoying because it is on my face. It is visible. That way it is a bit embarrassing. But apart from that it is ok. It doesn't look good.

This response gives us some insight into the thought process of the patient. We can see that appearance is important to him. But we need to understand this in context of the rest of the case, so we ask the patient to tell us about himself —

I used to be part of college team where we used to make aeroplanes so I had an airplane at that time. I have interest in aeroplane and aero design. How air planes fly? How do these massive machines fly? I had that curiosity for that. Airplanes are massive and still they take off the gravity. So, it is fascinating how they lift up the ground, in spite of being so large. It interesting and exciting. It is impressive. It is not something that you can easily understand. There are lot of complex physics and design involved.

It was a challenge. Trying to understand how the planes fly. It is not easy to understand. It is not truly complex. You break it down, approach it one thing at a time. Understand the whole thing.

It is exciting to see it. It is not something that is very common. We don't get to see it every day. E.g.: regular daily routine. It would be little bit boring. Doing same things again and again. You don't get to see or do new things. And you don't go out of your comfort zone and don't get to have new adventures and experience. Learning new things, trying new food, going to new places. That is interesting.

As we have discussed previously the phrase 'comfort zone' is very important for the 4th superclass. The 4th Superclass wants to be in their comfort zone they don't like to leave it. In this case the dynamic is somewhat opposite. Here the experience is that to be in the comfort is very boring. He wants to break the routine. To think outside the box is very important for this patient. We ask the patient to tell us about this comfort zone —

Comfort zone is something that you are comfortable doing, part of your routine, you don't think twice about doing it. Something new isn't. Having new experience. You get to grow as person as a result of these experiences. We are the sum of all our experiences. When you get to experience something new, you learn something because of it. You learn more things and become better. And you grow. Going to country. You learn new language. You learn new cuisine. That is what is most essential things to do. To be better tomorrow than you were yesterday.

Again, we can differentiate with the 4th Superclass which is about doing routine tasks, doing your duty… but here it is about something beyond that. You need to be better than routine, you have to grow.

We ask the patient about his dreams —

Dreams of witnessing a flight test. It was very happy. We as a team had made that aircraft and me being a part of them. And seeing that plane fly is like an accomplishment. Seeing your plane fly is a very happy feeling. When you set a goal and set a destination and you reach there, it is satisfying. First you need to identify your goal. You have set a reasonable target. You have seen what are steps you take and eventually you reach the goal. There are challenges along the way. Try different methods to face those challenges. Come with solution to overcome those challenge and take one step at a time.

This is a very interesting dream if we think of the Neurotransmitters and their relations to the Superclasses. We can see which neurotransmitter is best seen in this dream : Dopamine. Dopamine represents motivation, drive and pursuit of goals. And we can see that this patient is highly motivated and driven to set goals .

Thinking out of the box is his other quality. Here we can clearly see that the main action is to get out (mentally) there is no issue with flight or fight as in the 6th Superclass. So it must be the 5th superclass. This differentiation between 5th and the 6th becomes clearer as he continues with his description of the dreams —

> *They are not negative dream or nightmares. Like getting kidnapped. Lost and hurt somewhere. May be going somewhere and getting kidnapped. You are going somewhere and your car breaks down and you get lost in some jungle. Helplessness. You are stuck in situation and can't do anything to get out of it. It can get overwhelming at first. You don't have plan how to approach them. Fear how you are going to get out of this situation, how it is going to end. Animals are going to eat, infection or some disease, insects could bite you, you could run out of food or water. I am more process oriented. What work needs to be done and approach one thing at a time.*
>
> *When you have certain challenge, rather than getting overwhelmed by it, you try to figure out what you can do to overcome the challenge.*

In his words he is telling us, this is not a dream of the 6th superclass but a dream of the 5th superclass. You aren't getting kidnapped but rather you are stuck in a situation which you have to get out of. The emphasis is on getting out and overcoming a challenge. This is the 5th superclass.

We ask the patient to describe more about 'challenge' —

> *I like to take problems as challenges and find solution to it. That would be an interesting challenge. It could be anything that hamper you in your goals in the process of whatever you are doing. If you are running the race and you have hurdles and you have to get over that hurdles. It is satisfying of overcoming a challenge. It is much less of problem than before. Hospitalisation was the time where it was challenging. I had my exam going. It was definitely a challenge. I never thought I will have to face it. I approached the problem and gave my exam. Vindication. Happiness. You face a challenge; you are able to overcome it and you feel like you*

accomplish something. Meet a goal, accomplish a task or complete a task. It means like certain work or target that you have to meet. It is a target and you have tried and met that.

We are able to sort the information into its various categories. Firstly, we see the idea of a challenge and overcoming the challenge. This Dopamine-like motivation and drive which show us the shades of the 5th superclass. We can also see the perception of the challenge is through the lens of capability. It is about whether you are capable to overcome the challenge or not. This is the mineral kingdom. So, we can see that it is 5th superclass and mineral kingdom.

This could mean that we are looking either be the right-hand side of the 2nd row or the whole of the 5th row of the periodic table. Both correspond to the 5th superclass. The issue which he is discussing is about performance and out of the box thinking. These correspond with 5th row issues .

The patient then tells us his fears —

Fear of high places. If it is high place without railing, I feel I can fall over.

Fear of spiders and insects which I overcome to some extent. I might not be comfortable in narrow place. I would have claustrophobia.

We ask about any stressful incidences in the patient's life —

There was a phase, where I didn't do well in few exams. I wasn't getting into IIT's or Bits, great institutions. So, I repeated my entire 12th grade one year. Friends had gone ahead. Academically and socially things weren't good. Even my grand mom was diagnosed with cancer. But eventually I got through it. It was a challenging phase. It was something that you wouldn't expect that this would come up. I had to look at it one day at a time. Step oriented process. Chart out what needs to be done. And then you do one step at a time. Make sure you don't miss out of anything. You are doing it in most efficient way. You don't have to put huge amount of effort for huge amount of work. You can work smart. Put in lesser amount effort and do the task. It makes more sense. It is more efficient. Lesser amount of energy and time. There were lot of things to be dealt with. There was lot of uncertainty. You don't know how things are going to work out in future. It creates little bit of nervousness. But it just takes one step at a time. Cross the bridge when you are there, rather than worrying about it now.

We ask the patient what are his interests and hobbies —

> *I used to make Lego few years ago. You have all these different parts and you can make anything you want. Freedom for creativity. There are lot of different blocks and you can make anything whatever you want out of it. You can make anything that you can imagine. Opposite is being more constrained. Not having freedom. Only being able to do specific things. Helplessness. Being bored. Only having few things to do and being able to do those. Like during lockdowns. Online courses, learning new language. I started course on programming language. It was out of my interest. We weren't taught that. You can think of any challenge and the programme and does it for you. It finds the solution for the problem. In college, our competition was like creating passenger aircraft. We had to design the aircraft with certain other constraints. With those you have freedom to create any aircraft with any design that we wanted. It was very interesting. I learnt a lot of things.*

We ask the patient to tell us how confident he is. This will give us a better row which column he may belong to in the periodic table —

> *In confidence, on the scale of 10 I can range myself on 9 ½ . I am pretty confident when there is crisis and problem.*

We ask the patient what he is sensitive to —

> *Nothing specific. I am levelled as such. Flat. There is no change in terrain. Constant. Uniform. White sheet of paper which is flat. Blank white paper. It is convenient for travelling but again it is very boring, because it is constant and there is no change, stuck in the same situation. Don't get to experience something new. Bit boring. You can't do something new. Stuck in comfort zone. Good because you are in your comfort zone, but it is irritating because you can't do something new. You know your surroundings; you know how everything is. It is convenient. Like my house, my Air conditioner, my bed. I know number on TV. Its known convenient and known. Opposite is inconvenient, you have to put in more efforts to figure out things but that will be interesting experience.*

These were the generals of the patient —

- Desires – chicken burger, chicken pizza, pizza, French fries, pasta, Italian food, sushi, Thai food, Thai curry. Pav bhaji (mashed, spicy vegetable dish). Cheese

- Aversion – Gujarati food, eggplant
- Sleep – position on sides, sleep is good
- Sweat – scanty
- Thermals – hot patient, I like warm bathing and going out in sun but when it is not too hot

— End of Case —

All the information from this case can be put into the various boxes;

Diagnosis —	**Main complaint —**	**Generals —**	**Interests and hobbies**
Psoriasis	Scalp, Eyebrows and beard No itch Flaking, dry skin White flakes	Desires Junk food Aversion – Gujrati food, Eggplant Sleep – on sides Sweat – scanty Thermals – Hot patient	Likes learning new things Travelling to new places Getting out of comfort zone "Challenge"
Dreams —	**Sensitivity —**	**Kingdom —**	**Genius —**
Flight test, overcoming a challenge	Constant No change boring	Issues of capability Am I able to overcome any challenge	He has to prove and it's a challenge to go into something new, to learn, to create or to perform.

With the boxes complete, what have we understood?

Some words are repeated often, words such as 'challenge'. He likes to break down things and approach one thing at one time. Uncommon things are exciting. Daily routine is boring. Wants to be out of comfort zone. Adventure. Likes learning new things. Trying new food. Going to new places. Learn to be better and grow. Learning a new language, new cuisine.

To be better more than you were yesterday. Working as a team and seeing that plane flying is an accomplishment. There is a goal, a destination, target. You have to face the challenge. Come with solutions to overcome the challenge.

He is process oriented wants an efficient way. Taking one step at a time. Freedom for creativity. Blocks. Online courses. Learning new language. Course programming.

From all this information it is easy for us to understand that this is from the 5th Superclass. And from the Mineral Kingdom, the 5th Row of the periodic table. Now we have to understand which column this case belongs to.

If you refer my book on the mineral Kingdom "*Structure*' we can see that the themes of the 6th column are as follows;

> *The structure is complete and tested but feels compelled to face the challenge. Needs to prove himself. Daring, run, risks, show them.*

This describes our patient very well and makes our prescription very clear : 5th Row, 6th Column : Molybdenum

The patient was given Molybdenum 1M

Within 6 months of treatment the eruptions had reduced by 70%. No longer using allopathic cream for the psoriasis. The mind state is good, busy with online work and feels the need to do creative things.

The patient continues to do well on the remedy.

The summary of the classification of information is as follows;

Superclass	**5**
Kingdom	Mineral
Row	5th
Column	6
Remedy	Molybdenum

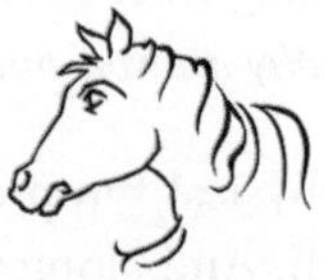

Case 16

This is the case of a 42-year-old female who was diagnosed with an Autoimmune hepatitis. This was quite a complicated case with a progressive pathology, so there were many discussions and interviews with the patient which we have summarised and presented in a concise and comprehensible format.

The patient had presented with complaints of jaundice. For one week she had been experiencing dark yellow urine and her son had noticed a yellowing of her sclera, so we suggested she have liver function tests done. She is also a known case of Autoimmune hypothyroidism.

The LFT's presented on 30/07/2020 as follows;

Hb: 12.6
Total S Bilirubin: 4.09 (Normal Up to 1)
Direct: 2.34 (Up to 0.25)
Indirect: 1.75 (Up to 0.75)
SGOT: 411.6 (Up to 40)
SGPT: 491.6 (Up to 40)
S. Alkaline phosphate: 140.5 (35-118)

She was also suffering from nausea and a strange taste in her mouth. She was complaining about her son, who she feels takes up 70% of her time. She has no time for herself, and all her effort goes into him. She describes having to wake him up, run after him and ensure he does all his homework, in doing so she describes him as an unwilling ox, when asked to describe this further, she says the following —

> *The ox is digging its feet in ground. I have to take it somewhere else; it wants to graze. I have to pull it, to drag it. It is being pushed against its will. It feels I don't want to go there, why are you pulling me there?*

Based on some characteristic physical symptoms like the nausea, sleepiness, jaundice, and taste in the mouth. And along with the symptom, "undertakes things opposed to her intention" the patient was prescribed Sepia 200 three times a day for 7 days.

The patient returned and said she had felt a little bit better after taking the Sepia. The pain in the liver was still there. There was also no change in her state. She continued to discuss the issues with her son and felt she was doing things against her will. Sepia 200 was repeated but now four times a day. After this prescription there was some change, the patient was feeling less drowsy. But no change in the liver symptoms. The potency was increased, and she was prescribed Sepia 1M every 3 hours. The state and physical symptoms were still covered by Sepia. She was also referred to a gastroenterologist for an opinion.

The nausea and vomiting have continued over the next three days, and we continue to repeat Sepia 1M. The Gastroenterologist has found no liver enlargement and is waiting for the results of the investigations he sent for. And he has prescribed no allopathic medicine as she is continuing with homeopathy.

The Ultrasonography was returned with no major changes found except for those correlating with an acute hepatitis. The patient says the nausea and vomiting is getting a bit better.

At this point she has been taking Sepia for about 10 days. We repeated the LFT's and unfortunately, they were still rising.

LFTs	30.7.20	6.8.20
Total Bilirubin (up to 1)	4.09	8.21
Direct (Up to 0.25)	2.34	5.37
Indirect (Up to 0.75)	1.75	2.84
SGOT/AST (Up to 40)	411.6	543.1
SGPT/ALT (Up to 40)	491.6	652.7

The patient's state is still indicating Sepia. There are no major characteristic symptoms except for her sleepiness. We continue with Sepia 1M every 3 hours.

The patient continued on like this for a few days, saying her appetite was a bit better. We had also advised in this time to get the ANA test. We continue with the Sepia 1M every 3 hours. This continued for 4 more days, at which point the ANA had come back positive (indicating auto-immune hepatitis). Her Gastroenterologist had advised complete bed rest. He also advised that she would require steroids and that if there was no improvement the prognosis was not good and could result in cirrhosis of the liver. She was also advised to undergo LFT's weekly and a sonography of abdomen every 3 weeks.

After 15 days of treatment with Sepia her LFT's came back showing the following;

LFTs	30.7.20	6.8.20	14.8.20	20.8.20
Total Bilirubin (up to 1)	4.09	8.21	8.77	11.18
Direct (Up to 0.25)	2.34	5.37	5.43	10.11
Indirect (Up to 0.75)	1.75	2.84	3.34	1.07
SGOT/AST (Up to 40)	411.6	543.1	662.8	648.8
SGPT/ALT (Up to 40)	491.6	652.7	619.9	595.6
S. Alkaline phosphate (48-279)	140.5	113.3	104.3	109.1 (35-105 U/L)
GGTP (5-61)			137.4	142.2 (3-40 U/L)

There was no improvement in LFT's. Here the patient was wanting to stick with homeopathic treatment. So, we prescribed Sepia 10M every 6 hours. We also referred her for a WISE review. This is for two reasons, firstly the WISE in itself can be a beneficial therapeutic process and secondly it would be able to get to the patient's deepest state and confirm if Sepia is still covering the case.

Dr Sarah Coutinho then conducted the WISE review with the patient;

The patient was sent some questions beforehand in order to prepare her for the session —

PRE-WISE QUESTIONS

1. Your Fears —

   Of being alone especially in the dark

2. What are you sensitive to physically and emotionally, what do you hate, how does it affect you?

   Physically- Sensitive to cold

   Emotionally - When I have to do something that I don't want to do I feel then, as if I am not free.

3. Interests and Hobbies- what do they do to you? —

   Mostly, I read. I like to paint. Sometimes, I watch movies. Of late, nothing much

4. Recurrent dreams

   None now a days. Years earlier, I used to get dreams of trains and railway stations- of me going somewhere, sometimes getting off at the wrong place, sometimes missing the train and everyone else on it etc.

5. Situations that affect / affected you and how?

   That my son shows no interest in his studies and is okay with not exerting bothers me. I feel like caught on a situation from where I can't run.

6. Preference in colours, smells, and aversions

   Usually pastel colours. Yellows. No particular preference in smells

7. Complete details of your past and current physical complaints, since when has it started, what makes it better or worse etc.

   Hypothyroidism and goitre since 2001. Now, thyroiditis. On eltroxin 100. Putting on weight makes goitre worse.

   Hepatitis since last month.

The patient is then shown the picture of a statue of a man and asked to describe all that is happening —

> *It seems to be some sort of a Greek person. I assume it is in those times when there used to be kings in Greece. Doesn't seem to be a king but must be an advisor. He has a worried expression, and he seems to be thinking. He found out that the king is unfit to rule, and he has to save the kingdom. Possibly there are certain qualities that a king needs to rule, and he has found the current ruler doesn't have the qualities. His loyalty is towards the kingdom, and he realises the kingdom needs someone to rule. Something core to being a king he doesn't have, the ability to have a vison, deliver and govern, it is not something trivial and that which can be overlooked. Something core to being a king. The advisor is very concerned for the future of the kingdom. And possibly his options are limited which is why he is worried. He has a question in his head, and he is mulling over it. It is like the question never leaves him. There is no interest in anything else. This is something that has to be resolved immediately so he cannot relax.*

You have described his situation very nicely. Now just see what his inner experience is to be in this situation. Take your time, no hurry at all. —

> *Always a tension in the body (HG- her fingers close to form a fist) when you sit in a posture you don't realise you are not sitting well and suddenly you realise that you were not sitting well. The body is very tense (repeats the same HG fist). It is like grabbing and holding. Some sort of a will, some force. It is like a pushing through which need not necessarily be in an ease state. It is pushing through. When I close my fist, I get in a state of extreme alertness. It is like how you become very alert to fight. It is as if there is a situation which needs a fight. Something needs to be done urgently. Breath becomes faster and I can feel my heartbeat, which usually happens when I am in a stressed state, and I have to deliver something. Push through force, something needs to be done and it is unconducive, so extra amount of force that needs to be applied to get that work done. So have to push it through. Enforce, and impose. (Pause- she smiles)*

Here we can start to see some of the Superclass features. The state of being alert is very important in the 5th Superclass. This is a good differentiation with the 6th superclass. In the 6th Superclass the response is as if the tiger is attacking you. In the 5th Superclass the response is as if tiger is around the corner and is about to attack you, so you constantly have to be on alert. We can see this in the representative Neurotransmitter of the 5th superclass: Histamine. The function of Histamine are to respond to foreign invaders in the body and mount a defence against them. We can see this characteristic alertness very clearly as a part of it. And in this case where part of the patient's dynamic is to be alert, and ready to get out at any moment.

Something is going on, you are smiling, what is it? Say a little…

(Patient laughs) —

> *It seems like grabbing a prey (laughs). HG (Moves her fingers slowly up and down and then makes a fist). Some tentacles and it reaches out to food. Like how snake charmers hold the snake like that. Under sea creatures like jellyfish, they eat their food like this. Tentacles look like fingers, white, like octopus or hydra like, tentacles seem to be squishy. As if there are stones and you go through the stones. Blue under water. Boredom feeling that this all that there is to it and there is nothing more. There seems to be no great experiences, the same thing again and again. One day seems like the next. Feels bored. Lethargy, slowing, Fatigued. Everything slowing. Just want to laze and lie around. Opposite is purposeful work, meaningful work.*

The patient goes very readily to a deeper level and gives us some very useful information. For example, we can see the features of the animal kingdom in this extract. The idea of predator and prey is the very key in the animal kingdom. We even see her talking about animals which are very similar to Sepia and belong in the same group of cephalopods to it like the octopus. So, we can see the relation to the source here.

And what would that be like? —

> *That would feel like HG (opens the palm) opening up and expanding HG (hand open). It would feel…. Expanding. Freedom, joy, happiness. Like blooming of a flower. It is opening up. Open is where there is movement happening (moves hands from side to side) things come in and go out ventilated. Breeze coming through and through (HG). Swaying. Moving from one extreme to another or one side to another. I am getting an image of one video they had showed…. in the storm one tree moving end to end. Fun and excitement. There is something happening which is exciting. It feels*

energetic, filling you with energy. Feels like you are in control. Like you are not failing. That you can do. Things are moving smoothly. Whatever planned to do moving smoothly. According to the plan, without any glitch. Without something that will need you to spend more energy or do more work to overcome. Not being in control is when things are falling apart. Too many things to pay attention to and each has a mind of its own and you cannot bring it together. It is like a riot kind of situation. Not much control, each act on own agenda. It would go out of hand, there would be agitation and tension. In the chest there is a sensation as if spreading outwards, of the same kind of feeling can hear your heartbeat and tension in the body.

We need to be careful when analysing the information from this extract. We could be misled and think that expansion and freedom could point to the 3rd Superclass. This is not the dynamic she is talking about. It is a sensation and therefore does not belong to the Superclass information. The important information which we can use to confirm the Superclass is the modality of amelioration from movement.

Describe this sensation as if spreading outwards —
(She closes her eyes spontaneously)

Like a heart which is like a sponge and when it pumps it releases blood and you can see it spread all through. Something which has a centre where intensity is maximum and as it goes outwards the intensity reduces. There is a red sponge ball with ink stained and when you dip it in water and squeeze it, it releases in the water and becomes dilute. In the centre it will be more intense and as it spreads it will dilute as it goes and then it is not there. Until it pumps again that ink and then release again. Like a writing ink… it is blue in colour. Squeezing of that ball which is saturated with ink. It colours the water around. To give something to the rest of the place, to communicate. It could be to transfer something from one point to another or just let everyone around know that the ball exists. I get the image of lot of exactly same colour things and then one is different. Everything exactly same and one different, eyes go to that. It doesn't realise that it is different. It can't see itself. It would want to explore and know itself.

Again, we come to the expression of the source of the remedy. This squirting of the ink is a clear link with Sepia's defence mechanism of squirting ink in order to escape from predators. When we have such a clear connection with the source of the remedy, we can be 100% sure the remedy we have selected is correct.

You had said something earlier about expansion and freedom. Can you describe this a little bit more? —

> *Expanding and freedom, it is like being outside. In an open place. You are one with it and you are that open. Feels free. When you can choose anything, you want.*

What would happen otherwise? —

> *The opposite having only one option and it is something you have to take. And if it is an option, I don't like I would not like it at all. I will try and escape. I will go through it grudgingly but will feel someone has clipped my wings. Feels restricted. As if someone has imposed on me. Like imposed their will on me and I am not ok with that, and I feel powerless. Like nowhere to run, nowhere to go. It's like going through a very narrow tube or place (HG- shows a small space with her hands), no way you can turn left or right. Only if the tube turns, but it is very narrow and only one way to go. Feels aloneness and boredom. Powerless feels like caught between the things. Like a fly caught between a tweezer. Like all your might you take to try but you cannot break through. Cannot fly. HG (Hands joined).*

This is a great differentiation between the 5th and the 3rd superclass. In the 3rd superclass there is no external force which is limiting you. You are the one limiting yourself for whatever reason. We can see this in the animal group of the 3rd superclass, namely the birds. Take the example of a falcon. Once Falcons are trained, they are no longer physically bound. There is nothing stopping them from flying away. They get trained into staying with their owner, they limit themselves. They are not limited externally. Whereas in the 5th Superclass they desperately want to get out of the situation. They feel as if they are being blocked or obstructed by an external force. This is what we are seeing in the dynamic of this case. She feels like she is under the power of some greater force which is not allowing her to escape.

Tell me about this HG —

> *Pair of tweezers and there is a fly in that unable to fly. It feels powerless. Something so big and so huge that all the strength of the fly cannot help it*

to escape. It was caught unaware. Going about its way and someone just caught it. To restrict in a particular direction. As if shackles tied on the feet. Wherever you are going there is so much heavy load you are carrying. Can't go as high as you want to. It tires you just doing a little bit.

Whatever you are saying is helping me to understand you better. Can you say what is the opposite of this? —

Opposite is flying freedom, movement, free movement, lightness. It's like how a butterfly soars and flies. Happy. Like an opening up, HG (fingers apart), Expansion, sense of belonging with everything around. Like the clouds which just move in all directions, and everything is open the entire sky is open for the clouds to move, and it just moves any how it wants to. Not like boxing in HG (Shows a box with her hands). Like you are fitted in, no other place to go only one. It would be terrible to be boxed in and fitted in. You lose the zest. Like you look for ways to escape. Feels anguish, sadness, and frustration.

And now we can understand this sensation of expansion and freedom even more. We can see here clearly it is the sensation (not the dynamic) and is an expression of the broader dynamic: namely to get out.

We now show the patient the picture of a statue of woman (the first one that we usually show) and repeat the process —

It looks to me that she is some sort of maid who has been turned out of her work and her clothes are wet. May be because of something she did but the shock and sadness in her face shows that she was not responsible for being turned out. A lot of worry ahead and sense of unfairness. Big turmoil for her. Worried about the future. She had planned a longer time with the job and that won't happen. She is worried because she is turned out and she will not get a job because of bad reference and the injustice and unfairness of the whole deed. It was a misunderstanding. Possibly she was at the wrong place at the wrong time. Things just pointed towards her, and it was convenient to remove her rather than take a risk. Her blood rushed to her face. Hands shaking. Perspiration, Lot of heat in the face. Some sort of sensation in the chest and abdomen. Like something squirting. Like a balloon which is squirting. Like a water balloon which is filled and squirts water. Like the ball in the previous example. Squirting is shooting of a liquid out like a jet from one or more places. When pressure is applied

> *the content inside would leak and will find a way to escape out and with a pressure it just squirts.*

Here again we come back to the source quality and reconfirm our remedy selection.

The next picture we show the patient is of the first tree and ask her to describe what is happening —

> *One tree standing, doesn't have too many leaves, birch tree and against the sunset; it is nice to look at. The blue and yellow of the sunset and small bushes around. Contentment. As being still. There is no activity, no great activity. Everything in harmony moving smoothly. Without any roughness. Like a nicely polished surface, of glaze, shine. Touching it is nice pleasurable cool. Being on it is like the causation of falling, slipping. Imagining walking on it there has to be caution. Experience of being very alert. All your attention only on walking.*

What does alert mean? —

> *Alert is when all senses are active, and you are constantly aware of many things in the environment and very heightened awareness. Like a tiger on a prowl. Or even a deer when it is sensing a tiger and is very alert. All its senses are alert. Like all your body is in a very tense state, not relaxed there, all parts standing up. Very alert. And scanning everywhere. Almost like you are stopping your breath-(HG) (fist -same gesture done previously), just hearing, don't make any unnecessary movement or sound, tenseness across the body and every movement is deliberate.*

What are you showing with your hand? —

> *Holding, grabbing. When you take something forcefully. I remember having seen snake charmers holding the snake and preventing it from striking. When they remove the snake, they remove it by the tail and then they hold by the neck, and they hold like this (HG). The snake will feel restriction of movement. If it wants to go wherever and it is not allowed to go. It would have fun going elsewhere, but it just gives in. People give in for peace, to avoid conflict.*

The features of the 5th Superclass are very clearly defined in this WISE process. We can recognise all the remedies which fall in this Superclass. Here

we can see the Anacardiacaeae type of restriction of movement which she describes about the snake. It is possible to see features of any of the remedies of a given Superclass in a case of the same Superclass.
In this case we could see the clear animal kingdom features. We know that it cannot be an Anacardiacaeae remedy. Even though we recognise some features of the family.

We show the patient the picture of the second tree and repeat the process —

Looks like the tree is in full bloom. It is very eye catching. Very attractive and pleasant to the eye. It gives me joy to see this. It feels as if everything is in harmony.

Where everything is exactly where it is supposed to be. Become one with the scene. Everything has a place and perfect piece in jigsaw.

What would be the opposite? —

Opposite is chaos. Too many things cannot figure out. Everything all together, giving up just too much chaos. Lots happening within, cannot relax and find quietness. Unpredictability. When you cannot be prepared. Like lightening or climate. You don't know how the weather is. If raining one cannot predict when lightening will strike, its erratic.

We move on to the next picture and show the picture of the Swans —

It looks like two swans. One of them is actually scolding the other, the other is feeling guilt ridden and hanging head in shame. That swan didn't listen to the 1st one. It did whatever it wanted to. Didn't listen, wanted to do what it wanted. But it didn't work out according to the plan and something must have happened which is not good. Sad for being scolded but not for what she has done. It is the feeling you get when you want to do what you wanted. Even if it doesn't happen according to you. You won't blame self. Feels good that you can explore, create own experience. The opposite is being told what to do. Imposed on, it is as if someone is always directing you poking you, someone sitting on your head all the time. Making you go where they want to go. Like mahout sits on top of elephant and directs him and pokes it and he has to do what mahout wants it to. Total lack of freedom and powerlessness. Of giving up. Everything falling apart getting scattered. It is like a set of marbles in a formation, and you put a ball and it scatters you don't know where it has gone. Going in every

> *direction in which you cannot predict. At various speeds. Failure, giving up, tired, feels as if he is of no use, feels there is no purpose of his being. Failing in one thing is ok, failing in everything is like you are of no use. Feels he cannot do anything.*

This scattered sensation has also come previously in the case, and it is interesting to note that the Fabales fall within the 5th Superclass where we can find the sensation of being scattered.

Next, we show the picture of the baby goat —

> *Grazing in a meadow or some place. Just happy. Content. He is exactly where he is supposed to be. It is a pretty open place and that is what he is meant to do. If they put him in a cage, he will be unhappy. Right now, it is the open place which is contributing to his happy state. He will feel in a wrong place. There will not be enough space for him. Because it is a small cage. A cage is much, much smaller than an open pasture. And it will not be beautiful or pleasant to the eyes. Cage is an artificial place; it is not nice and green and with flowers.*

Imagine this situation you have just described. Take your time and imagine it fully.

What would be the experience to be in this situation?

> *Crowded (HG) too many things in the same place so not much place to move. Lots of things compressed in one place. Feeling of compression, of restriction. Tight, Heavy tense.... Everything being alert and tense. Fight at any moment kind of state. Alert as if a fight will happen and how you are alert. Like I said I feel something oozing, like in my stomach HG (hands slightly apart), something oozing, something is releasing. Coming out like liquid, from something which is permeable. Coming out of liquid. Like squeezing and releasing. Squeezes and something ooze out. That ball image comes to me, when you press it, the ball has some different colour liquid and when you press it, a different colour mixes in the water. Ink red in colour. Last time blue colour I saw, royal blue. Blue black in colour but now it was red. It slowly diffuses like that. Presses from all directions, get compressed, and when releases come back to original shape.*

Again, we see the features of the 5th superclass: this feeling of restricted movement, and tight like the Anacardiacaeae and Euphorbiaceae and the need to be alert as if a fight is about to happen and along with source qualities of the ink in the water, we are again confirming our remedy and can be so confident that it cannot be any other remedy.

Anything else you would like to share? –

> *My biggest issue is when I don't spend time with "me" doing things what I want. When this happens, my problems start kicking in. I feel I should first give all time for me and then give to him. My son is extremely strong willed. There are several things that affect me - That I am not allowed to do what I want is definitely one. How stuck I am in a thought, that only if you do this you are successful and worthy. Otherwise, worthless, useless. I locate a worth for an activity. I experience it at one end of spectrum and at the other end I do it. I make my son do this, you have to do it, borders have to be like this. He may just want to explore. I want him to do what I want to do. My younger one feels like me, there was an incident once when I forcefully made him wash his hair when he didn't want to and next day, he got fever. I know it was because I made him do it. I realised that was the cause, this is similar that he felt there is no other way and then he gave in to me. And I feel this way too. Elder one he gets angry and throws tantrums, like how I used to throw tantrum like how dad used to be with me. My father was particular about studies, slept at 8.30 till my marriage, very disciplined rhythm. I used to burst out in anger. Throw tantrums, hit him, scratch him once he cools down. I was a bit reined in by my dad. Controlled. HG (hand in fist moving back) Pulling back. Recently I was thinking he should not feel like this or make himself sick to get out of situation. I feel at some level I have brought it out on myself, this disease so that I can escape the situation.*

This is the power of the WISE process. We can see the awareness that we are able to bring out in the patient. Even the description to escape the situation is the exact context of the Superclass. She has realised that this disease is the expression of her Superclass. This awareness on its own can have therapeutic value.

We are also able to see how in every situation she is only able to describe her own inner state. Even when she is talking about her son, she is describing her own inner pattern. We can see the exact characteristic symptoms of Sepia in this description of her son.

She continues —

I was working for 10 years then quit. Had to stay away from son. Was not able to relax in work. Fly every Monday morning and then go home on Friday. Only for weekends. Work was extremely demanding. Before this I was in another company and it was nice there because I had my "me" time, here I didn't get I was managing so many projects, all the time. No time for me. So, I realise I like when I work and then can chill and then work again. So was not enjoying, Also, there was the angst of leaving my child. I am happy with the decision of not working. I felt sorry for my parents. They had done so much for my studies. Moved to Mumbai to care for my son so that I work. They knew I was doing well, and they were proud. I was feeling bad of letting them down. That was my conflict.

What are your physical complaints? —

No symptoms as such, just urine yellow and eyes yellow. I feel tired all the time. Slight stiffness in finger joints. They have advised me bed rest. Even with the thyroid issue, no symptoms only swelling.

— End of Case —

Following the WISE process, we continued the patient on Sepia 10M every 6 hours. 5 days after starting the Sepia 10M the LFT's were repeated;

LFTs	30.7.20	6.8.20	14.8.20	20.8.20	27.8.20
Total Bilirubin (up to 1)	4.09	8.21	8.77	11.18	9.23
Direct (Up to 0.25)	2.34	5.37	5.43	10.11	8.16
Indirect (Up to 0.75)	1.75	2.84	3.34	1.07	1.07
SGOT/AST (Up to 40)	411.6	543.1	662.8	648.8	576.5
SGPT/ALT (Up to 40)	491.6	652.7	619.9	595.6	489
S. Alkaline phosphate (48-279)	140.5	113.3	104.3	109.1 (35-105 U/L)	102
GGTP (5-61)			137.4	142.2 (3-40 U/L)	131.1

Here we can see some improvement in the LFT's however according to the sonography there were cirrhotic changes to the liver. This was the day which the patient was scheduled for the WISE review. Following the WISE review we had the confidence to continue the Sepia 10M in spite of the liver changes. Following this we repeated the LFT's 5 days later and saw even further improvement.

This patient had a very long follow up as this was a very severe progressive pathology, but from this moment on we continued with the Sepia 10M 6 hourly and daily there was improvement physically and emotionally. The shrinking of the liver was halted and eventually it regained the normal size. See the before and after reports;

USG UPPER ABDOMEN

LIVER:
Liver appears slightly shrunken in size, (10.2 cm) with normal shape and echotexture. There is no intra-hepatic biliary radical dilatation. No evidence of any focal lesion.

Three months later —

USG UPPER ABDOMEN

LIVER:
Liver is normal in size,(11.4 cm) shape and echotexture. There is no intra-hepatic biliary radical dilatation. No evidence of any focal lesion.

The LFT's were also repeated for a long time to track her progress and we can see the continued improvement below;

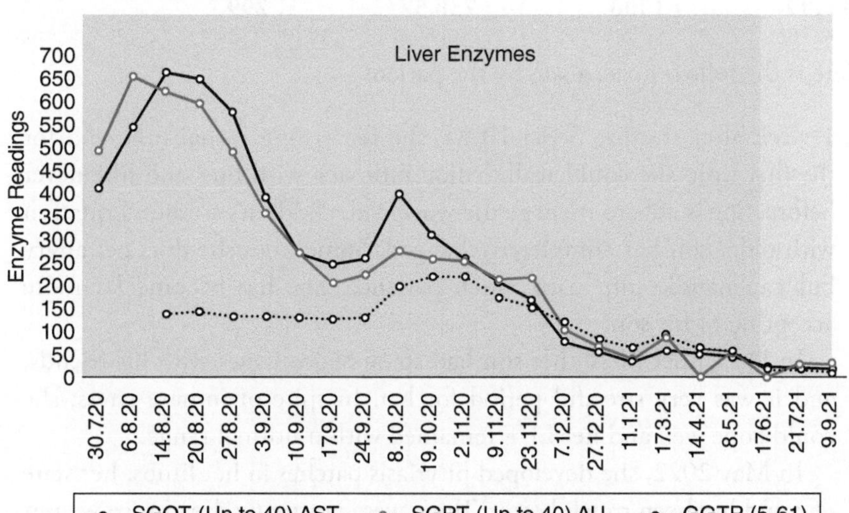

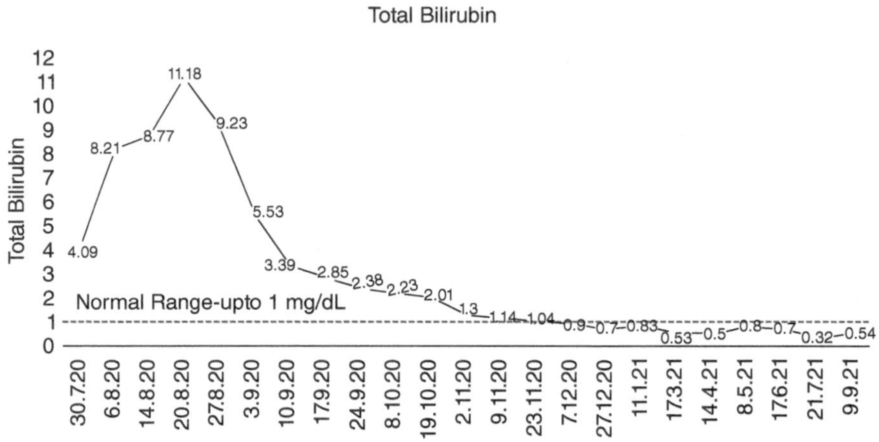

The Patient's thyroid levels were also monitored, and we can see the improvement in these —

	17/02/2019	30/07/2020	11/01/2020
Total T3		183.2(69-215)	—
Free T3	2.69 (1.50-4.10)	2.90 (2 – 4.4)	5.30 (3.5-6.5 pmol/L)
Total T4		**13.87 (5.2-12.7)**	—
Free T4	1.15 (0.80-1.90)	1.23 (0.93 – 1.7)	19.3 (11.5-22.7 pmol/L)
TSH	1.38 (0.40-4)	2.41 (0.32-4.35)	—
Sensitive TSH			0.703 (0.35-5.5)
ATPO	**>1300**	**738.57**	**299**

Here is the follow up as given by the patient –

> 1 week after starting Sepia 10 M, she felt strong sexual urge and for the first time she could really enjoy intimacy with husband like never before. She is able to manage the workload, children's studies. Equation with older son has completely changed. Sometimes she does get angry but can handle him with much patience. She has become far more accepting of his son.
>
> In December 2020, her son had some major issues with his friends, and it was very stressful period for her. In spite of intense stress, she could cope well and her LFT remained within normal range.
>
> In May 2022, she developed pityriasis patches in her limbs, her state of mind has been much better. There were not many dreams, so we put her on Sepia 200 and LM 6 and she continues to be doing well.

Case 17

To better illustrate the features of the 6th superclass we can look at a case example.

This is the case of a 45-Year-old male who was suffering from vertigo and nausea. He begins to narrate the complaints —

The vertigo started in 2014 very suddenly. I had drunk a lot of alcohol that night and following day the ear pain and vertigo started. What bothers me the most is the vertigo. There is also mild hearing loss in both ears, right-side more than left. It is very severe. The vertigo starts suddenly and the surroundings rotate it is worse when I am sitting, standing, making any movement, loud noise, cold things, exertion, looking out of the window while travelling, looking at the computer screen. It is better when I rest and sleep. Along with the vertigo I get vomiting. At that time, I want darkness and silence. I cannot bear noise or light. There is also this ringing in the right ear.

We ask him what the effect of this complaint on him is —

There is an imbalance in my life. I am not able to go out or attend social gatherings. I have a fear that I will not be able to go out because the complaints may come on.

Before the complaints I used to work a lot, all the time. Apart from my main job I had a side job for extra income. I would never rest at all. It was non-stop work. Since the complaints became worse, I have reduced my work a lot because I am afraid that I will get some problem and it will ignite something worse. I am afraid it may start during a meeting. There is a constant fear about that. So, I prefer to avoid it.

The patient also has some other complaints which he tells us about —

I suffer from constipation, there is an unsatisfactory feeling after passing stool. My appetite is reduced. I have heaviness and bloating in the abdomen. It feels tight. I feel better when drinking warm water but I am worse when I eat non-vegetarian food or heavy food.

I have been having a fungal infection since 4 years. It is on the face and neck mainly. Also, on the right leg and right toe there is a blackish discoloration on the face, it gets worse from exposure to the sun and starts to itch.

I have backpain in the lumbar region it is worse when I have been standing for a long time and feels better when sitting or lying down.

We also elicit the following physical generals of the patient –

Desire- sweets +++, meat, spicy food, rice, cold water
Aversion-Tomatoes, sour food +++
Thermals- hot ++
Sleep- Unrefreshing. Sleepiness after eating
Agg- sun +++, *I never go in the sun. I cannot bear it. I get weakness in the sun, uneasy feeling. I like rains, going in the water, in the cold breeze.*

Noting all the physical complaints, we ask the patient to tell us about himself —

I used to be very aggressive earlier. Now I bear and accept things. I used to be very social and didn't like to stay alone. I used to always be travelling and going out either with family or with friends. Since the vertigo I am avoiding it completely. I like things to be neat and clean, kept in their correct place or else I get very irritated. I feel that work should be completed on time. While working I feel an intense anxiety just to finish my work and get free. There are other times when I am very lazy. A certain standard should be maintained even if it takes a lot more money. Whether it be the place I stay or how my family behaves, it should be maintained very well. It should not be cheap at all.

I don't like black and dark colours. It is not that I am afraid. But lighter and brighter colours make me feel relaxed. I like nature, farms, greenery. I want to live in such places which are very peaceful and quiet.

We ask the patient to tell us what he is afraid of—

I get so much anxiety and so much tension when I see a fight. It could be anywhere in the world. If I hear of it I get very tensed. Same with any accident on the road, if I just get the news of it, I get a lot of anxiety. I am fearful that it might happen to me. I am too scared of quarrels and accidents. It is like a constant fear that if I go and intervene in fights then they might hit me. If there is a quarrel in my area they might damage my family members. They will use swords and knives and I will be beaten up when it is not my mistake. I have a fear of heights since getting vertigo

We can start to see some of the patient's individuality here in his fears, especially in the sensitivity to violence and injury. In order to take it further we ask him what he is sensitive to —

Rape of minors and other such things which are torturous. A mob is attacking a small family with swords in their hands and they will kill them.

Again, the theme of violence and injury comes strongly in this case. It is important to understand that this is not the sensation but the theme of the Superclass. We must be very careful when sorting our information. We must be able to differentiate between the two. This is often easier done in retrospect.

So, when we are taking the case we don't have to jump to conclusions. We can just listen and keep everything in the back of mind. When the next piece of information comes it often puts the previous information into context. We will be able to see that in this case. When we study this case we can see that his basic dynamic is that of violence and injury, this indicates the Superclass.

We can also see that there is sensation and the reaction thus indicating the plant kingdom. When can see in this case the main features of Asteriidae (6th subclass of the Dicotyledons).

We need to see the other features and aspects of the patient that can indicate the specific order and remedy characteristics...

We ask the patient to tell us about his dreams —

> *I am not sure if you can call them dreams because I don't get them only at night. I imagine all the time even when I am awake. I imagine things like Mukesh Ambani (Indian Billionaire businessman) will become my friend and business partner. He is investing in my ideas and my plans. I imagine that I have got some super powers and even the prime minister is under me. I will kill all the enemies of India and will kill them in public. Nobody can see me and if I touch someone he becomes invisible.*
>
> *Some more things which I keep imagining are that I will construct a home in 5-10 acres of land, in a posh mountain area with huge rooms. It will have all the luxuries one can imagine. Everyone is working for me. I will have my own school and my own industrial estate.*
>
> *Everyone will listen to me and ask me for solutions. I will have a lot of money. Everyone would be under me. I am constantly working on ideas for this and planning how to make this happen. I will build a campus and a huge school committee and will give high posts to all my relatives and then I will see them growing. I keep planning these things in finer and finer detail. I discuss these ideas with my wife. My brain is full of ideas especially at night, while I am in bed and trying to sleep. Many nights I fall asleep thinking all these things. I try to do all this but because I am lazy and tired, I have not been able to do them yet. Then I think what am I going to get from all this? I feel sometimes that human beings are just running behind money. It would be better if I just enjoy my life and rest. What is the point of this rat race anyway?*

When we come to study this case we can see there are two aspects —

1. 6TH SUBCLASS

We can see the features of the 6th subclass, such as his fear of dark colours. He talks of accidents, fights, mob killings, rape and torture. There is the fear someone will beat him and use violent weapons such as swords and knives.

Within the subclass features we also see the Rubiales and Rubiaceae themes. Then within the Rubiaceae family we see his constant imagination and vivid fancies such as having superpowers, being friends with billionaires, killing all the enemies of India, and of people he touches becoming invisible. This begins to point to the remedy China. Later we will also discuss the features of the miasm which are very helpful in also confirming China as the remedy from the Rubiaceae.

2. SULPHUR

There is a second aspect to him which does not belong to 6th subclass or the Rubiaceae or to the remedy China. This includes his qualities of being lazy, image conscious, egoistic. He speaks of the standard that must be maintained even if it takes more money. He is particular that the image his family portrays mustn't be seen as cheap. This aspect belongs to Sulphur.

The Miasm of the case is also clear, we can see that the effect of the complaint is that it hinders his life. He is constantly anticipating and avoiding. This is the Malarial miasm. When we look at the Rubiaceae family and the corresponding miasms we will also note that China and China sulph are both remedies of the Malarial miasm.

We also make sure that we cover every aspect of the case when check the 8 boxes;

Organ affected	Symptoms	Physical generals	Effect of complaint
Ear Back Skin	Decreased hearing Tinnitus Vertigo Vomiting Pain Fungal infection, blackish discolouration on the face	Sun agg Alcohol agg Sweets desires Hot patient <sitting, standing, movement, loud noise >rest, sleep	Afraid to go out, avoids it, anticipation that if he goes out or works too much complaints will agg
Nature	**Delusion**	**Kingdom**	**Miasm**
Earlier aggressive Fastidious Lazy Wants to maintain a certain standard Family should not behave in a cheap manner	Constant imagination, fantasies, planning, Fantasies but doesn't put into action Fear – Fights Accidents Beaten, attacked with swords and knives Rape and torture Mob killings	Plant Kingdom 6th Subclass	Malarial Anticipation, avoidance, hindered

We can also see the exact symptom in the materia medica —

Phatak's Concise MM ✖

EARS.

Tinnitus. Deafness. Meniere's disease.

Rubrics;

Generalities —

	Sulph.	Ars.	Lach.	Nat-c.	Nat-m.	Phos.	Psor.	Calc.	Lyc.	Con.	Tax.	Chin.	Arg-n.	Bry.	Carb-v.	Graph.
Total	23	19	19	19	18	18	18	17	15	14	8	20	18	18	18	18
Rubrics	6	6	6	6	6	6	6	6	6	6	6	5	5	5	5	5
Kingdom																
CR19 - Generalities; Closing; eyes; agg.(218)	4	3	4	3	3	4	3	4	1	4	1	4	3	4	4	3
CR19 - Face; Black(78)	3	3	3	1	2	2	3	1	1	1	1	4		3	3	3
CR19 - Generalities; Food and drinks; sweets; desires(295)	4	2	1	3	2	3	3	3	4	1	1	4	4	3	3	4
CR19 - Generalities; Warmth; agg.(637)	4	4	4	4	4	4	4	4	4	3	1	4	4	4	4	4
CR19 - Generalities; Weakness; warmth agg.(59)	4	3	3	4	3	1	1	1	1	1	1		3			
CR19 - Generalities; Exercise, exertion; agg.(736)	4	4	4	4	4	4	4	4	4	4	3	4	4	4	4	4

Vertigo —

	Chin.	Cocc.	Kali-c.	Glon.	Petr.	Bell.
Total	16	22	21	20	18	17
Rubrics	8	7	7	7	7	7
Kingdom						
CR19 - Vertigo; Sitting; agg.(164)	3	4	3	3	3	1
CR19 - Vertigo; Lying; amel.(119)	3	4	3		3	3
CR19 - Vertigo; Vomiting; with(92)	1	4	3	3	3	2
CR19 - Vertigo; Hunger, fasting agg.(10)	1		3			
CR19 - Vertigo; Motion; agg.(215)	3	4	3	3	1	3
CR19 - Vertigo; Motion; agg.; head, of(98)	1	1	3	3		3
CR19 - Mind; Alcohol, alcoholic drinks; agg.(53)		1		3	3	1
CR19 - Vertigo; Nausea; with(246)	3	4	3	3	4	4
CR19 - Vertigo; Violent(56)	1			2	1	

Mind – (Note the 6th superclass remedies)

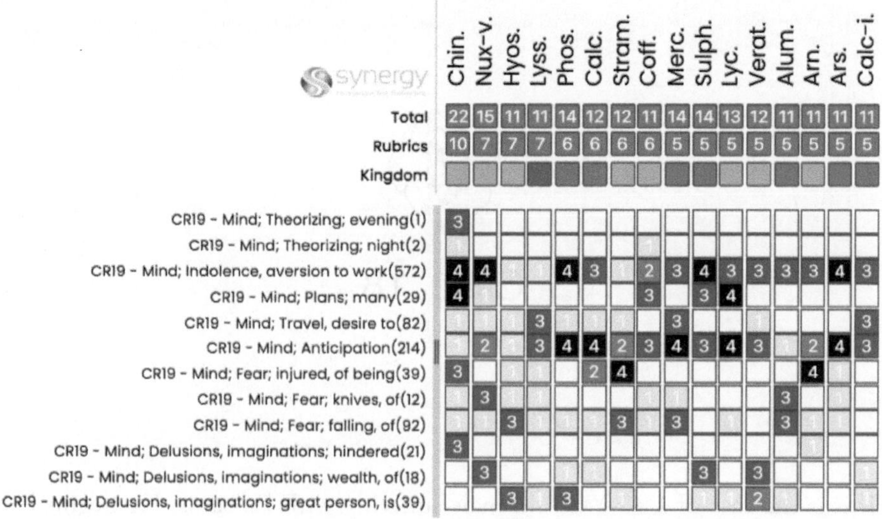

Based on the all the information that we have analysed we prescribed to the patient China Sulph 1M. This is the patient's follow up after 2 years of treatment —

> *I am feeling fine now. No vertigo at all now. Vertigo is 100 percent better. No vomiting, no tinnitus. Ringworm has almost disappeared completely. Fears and anxiety much better. No dreams of late. My normal life has been restored to me.*

For this case we have the summary of the classification of information —

Superclass	**6**
Kingdom	Plant
Subclass	Asteridae
Order	Rubiales
Family	Rubiaceae
Miasm	Malarial
Remedy	China Sulph

Case 18

This is the case of a 38-Year-old male suffering with Psoriasis. He begins his case narrating his complaints —

The Psoriasis started in 2011 It comes every 7-8 months. Started from the scalp. After my father's death in 2012, it increased a lot. There were many circular patches on my scalp. The skin patches soon spread to the whole body. There is a lot of itching, I would scratch it until it would bleed. Little white flakes would be there on the patches.

Also having joint pains which started around the same time. Swelling in the finger joints. There is swelling in the right leg. From the time the complaints increased, I am not able to run or do things. I feel I need to be cautious. Since November 2020, there is swelling in the right toe and slight pain has started.

We ask the patient how his complaints started —

At the time when it first started, I was working in a bank. I was trying to get into a government bank. I was the assistant bank manager in the bank and there was a lot of stress at that time. Also, my father was sick during that time, and I had constant stress about it. He was suffering from cancer. Fear of losing him was constantly there. It was cancer so we never knew if he is going to survive or not. Just hearing the word cancer –you feel scared. So, if your father is suffering then he will die.

When you have a parent, there is a guardian. You would be free. I didn't have responsibility. I used to take all his guidance. I used to take his advice. Now I feel as if everything is on me. All the responsibility came on me. No one to guide or support. Father was like a support.

I was 29 when he passed away. People are enjoying their life at this age. But then responsibility came, and life changed completely. Sudden and unexpected responsibility on me. I have to take responsibility of the house and family. When my father expired in 2012, I was with him a lot of the time. I never thought I would have to take responsibility of the family. Even though at that time I was single, unmarried.

I wanted to leave my job at that time. In my family everything had to be managed.

Feeling of loss was very severe. I used to keep thinking if he was alive things would have been managed. He would have managed as an elder of the family. But then everything came on me. It was very new to me. Whatever happened I had to involve myself in that.

It was very unexpected. It all came suddenly. But I managed everything. I managed my professional life, followed by managing my brothers and sister's wedding.

We ask the patient to tell us about his nature —

I like doing social service and involving in society. I manage my personal and professional life nicely. Whenever customers come, I try to help most of them. Even for my villagers I try to do some or the other thing. I am easily adjustable. I get angry when people do wrong things. For example: When people hate Narendra Modi (Prime-minister) and comment about him.

I feel like it is a respectable post so you shouldn't say like that. He didn't just reach there; he has reached there with our votes only. I only get angry if people say stupid things. Most of the times, I try and manage it coolly. I don't like people when they don't respect or say anything foolish. It really makes me angry.

The patient proceeds to tell us about his job —

I like my job a lot. In my job I am responsible for everything. I am like the branch head so I must take all responsibilities. I don't keep my work pending. I try to solve all the problems. I have worked a lot in my life and satisfaction is there.

We ask the patient to tell us about his interests and hobbies —

I like to do Yoga, walking, going to different places. I like listening to music - traditional, old 90's songs. I am more interested in politics. Like political debates. I like discussing about politics. I want to become a politician also. For whatever you want to do, you need power. If you are in power, then you can help a lot of people. I have been involved in politics. When we go to villages where people don't have basic necessities. I try to give them, but I can only give 5-10 people. I really feel good about it, but I feel If I help 1000 people - how happy I would be.

We ask the patient to tell us about his childhood —

I was playful. I used to study also. I was very mischievous. I used to mingle, and I had many friends. Childhood had dreams of flying. I was enjoying. I enjoyed reaching very fast from one place to another.

The patient then tells us about his fears —

Mostly about ghosts and snakes. Fear of darkness. They will kill and attack. Then we will die. There is a sudden noise, and some ghost is there. Fear is more at night, in the darkness, when alone.

We ask the patient what the effect of this complaint on him is —

I feel it is kind of irritating, is it going to stay with me whole life or not? It is like continuous. My future generation can get affected by it. I feel whatever troubles I am facing my kids shouldn't face.

Next, we ask about the dreams the patient gets —

Rarely get dreams. Mostly about office work. I don't get negative or fearful dreams like you are drowning in water. I don't get bad dreams like you are travelling, and you meet with an accident. You feel anxiety and palpitations with these kinds of dreams. Like they can cry in dreams like these. There is shivering, shrieking and kind of fearful voice. Dreams about my father. He would be scolding me. Dreams of losing loved ones.

We ask the patient what he is sensitive to —

When I saw my sisters bidaai (ceremony where the female leaves her father's house after marrying), I was emotional. Also, I am sensitive about memories of my father. If someone in the family is crying, then I feel like crying. If family gets affected, then I feel sad. Mostly about covid, about death of people, cremations. I feel when will things would get better. There is a kind of fear, anyone can die. If someone just speaks too much then I get irritated, like if someone is speaking something irrational.

The patient's physical generals are as follows —

- Appetite: good
- Desire: green vegetable, non – veg - chicken, mutton, red meat, fish+++, spicy, sweet like jalebi and rasgulla.
- Thirst: 4-5 litres, normal water, I take 1 glass at one time
- Sleep Position: on left side
- Urine: NC
- Stool: NC
- Sweat: forehead, axilla
- Thermal: Hot patient, likes more chilly

— End of Case —

Firstly, before analysing this case, we can sort all the information into the 8 boxes.

Diagnosis –	Local symptoms –	Physical Generals –	Mental symptoms –
Psoriasis Joint pains/ Psoriatic arthritis?	Severe itching until it bleeds Scaling in flakes	Desire- Meat, fish, sweets Thirst-4-5 l/day Sleep- left side Sweat-Forehead, axilla Thermals- Hot	Sadness death of father Felt responsible for everything. Angry when people don't respect others position Hardworking
Fears –	Dreams –	Kingdom –	Genius –
Ghosts, Snakes, Dark They will attack and kill	Losing loved ones Father scolding Sister's wedding Accidents	Mineral- Support, Capacity, Losing,	Very high sense of responsibility Loss of parent agg

Starting with the Superclass in this case which is coming? We can see him talking of the following things;

- Sudden, unexpected
- Ghosts
- Snakes
- Darkness
- Kill
- Attack
- Die

Here we can see the elements of the 6th Superclass.

The kingdom is quite clear. We see issues with support, capacity and losing. From this we can see the mineral kingdom in this patient.

Within the mineral kingdom, identifying the row is easy. We look at the main issue in the case : responsibility. We can see this in the stressful situations for the patient —

When father died – "I feel as if everything is on me. All the responsibility came on me. I was 29 when he passed away. People are enjoying their life at this age. But then responsibility came, and life changed completely. Sudden and unexpected responsibility on me."

"But I managed everything. I managed my professional life, followed by managing my brothers and sister's wedding."

We can see the same issue of responsibility in his job —

"In my job I am responsible for everything.
I am like the branch head so I must take all responsibilities."

Issues of responsibility belong to the 6th row of the periodic table. Reading from VitalQuest we get the following information about the 6th row —

> In Row 6 the issue is about taking up responsibility and leadership, the need for power and the ability to withstand high pressure of this responsible position. The attack at this level too is of a very high degree; their perception is that people are going to finish them because of their leadership.

Then looking at Column 11 —

- The structure stands by itself
- Will maintain itself in adverse circumstances
- Repeatedly facing attacks and challenges
- He has to maintain his/her successful position, hold on to it and defend it against any attacks

From this we get to the remedy Aurum. Are there any other aspects to the case? We see the following :

He is greatly affected by the death of his father. There was much dependence on his father.He says, "Even for my villagers I try to do some or the other thing. I am easily adjustable." "When I saw my sisters bidaai (ceremony where the female leaves her father's house after marrying), I was emotional. If someone in the family is crying, then I feel like crying. From this we can see that he also has a soft, sensitive, caring quality that we associate with the 3rd Superclass. Therefore he may need a salt of Aurum with 3rd row elements.

Key word for Aurum:
- Responsibility.

Pathology: Ischemia, stroke, apoplexy.
Excerpts summarized from earlier books:
Aurum is a syphilitic remedy. It is one of the heavy metals of row 6. In Aurum the feeling is that the person must perform tasks which are impossible or much beyond his capacity. He demands of himself industry and responsibility, conscientiousness and duty of the highest degree, uncompromising principles or goals that are beyond the possible.
He almost destroys himself in trying to achieve these goals, because if he does not achieve them, he gets the feeling of failure, guilt and despair of salvation. It is as if his very survival depended on his ability to take on these huge responsibilities. He is afraid of losing the confidence of others and of himself. He has a feeling that he may fall down from this high position. This can make him suicidal.
They are usually relieved tremendously by music. One of my early observations was that Aurum patients like to hear Bhajans (religious, devotional songs). Bhajans are Indian religious songs, which are sung with exact meter and with a lot of devotion. The combination of the following three components is only found in Aurum :
- Religiousness
- Music ameliorates
- Exactness

When we look at the rubric : Death, ailments from, we see Aur-mur-nat. The other rubrics of the case confirm the remedy.

Complete 2019 Repertory > Mind

Mind;Death;ailments from, agg. (65) : Acon., alum., ambr., ars., astac., aur-m-n., beryl., calc-ar., calc-sil., calc., caps., carc., caust., clem., con., cupr., erb-c., gall., garden., gels., germ., haliae-lc., hippo-k., hoch., hyper., IGN., Kali-br., kali-c., lac-c., lac-f., Lac-h., lach., lant-p., lat-m., lim-b-c., lyc., med., merc., nat-c., Nat-m., neod-p., Nit-ac., nux-m., nux-v., Op., par., pass-d., peg-h., Ph-ac., phos., plac., plat., rhod., salx-f., scorp., sile-c., spig., stann., staph., sulph., thul-o., uran., urt-c., urt-u., verat.

We can see the mind symptoms —

	Aur-m-n.	Ars.	Caust.	Aur.	Nat-m.	Merc.
Total	7	9	14	11	8	4
Rubrics	7	5	4	4	4	4
Kingdom						
CR19 - Mind; Death; ailments from, agg.; parents or friends, of(39)	1	1	4		3	1
CR19 - Mind; Responsibility; ailments from, agg.; unusual(4)	1			2		
CR19 - Mind; Anxiety; family, about his(73)	1	3	3		1	1
CR19 - Mind; Delusions, imaginations; neglected; duty, his(32)	1	1		4		
CR19 - Mind; Fear; alone, being; night(18)	1	1	3			
CR19 - Mind; Music; amel.(46)	1			4	1	1
CR19 - Mind; Sympathetic, compassionate, too(179)	1	3	4	1	3	1

The physical generals —

	Aur-m-n.	Carc.	Nit-ac.	Calc-p.	Nat-s.
Total	7	7	7	6	6
Rubrics	3	3	3	3	3
Kingdom					
CR19 - Generalities; Food and drinks; fish; desires(68)	1	1	3	1	3
CR19 - Generalities; Food and drinks; meat; desires(163)	2	3	1	4	1
CR19 - Generalities; Food and drinks; sweets; desires(295)	4	3	3	1	2

Skin and joint symptoms —

synergy	Aur-m-n.	Sulph.	Graph.	Lyc.	Calc.	Puls.	Sep.	Led.	Mag-c.	Merc.
Total	21	34	33	33	32	32	32	29	29	29
Rubrics	10	9	9	9	9	9	9	9	9	9
Kingdom										
CR19 - Skin; Eruptions(1167)	4	4	4	4	4	4	4	4	4	4
CR19 - Skin; Eruptions; itching(494)	3	4	4	3	4	3	4	4	4	4
CR19 - Skin; Eruptions; psoriasis(167)	1	3	3	4	3	3	4	2	2	3
CR19 - Skin; Itching; intolerable(48)	1	3	3		3	4				3
CR19 - Skin; Itching; violent(244)	1	4	4	3	3	4	3	3	2	3
CR19 - Extremities; Pain; joints; right(109)	1			3			3	1	3	
CR19 - Extremities; Pain; fingers(525)	4	4	4	4	4	4	4	4	4	4
CR19 - Extremities; Pain; fingers; joints(298)	1	4	4	4	4	3	4	3	3	1
CR19 - Extremities; Pain; joints(1005)	4	4	4	4	4	4	4	4	4	4
CR19 - Extremities; Swelling; joints(286)	1	4	3	4	3	3	2	4	3	3

Based on the conjunction of all this information we can be very confident in giving Aurum muriaticum natronatum 200. His follow up shares how well he has done on the remedy —

> *After taking the remedy there was a slight aggravation, then there was relief and it started coming down. I only needed to take allopathic medications twice. After that I haven't had to take again and I am completely fine thanks to you and the medicine. Wherever there were spots they have cleared and there is no irritation. Mood wise I am also better, I used to be stressed because of the condition, but now it is all good.*

The classification of the information is as follows —

Superclass	6
Kingdom	Mineral
Row	6
Remedy	Aurum mur nat

Case 19

This is the case of a 35-year-old Female, she is a theatre artist suffering with polyarthritis.

She begins with her current problem —

> *Right now, I am staying in K, but I can't deal with the cold weather. I have pain in the joints (knuckles), and every joint, back to neck. I have a different kind of headache and I can't figure out the location exactly. It is somewhere inside my brain. It's very painful and it just squeezes all my energy. It stops me from doing things. I don't feel like eating and it makes me sleepless. I have a lady who would massage me. She was very upset because she massaged and massaged with hot oil and put socks on me, but my feet never were warm. They would still be cold. I am always under tension. I feel very anaemic. Again, I find the root is there because I spent sleepless nights there. Whenever I come to warm weather I am sleeping well, so I have no problem.*

So what's the main problem at the moment?

> *I need energy; I feel so energy-less. I feel right now also kind of feverish, though the thermometer will give me the reading of 36.7 C. I can't take the strain of reading. I love to read, but after 1-2 pages I have to close the book.*

What happens?

> *It starts (head) paining. It starts moving to the ear, it's cramping (HG: opens and closes the fist). Everything is moving inside (same HG). It is stretching out, coming out and it's really happening inside (same HG).*

Describe this hand movement a little bit —

> *It's vague and then it's fullest, it's stretching, stretching and when squeezing, it's squeezing like anything, (HG: when she say's stretching her fist opens slowly but with force and when she says squeezing, she slowly closes her fist). So much strength is there, it's very pressured, (HG: tightly closing the fist), squeezing. It's like pumping. (HG: same opening and closing the fist). It's hot inside, like something boiling, like while cooking something. Before it dries up totally, (HG: hand movement indicating boiling) there is a point where that portion becomes hot (HG: starting from the head. frontal portion and pointing down). It comes down to the neck and shoulders. The pain comes to this point, (HG: middle canthus of eye) and then it comes to the eye, (above eye; moving fingers on the eyebrow), and the eyes are very tired. Somehow, I feel that these eyes and my inner energy are forcefully withdrawn, (HG: moving her hands, and pulling away from her). I don't want to close my eyes, but I need to close my eyes. Yet I am not sleeping. I am completely awake, but I am not responding.*

Describe this, what you have shown. Forcefully withdrawn, just that sensation.

> *Inside the whole energy is just squeezed, (HG: closing eyes and moving fist away from her as in squeezing). So much so, that hardly any energy stays with me.*
>
> *It is like while washing your clothes, the way you squeeze, (HG: squeezing clothes) every single drop. It's happening like that throughout, to the last point, (HG: same). Maybe the next step would be like this, (HG: opening her hands, as if blowing up). (HG: squeezing) Pressure and maybe this is the last capacity that the elastic can take, (HG: moving her hands away from her as if pulling a rubber). After that, will it open up at some time? (HG: hands going outwards from centre as if bursting). Maybe the cerebellum of the brain will come out.*

Just describe this movement a little bit more —

> *Speed you know, one thing comes out, bursts out, like a volcano. It's very much like an abstract painting, with so many colours, (HG), blood and basically the destruction, the pain.*

Describe the destruction a little bit more —

> *The destruction is destroying my existence. It's destroying everything; my peace, and my ability to work. When and how a sound sleep comes and the pain goes off, I am not in a state of mind to follow. Then I feel free, relieved.*

Describe the feeling in the joy, the experience of that feeling —

> *It's joy, simple joy. Joy in every level. I love to sleep. I love to eat. I love to sing. I love to listen to music. I love to talk to beloved persons. I think that is the way I enjoy. It's not restless inside. It's calm and quiet and it's very settled. It reacts to situations in a positive way. I love being a very quiet and calm person but actually I am not, I am very aggressive, (protrudes her tongue).*

What is very aggressive? —

> *If someone is harming another person, I will protest. I will go and jump into the trouble. I am very impulsive. I always listen to my heart. I am willing to do that. What will be the next result, next effect, I don't care about that. I think one person should care about that. That is the one problem. If I am very calm, quiet, and settled, then I also will jump in, but my process of jumping in it will be different. It will not be that aggressive.*
>
> *If I feel I should beat the person, definitely I will hit him. In a way, I will also keep it in mind that hitting him is only to protest to him or to make him understand that this is not good and there is no other way. But if I am not in that steady, quiet or calm state I will hit the person like anything. I will kick him and beat him, (HG: shows punching).*

(Important to note that while she says this, there is not much aggression on her face, with more or less a straight face.)

We have received some information about the main complaint and then the patient describes some aspects of herself. We can see that she is a very aggressive person. She is not timid or shy but extremely confrontational to the point of violence. With this it is easy for us to consider the 6th Superclass. She also describes how the pain in her headache is very destructive. This is an important theme in the 6th Superclass. This destruction is also matched by her physical violence. She also describes herself as impulsive. This is more a quality of the 5th and 6th Superclass.

Describe the kicking and beating, just that action —

> *I will hold the person (HG: shows the action of holding). I will kick, and I will give him a good punch (HG: shows the action of holding and punching). I can't bear injustice or humiliation without any reason; if all of a sudden, a person, without rational logic, tries to harm anyone.*

When you say physical harm, what do you mean by this? —

> *Simply torturing. Simply beating a helpless person, hitting them with objects, throwing objects arbitrarily, using sticks, even weapons, like rustic things which are normally used for cutting trees. Whatever the person gets within his reach to torture the other person, because the other person is helpless.*

Describe when you say torture. What is the picture that comes to your mind as an example of torture? That whole process, that action —

> *One is the violent face of the one who is torturing. The other is the helpless face of the person being tortured. Two faces; the violent face has a sadistic kind of pleasure, and the innocent, tortured person can't help it. I think the violent face also can't help, because if he understands how much harm he is doing, maybe he wouldn't like to torture the person. And the innocent, silent person, who is bearing the torture, I think this person is more in peace.*

Torture for her is one doing something to another. It's a victim-aggressor phenomenon. So, her main sensory experience is a strong person doing something to a weaker person. This is one soft clue towards the animal kingdom. The other is that it's a process, i.e., one thing follows the other thing in a sequence. So, we know we need an animal remedy from the 6th Superclass. These are the snakes. With this information it also becomes easier for us to understand some of her earlier descriptions of the main complaint of squeezing in relation to the sensation of the snakes. We can also see along with the victim aggressor themes from the torture and violence but also further confirmations of the 6th Superclass with the intensity of this violence.

Tell some dreams —

> *When I was an adolescent, I used to dream of snakes. Beautiful, colourful snakes, playing with me and so multi-coloured! It's like they could be paintings of Picasso, its painful and very fearful, but still there are colours of joy too. In one dream there is a multi-coloured and huge snake, (HG) which can uplift the world. I am floating, I am playing, and he is not doing any harm to me. I am so pleased and charmed by the beauty of the snake, that I fall in love with the snake.*
>
> *I grew up in a countryside home. There were snakes in my house, ferocious snakes like the cobra. Many times I encountered snakes. Once I woke up at night thinking a snake is coming and I really used to search for the snake, but there was no snake. But snakes never do me any harm. One day I was sitting on the roof and a snake came close, looking at me. I looked at the snake for a long time. Then I went away some distance and kept watching. It just went away.*

You showed this with your palm, what is that? —

> *This is that fanna (HG- shows a hood). It's like sshhhh, (makes the hissing sound of a snake). They hit like that only. I was there and it was hitting a drain, this sound was coming, (HG: hits around and hits the chair). It was a black cobra, (HG: sign on the head). That snake was beautiful, long and parrot green, with a two-shaft split tongue, (HG: shows her tongue). I feel if you keep eye contact with any living object, it reacts. So, the snake also reacts warmly.*

So the dreams are also confirming our analysis. We had seen the features of the 6th Superclass, the Animal kingdom and some subtle hints of the snake sensation. Now the dreams give us a lot of confidence that we are looking for a snake remedy.

What is warmly? —

> *You feel warm, like when a person is very warm, and you feel good to see him or her, just to meet her. In my dreams I see my grandmother and great aunt who loved me and cared for me. Sometimes they try to scare me, but most of the time they are living with me, eating with me, chatting with me. They are staring at me from a distant place. While I was pregnant I dreamt*

of an accident of my husband. Every night I would see his dead face and that he is saying goodbye to me with passion and love. All of a sudden in the night I would wake up and cry, pray to God. The next morning I would phone him and ask him, "How are you? Don't ride the bike again." It happened when I got pregnant for the second time as well.

Here we can see dreams of accidents as well. Another important theme in the 6th Superclass.

We ask the patient to describe her experience during the pregnancy —

Very helpless. I felt mentally tortured. I wanted to run away. I had anger, destructive anger. I felt like hitting my mother-in-law. I used to think that if she dared to do this or that to me again, I will hit her. I will just bang her on the wall. But I didn't actually hit her because it is like torturing. I don't want to torture a mother. I can accept her torture of me, but I don't wish to torture her. My mind would get this plan every time, and most of my energy went into rectifying the mind, "Oh, stop it!"

You said that in other situations you get very aggressive when you see injustice happening. Give me an example of when it actually happened —

(Protrudes her tongue). In trains or buses there are some people who misbehave with girls. One day I was going to school. I used to teach dramatics in school and colleges. I was passing with an umbrella. The place is thickly populated, still there is enough place to go comfortably. An elderly man just pushed me. I just passed a look at him, so that he would realize. If he would realize, he would say sorry. He didn't say that. Again, I kept continuing on that same road. Then the man used a slang word. I just closed my umbrella. I always love to wear sports shoes, and I gave him a two- three. I threw him in front of a bus and a mass of people came. The bus was standing at the bus stop. I knew it wouldn't start. I beat him very badly. I grabbed his shoulders and forcefully kicked him in his back, since I was behind him. I broke my umbrella hitting him.

So first you told him something. What did you tell him? —

"Why did you do that? There was enough space. You should not do that to a girl or to woman." Then he used slang. Then I started.

So why did you tell him that first? —

> *Because he may be a good person who unconsciously did it. We should give him a chance to realize. He didn't take two of my signals.*

When you say take my signals, what do you mean? —

> *'Signals' mean I am trying to understand, and should I go for my extreme? (HG: palm facing outward, resembling the hood). If the person has unknowingly done it, there is nothing to be angry about. I asked him, "Why did you do that?" I point this out to the person, (HG: pointing with her index finger). "Are you intentionally doing it? If you are intentionally doing it, then I am going to teach you a lesson, (same HG). If it came unintentionally, then there is no harm."*

And when you beat, what is your feeling inside? —

> *Very wild anger and in a way, "Look at me, be scared of me." Then he will be afraid and will carry this fear. He will be not able to do this to any other girls in future. Absolute fear.*

This is the Elapidae theme—of giving a warning, a signal: I give you one, two, three chances to prove you're an honest person, and then I do such a thing that will cause intense fear, which you will never forget. It will scare the hell out of you.

— End of Case —

In this case there is a beautiful information which funnels our thought process into the final analysis. Firstly, we could see the Superclass information from the basic nature. When we go deeper into this, we start to see the patient's perception which shows us the Kingdom themes. With the 6th Superclass and the animal kingdom we were already on the lookout for a snake remedy which was confirmed in the description of the main complaint and also in the dreams. Going further in the case we can then see the sub-group understanding of the Elapidae. This is a very simple analysis and makes an intense case taking experience easy to understand.

Based on this information the patient was prescribed Naja 1M. The patient followed up with us two years after taking the remedy –

> She was feeling much better mentally. Feeling very happy. She no longer gets any dreams. The pains in the body are much less compared to earlier. She felt that her health had developed very positively as if there was something magical happening inside her. All the negative things which come she is able to bounce them back.
>
> In a further follow up she mentioned how she had found her husband was in a love affair with another woman. She feels that earlier she would have killed both of them. But now because of the treatment she has accepted it and is focusing on raising her daughter and living her life. All thoughts of jealousy and revenge are gone.

We can show the hierarchy of information in this case as follows —

Superclass	**6th**
Kingdom	Animal
Class	Reptiles
Family	Elapidae
Remedy	Naja

SECTION FIVE

Superclasses as portraits

While working on these ideas of Superclasses we were contacted by a homeopath Monica and her artist husband Momchil who is a painter. They reached out to us with the idea of whether we could create a painting based on the Subclasses. Which could also be applied to the superclass. A lot of time was spent on the discussion around these ideas and based on this he produced some sketches around this, and we discussed further and modified them. The idea was to create an app and we would jumble the paintings and let people choose a particular painting according to their inner sensation and if they consistently chose the same subclass/superclass we could use that app to deduce their superclass. This experiment was not very successful. The fundamental premise is that any given painting does not elicit a specific response from all those who see it; the response is specific to the individual. So, the application was not consistent. However, the paintings are quite evocative and could be used to illustrate visually the Superclasses. So, we are using them in this book as a visual description of the superclass. With this introduction in mind if you look at the paintings, you will be able to appreciate the meaning of these paintings and come to a greater clarity regarding the Superclasses and their dynamic.

Superclass 1

The Lotus eater

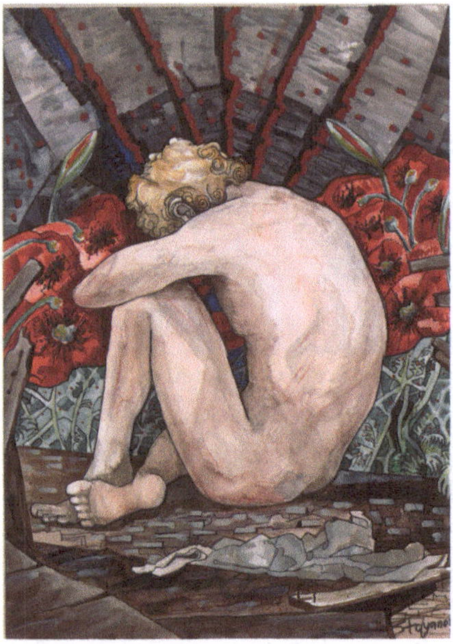

Pandora

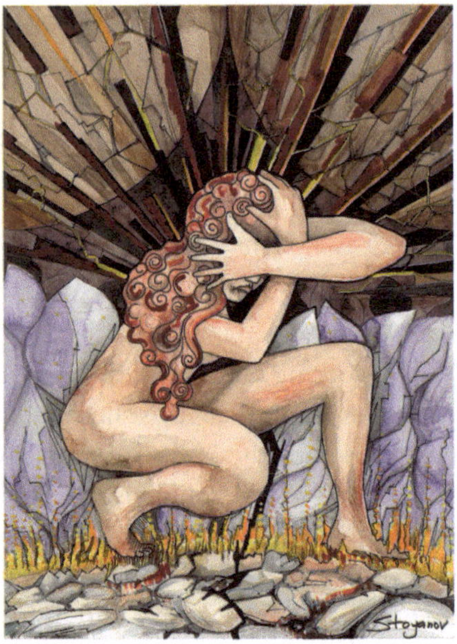

Demeter

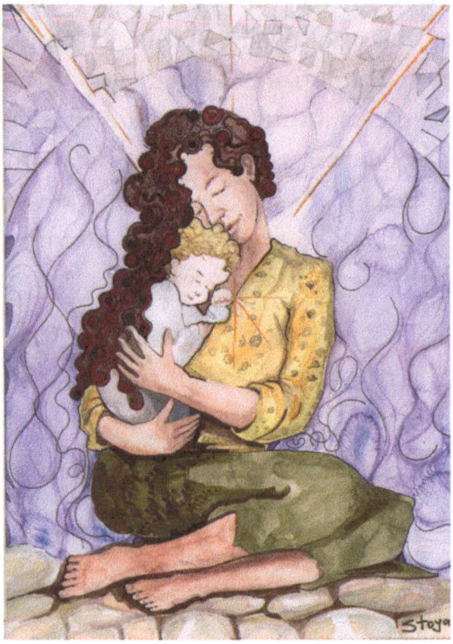

Dervish

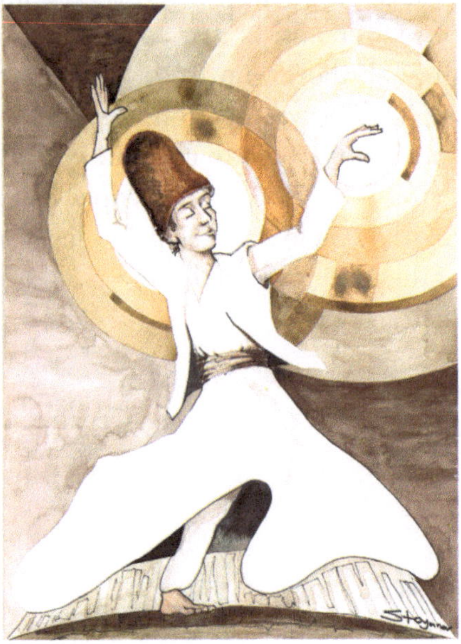

Superclass 2

Hamamelidae

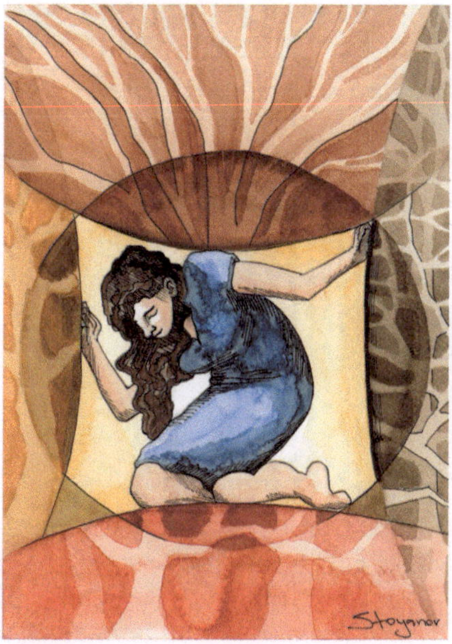

Hollywood

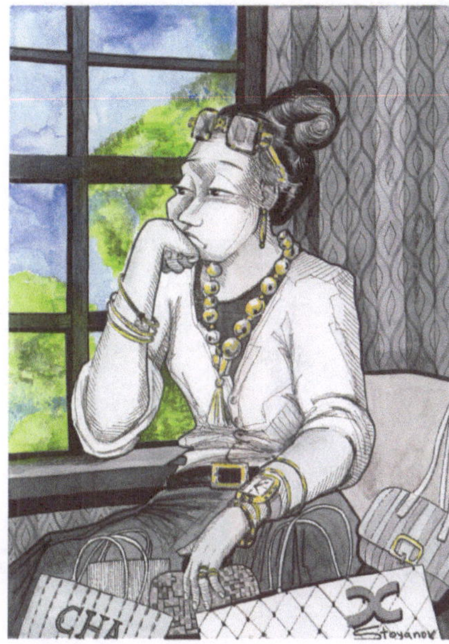

English Naval blue

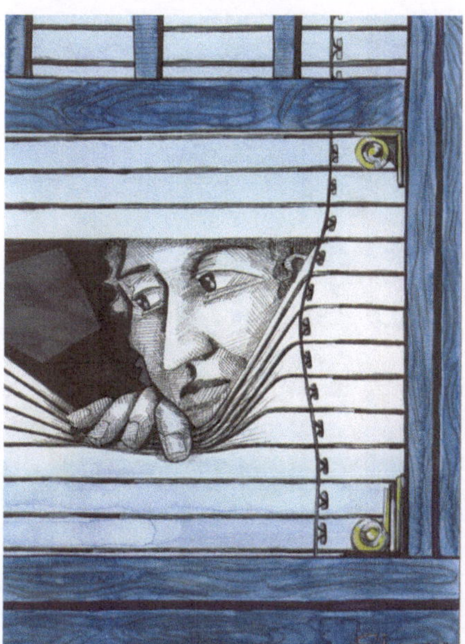

Well done

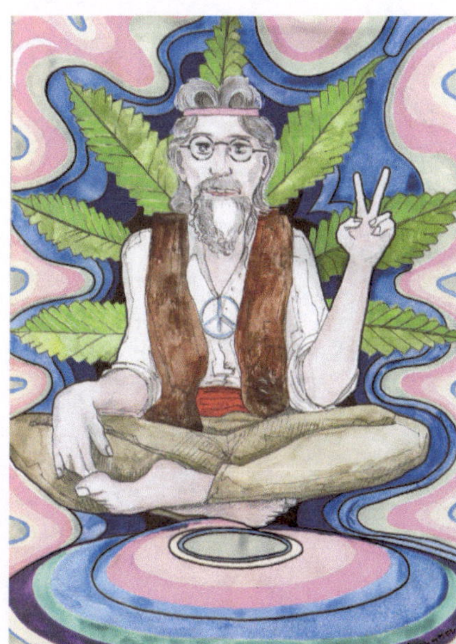

Superclass 3

Copil

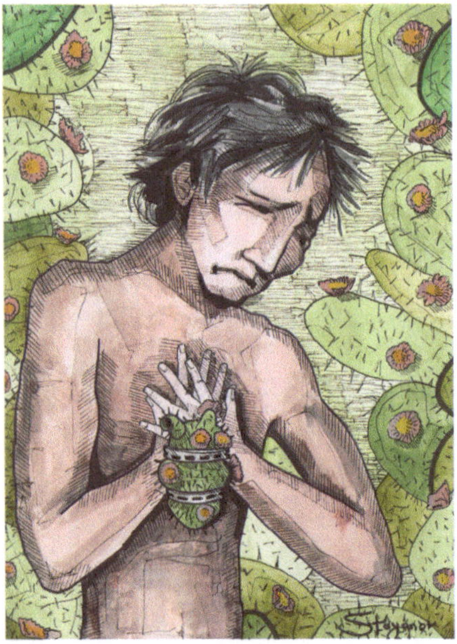

Hermes

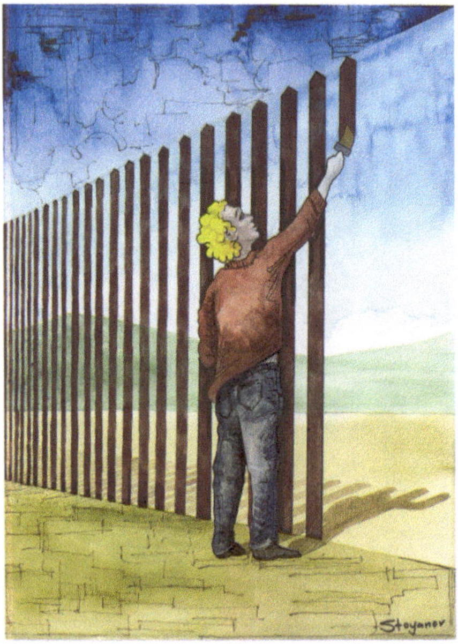

Within castle walls

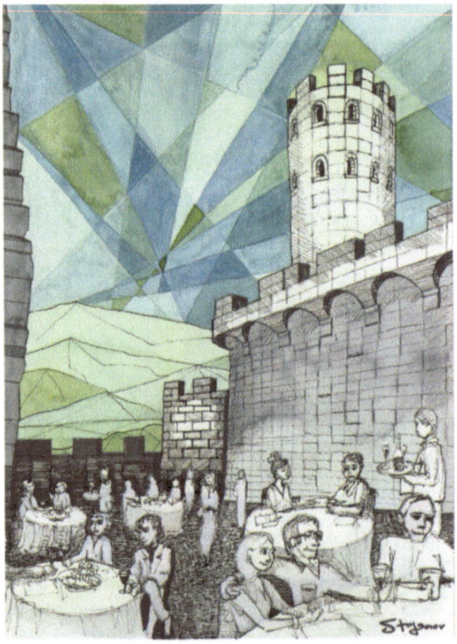

Limit and expand

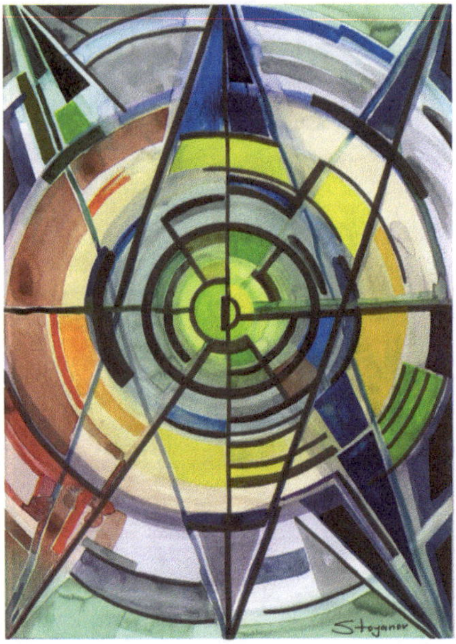

Superclass 4

Apollo

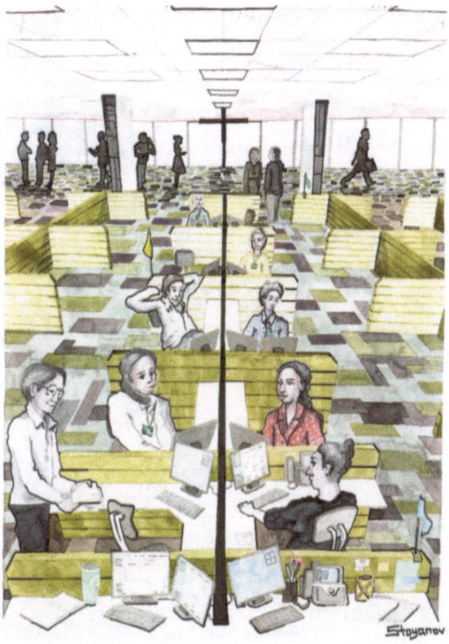

Countryside

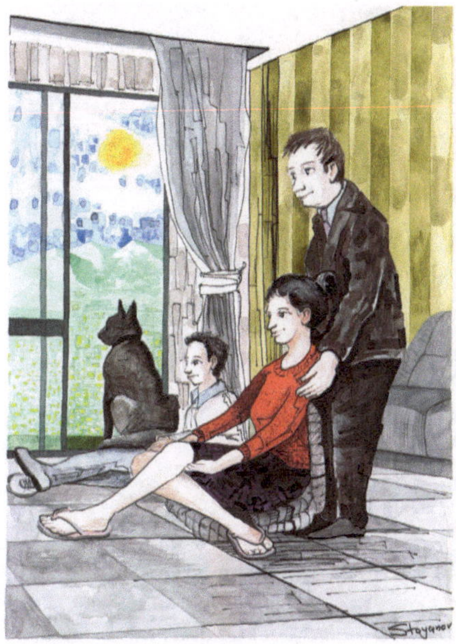

Good morning

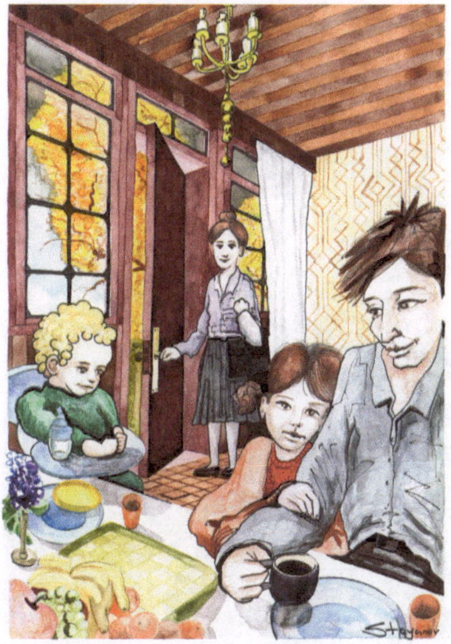

Do not disturb

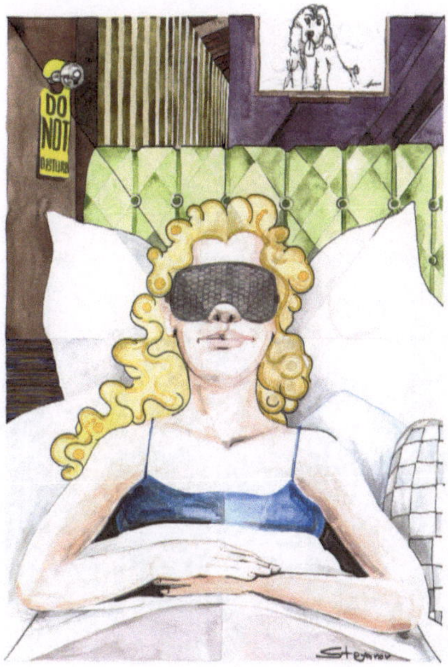

Superclass 5

Shipka

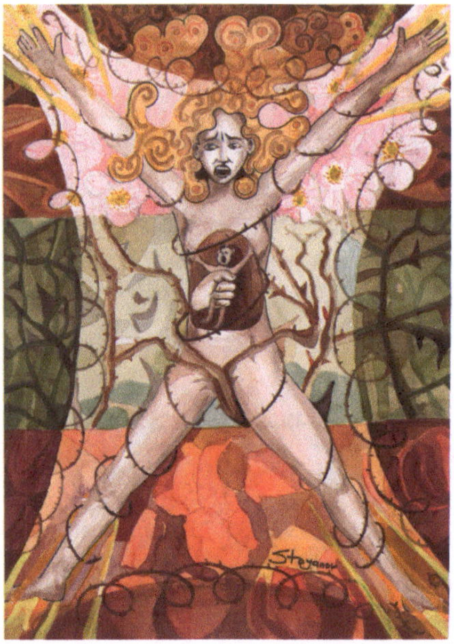

The last one

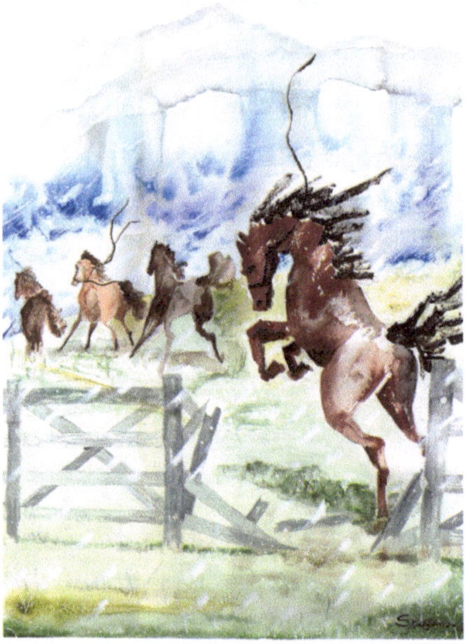

Must get out

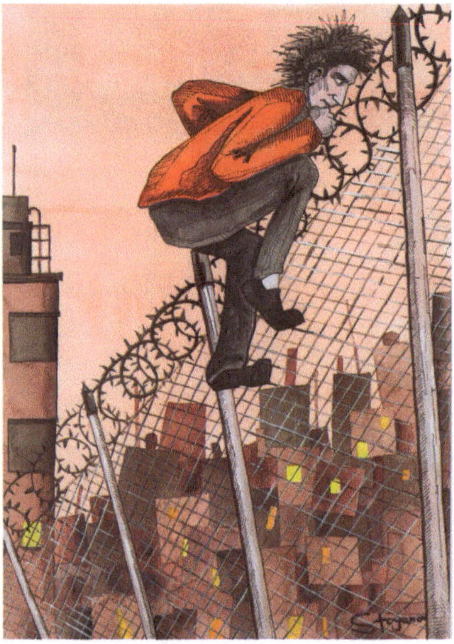

Sapindales

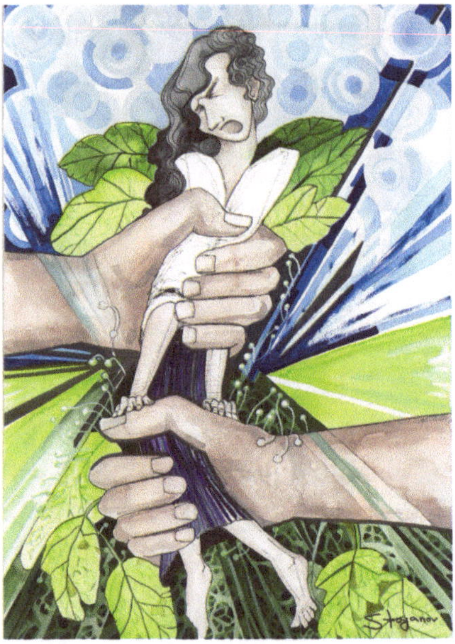

Superclass 6

Leo

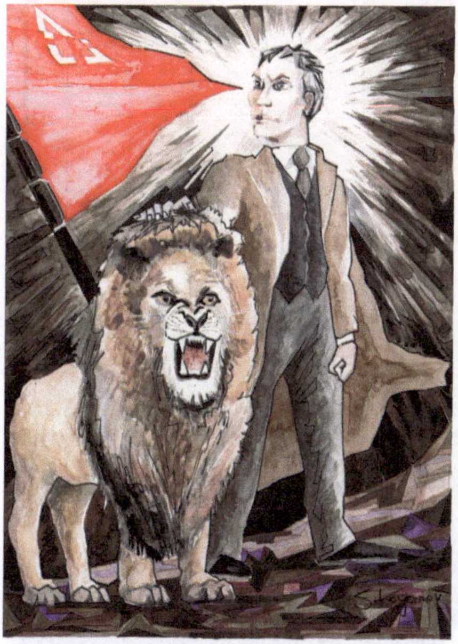

Umbellifers

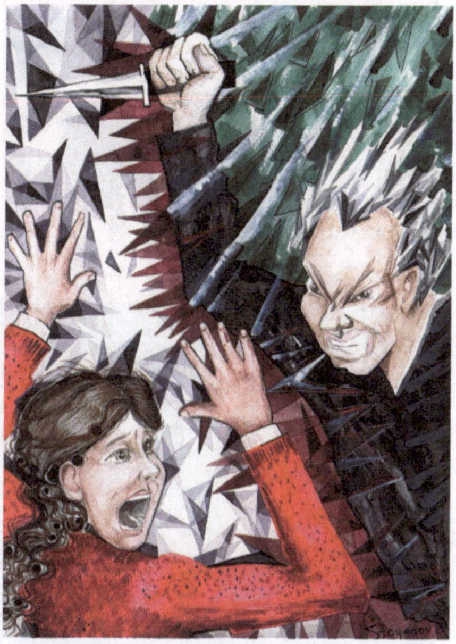

Asteraceae

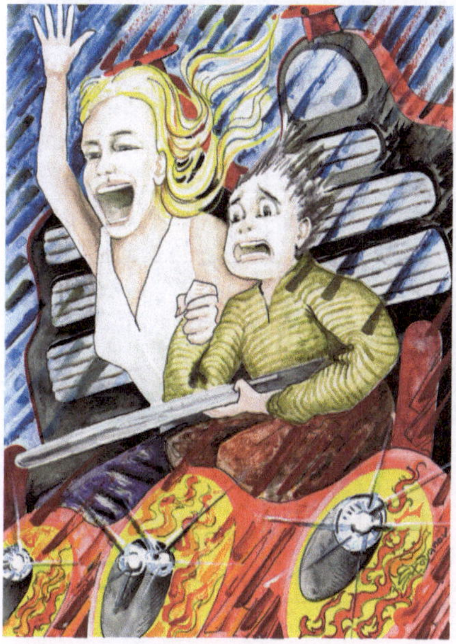

Stramonium

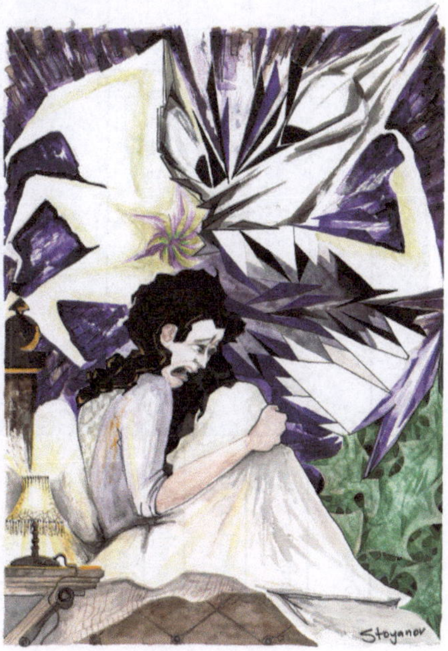

Superclass	**SC 1**	**SC 2**	**SC 3**	**SC 4**	**SC 5**	**SC 6**
Dynamic	Withdrawal & Clinging	Open & Shut	Limit & Expand	Stability & Security	Restless & Must get out	Fight & Flight
Animal group	Bivalves	Gastropods Fishes	Birds Lac humanum	Lac caninum	Cephalopods Spiders Insects Lac equinum	Reptiles Lac leoninum
Mineral group	2nd row: Left hand side	Carbon	3rd row	4th row	5th row & 2nd row: Right hand side	6th row
Dicotyledons	Magnolidae	Hamamelidae	Caryophyllidae	Dilleniidae	Rosidae	Asteriidae
Other plant	Mosses	Ferns		Gymnosperms		Fungi
Neurotransmitter	Endorphins	Serotonin	GABA & Glutamate	Acetylcholine (Parasympathetic)	Dopamine Histamine	Noradrenaline (Sympathetic)
Hormone	Melatonin	Oestrogen	Oxytocin	T3 (Triiodothyronine)	Testosterone	Cortisol Adrenaline
Nosode			*Ringworm*	*Medorrhinum*	*Tuberculinum Carcinosinum Leprominium*	*Syphilinum*
Drug	Opioids	Cannabis	LSD Mescaline Alcohol	Diazepam	Cocaine Nicotine Caffeine	Methamphetamine
Typical remedy	*Opium Mytilus Borax*	*Cannabis indica Helix tosta Graphites*	*Cactus grandiflorus Falco peregrinus Phosphorus*	*Bryonia alba Lac caninum Calcarea carbonicum*	*Anacardium Sepia Argentum nitricum*	*Stramonium Naja Merc sol*
Reaction type	Oyster type	Snail type	Bird type	Dog type	Horse type	Lion type
Keywords	Sleepy Shut off	Enclosed Excited	Love Limit	Health Home	Achievement Aggression	Violence Vehemence
Fairy tale	Sleeping beauty	Alice in Wonderland	Little red riding hood	3 little pigs	Rapunzel	Hansel Gretal
Movie		Charlie and the chocolate factory	Titanic	The pursuit of happiness	Cliffhanger	Schindler's list
Crisis Response	Panic	Inertia	Striving	Coping	Mastery	Leadership

Similar to different aspects

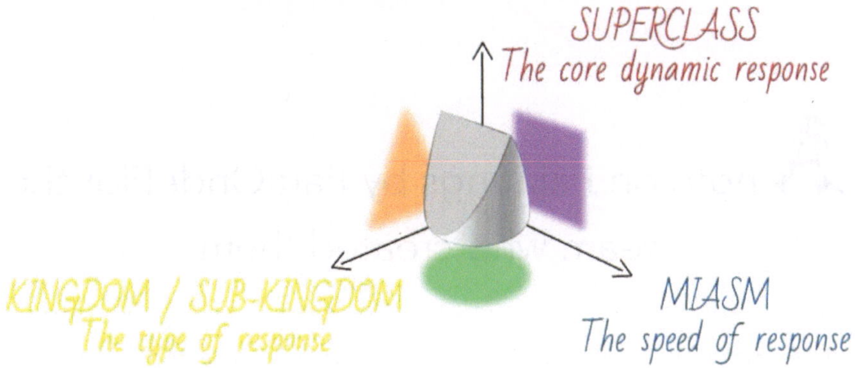

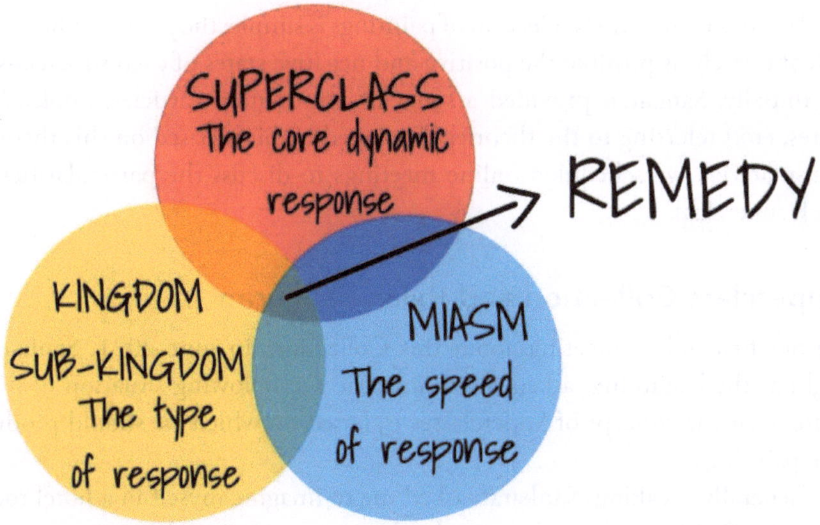

A note on Paintings by ParaOndeFlor the team who created them

We are Mônica and Momchil Stoyanov, pharmacist and architect, parents of Ana, Caterina and Daniel.

The idea behind this collection of paintings is simple: the paintings illustrate as completely as possible the positive and negative states of each superclass.

Initially, Sankaran provided a series of information (articles, books, lectures, etc.) referring to the theories developed by him. Based on this theoretical material, we scheduled online meetings to discuss the particularities of each superclass.

Superclass Collection and Rajan Sankaran

At our first online meeting about this Collection, in June 2021, Sankaran, right at the beginning, asked me to imagine the following situation to illustrate what the concept of Superclasses is, based on which we should produce the paintings.

Generally speaking, Sankaran asked me to imagine myself in a hotel room at night. Suddenly, from the outside, there are explosions, shouting, a mess. The question was: what would I do in this situation?

My answer: I would look out the window first and then I would evaluate what to do.

Based on that answer and some background information, Sankaran and Sarah concluded that I was probably the type that falls into Superclass 2.

Sometime later, with the production of paintings, we made Painting 11, English Naval Blue, which coincidentally illustrates my answer very well.

We formulated the following concept for the paintings:

- In the middle/ center there is a human/ animal/ plant or mineral figure which can be entire or part/ element (ex.: human body, part of a body or a portrait) and also could be abstract.
- Bodies position, face's expression, the feelings, the actual situation or action of the person or the graphic elements expresses the dynamic typical for the Superclass.
- The background is relevant also. Typically, it is divided in regions for each kingdom: animal, plant or mineral. Elements of each kingdom are represented: colors, textures, geometry, parts, etc.
- Each drawing represents a positive or negative dynamic of the Superclass. And there are differences in all aesthetic elements according to the positive or negative character of the drawing.
- There are geometrical elements of the composition configured in such a manner, that allows to rotate the drawing and in each position find a new meaning.
- Complementary elements could be added in the drawings such as texture appliques, words/ phrases, real plant parts such as flowers or leaves, etc.

In parallel, we conducted interviews with project participants. The questions we asked sought to obtain information regarding personal, aesthetic, cultural tastes, favorite places, among others. We found that there was a correspondence between the superclass that best described the respondent and the responses we obtained. This suggested that the elements we would use in the paintings could include a much larger horizon. Thus, we relate elements such as colors, favorite brands, clothes, places, animals, authors and personalities, with each superclass. An example of this was the relation of colors with the Superclasses, where for Superclass 1 we related light, illuminated, white, pastel colors.

One of the goals of the project was to produce paintings and other graphic elements for a potential app project referring to the Superclasses. So, in addition to the paintings, we produced other sketches that could be used for graphic elements such as the application's logo, icons, background colors, among others.

Afterwards, several situations and scenes for each superclass were discussed. The first sketches were produced in this way. In addition to the drawings, we set up a story board containing the sketch and the various elements we selected. The tables were presented and discussed in the meetings. Sankaran and Sarah commented or approved the board and then the painting was produced. Eventually, with the painting ready, new comments and corrections were made. The result was more than 40 sketches and 31 paintings.

As Sankaran's suggestion, the meetings and production of paintings started with superclass 1 and 6, followed by 2 and 4, and ended with superclass 3 and 5. The whole process lasted practically a year and coincided with our move from Bulgaria to the United Kingdom and finally to Brazil.

SECTION SIX

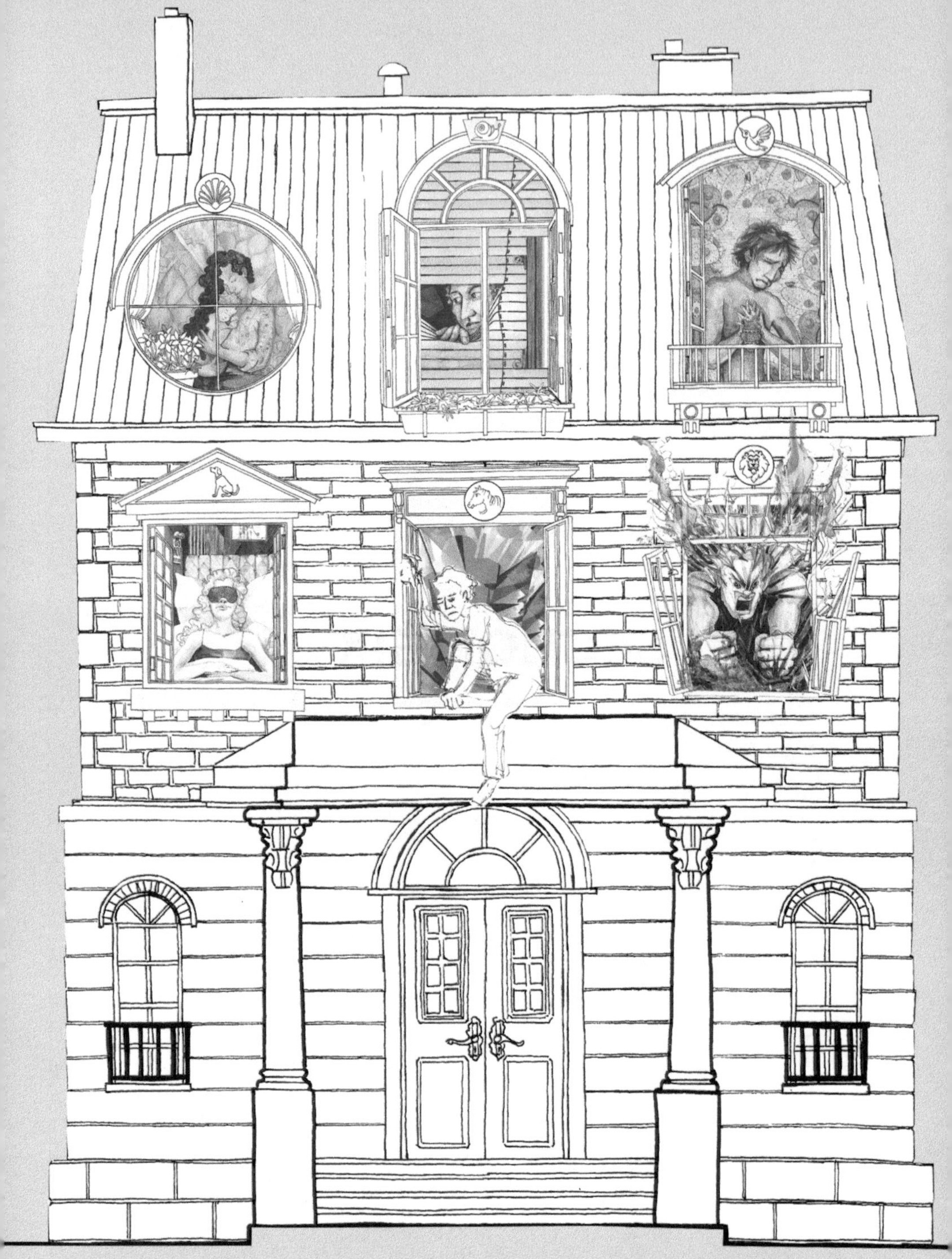

The Superclasses help us in differentiating between remedy groups

The Superclasses can assist us distinguish across various remedy groups and make sense of their fundamental ideas. To achieve this, one must align them with the Superclass's dynamic.

We can take the 3rd row of the Periodic table as an illustration.

In this row we can see the elements Natrum, Magnesium, Alumina, Silica, Phosphorus, Sulphur, and Chlorine. The primary theme in this row is the need for nourishment, love, and care. Love and care come with their own restrictions. One gets constrained. The freedom of choice is curbed. This feeling of restriction or limitation aligns with the dynamic of the 3rd Superclass

In this row one can observe a step-by-step transition from inside to outside. In the initial elements such as Natrum and Magnesium, one remains within and accepts the lack of freedom of choice, while as we go to the right one dares to step outside. Phosphorus declares, "I want to choose my own clothes, my own friends and want to have my own freedom of choice. Your decision for me will not constrain me."

The fourth row of the periodic table aligns with the dynamic of the 4th Superclass , namely the desire to be stable and settled. Kali, and Calc want the status quo and are anxious about losing it. Money, home , family, health, etc are the issues now, not love, care and identity as in the 3rd row. Arsenicum is very frightened with the change in the status quo.

Antimonium lies in the 5th row which is aligned to the dynamic of the 5th Superclass. Here the issue is about stepping into the new, be a performer.

Antimonium, lying on the right side of this row feels that he is losing his ability and feels discarded.

The Malvales are also a part of the fourth Superclass. Malvales have the sensation : together and apart. This is similar to that of the Conifers: joined and unconnected. The Scrophulariaceae (in the 6th Superclass) uses the terms "bonds, connected and disconnected."

All these terms sound similar. However, the Superclass dynamic differentiates them. Stability is a major element in Malvales (being in the 4th Superclass). Together, we are secure. It is unstable to be apart. The sensitivity to quick change from stability to instability is centre of the Malvales. Jeremy Sherr carried out the Chocolate proving. In this proving the image of the hedgehog prominently surfaced. The Hedgehog is a mammal which has an interesting feature. The mother hedgehog breast-feeds the baby for a period and then abruptly turns her back, exposing the baby to the jagged spines. The baby finds that its stable, familiar position has abruptly changed. This aligns with the idea of the 4th Superclass.

The Fabales in the 5th Superclass has also the theme of being split apart and going in different directions. However, this is in line with the dynamic of the 5th Superclass. The splitting apart here is an expression of wanting to get out, to break away.

The experience of breaking apart in the Scrophulariaceae (6th Superclass) is one of major assault, horror. Whereas in the Malvales (4th superclass), separation is experienced as a change and loss of stability, in the Scrophulariaceae it is seen as a traumatic one.

Thus, we can see that families or groups with similar sensations can be differentiated if we see them in the context of Superclasses.

We can compare the remedies China from Rubiaceae (6th Superclass) and Cannabis ind from the Hamamelidae(2nd Superclass). They both have the Theorizing or fantasising. However, in China there must be the topic of dread and fear like the remedies of the 6th Superclass. Many of the rubrics of China and Stramonium are identical. In Rubiaceae, dread and panic are the backdrop for the concept of stimulation. Such a stimulation spurs activity. Adrenaline is the operational hormone.

There is not much action in Cannabis. Inside your own enclosure, you are ecstatic. Nothing happens, there are no plans to do anything. Basically, it is about sensory stimulation. Serotonin is the operational hormone.

One can see how the context of the Superclass can provide a context to differentiate similar remedies and groups.

The Superclasses are different from one another

The dynamic of the first Superclass is one of withdrawal. To stay inside while keeping herself shut off. She doesn't want to be exposed even slightly. She can become numb/anesthetized. Whatever she does, entertainment or addiction or even meditation and spirituality is done to cut herself off from the world. This cutting off can also be achieved by remaining inside a womb, shell, or cocoon to which a person clings. Everything is internalised.

The desire to experience what is outside this cocoon starts in the second superclass. But the fear of going outside endures. They open a window to the outdoors while still inside the protective zone. When threatened, this can close swiftly such a window that opens to the outdoors. Indulging in fantasy is a way to stay within the safety zone. There is a lot of sensory excitement in these 2nd Superclass fantasies, such include colour, movement, excitement, and thrill. They are frequently only visualised rather than being acted upon. It is a window that they are momentarily gazing out of rather than one that they are opening and exiting. I have mentioned a talkative side of Graphites in my description. They get annoyed easily and also laugh readily (like Cann-I). Another side of Graphites which George Vithoulkas described is one of being drab, ponderous, and slow. Carbon is dual-sided. Coal and fuel are both carbon.

Cann-I has two sides in a similar manner. One is like a soda water bottle that is bubbling and about to explode, while the other is like a vegetative existence. And these switch off, though usually not in terms of activity but rather in terms of mental state. The inertia is substantial. We can refer to it as moving at a snail's speed. The pace of the action is rather sluggish.

This is something one can relate to Hollywood and television. Our window is television, but the fundamental distinction is that with television, you can at least go outside virtually. Once can relate to superhuman fantasies, like Jurassic Park or Superman. Cannabis take part in these fantasies. They can also discuss bliss and spiritual escapades. There are those who adore drumming, enjoying enormous bliss and pleasure while sitting inside the boundaries of safety.

What is expected of a person is crucial in the third Superclass. What sort of role, image, identity does one need to have to feel a sense of worthiness, becomes an important question. It is extremely constricting or restricting to feel as though the only way one can be good enough is to live up to this expectation. Despite these restrictions, mobility is possible. Get particular grades on examinations, talk a certain way, and wear a certain outfit. As long as it stays within that range, one can do whatever. By crossing the line, one runs the risk of losing the protection and security that conformity offers. The Third Superclass experience does not provide much in the way of sensory stimulation. It is more important to go past one's limitations and feel some degree of expansion.

There is a sense of restriction in both, the 3rd and 5th Superclasses. While in the 3rd, the restriction also offers safety, the fifth Superclass experiences the restriction as stifling, the interior is dangerous; it is stifling and constricted. The dynamic is a one-way push to go out and leave the place.

The fourth Superclass has some similarities to the third, but there is a sense of stability rather than limitation. The fourth also includes a longing for change. Bryonia has this symptom but it also wants to return home. In the fourth, owning a house gives one a sense of stability rather than a sense of safety. Change entails having the flexibility to leave the house now that you have a secure residence, home, family, etc. A woman who has three kids, a spouse, a family, a home, etc. feels like she is stagnating. The secure location also seems unchanging. The predominant sensations in the Cruciferae are flow and stagnation. She leaves the house and will soon find employment, indulges in a hobby, such as music or art, which creates the impression of change. However, there is always the need for stability, the desire to go back to. She can go outside as long as the base is secure.

What makes the fifth Superclass different? The fifth needs to leave immediately. There is no way back. There is too much internal pressure. This is how Carbon (2nd Superclass) and nitrates (5th Superclass) differ from one another. Carbon continues to long for the security of the interior, while assessing the state of the outer world. But there is too much pressure on the Nitrogen and Oxygen. There is just one way out of here. They are active individuals. Unease is present. There is no 2nd Superclass sluggishness or lethargy. Unlike in the third, there is also little desire to adhere to social rules as expected. There is a perpetual demand for rebellion and change. They grow to dislike the current situation. It is as easy to understand as the distinction between Tuberculinum and Kali Carb. Kali carb gripes about his doctor all the time, yet he will not leave. Unlike Tuberculinum, who desires to switch doctors frequently. Arsenic is in the fourth and stays with the same doctor as well. The long-term clients of your clinic are often in the fourth Superclass.

The sixth Superclass is one of extremes. While the 5th Superclass perceives threat, the 6th Superclass is already in the battle. While the 5th superclass is gearing up for action, the sixth superclass is already in the midst of it. They can demonstrate extreme terror and extreme courage in the midst of danger.

The Superclasses and the categorisation of information

The classification of information into the various categories is what matters. Superclass, kingdom, subkingdom, miasm, characteristics, rubrics, keynotes and source attributes are a few examples. The results will be good if this categorization is done correctly; else, there may be confusion.

As an illustration, we had a case of a patient who gave all the features of the mineral kingdom. There were features of the 3rd row and especially of the remedy Silicea. Yet, when we explored his experience especially through the WISE process, we came across the experience of limiting and expanding or shrinking and expanding. Which one could easily confuse with the remedy Cactus grandiflorus. One could not give him Cactus for the simple reason he had every feature of the mineral kingdom. Especially of the 3rd row and especially of the remedy Silicea.

This confusion can easily be resolved. We now have the awareness that Silicea belongs to the 3rd Superclass. It will share the dynamic of limiting and expanding with other members of the Superclass including Cactus. A remedy lies at a particular point. This point has three co-ordinates, Superclass, kingdom and miasm.

The remedy is not divided into these. When you describe a tall fair boy you are not describing 3 people. You are describing the three co-ordinates of a single person. At the co-ordinate of height, he is tall. At the co-ordinate of gender, he is male and the co-ordinate of skin colour he is fair. But it is all one person.

Similarly, when we say Silicea belongs to the mineral kingdom, 3rd Superclass and the sycotic miasm, we are describing 3 aspects of Silicea. You need to match these co-ordinates in order to find the remedy. These co-ordinates relate to the 'system' aspect. Once we plot the remedy in these co-ordinates then we can look at the factual side which includes the pathology, local symptoms, peculiarities, general symptoms and modalities, keynotes, genius of the remedy and source qualities.

When the patient narrates the history, information regarding all of these aspects comes to us in a rather jumbled form. If we ask the patient "What are your cravings in food?" he may say, "I crave potatoes. But the potatoes cause a lot of flatulence. Because of this I am not able to eat what I really like. I feel very unfortunate and I feel as if God has cursed me to not enjoy life, I feel deprived, I must just accept it. I feel limited and small. My whole world has shrunk."

In this one reply we are getting information about his cravings, generals, mental symptoms, miasm (avoidance and acceptance) his Superclass (shrinking and expanding - 3rd). Similarly through the various parts of his history you get all these aspects. It is up to us to analyse and categorise this information. Wherever information is missing , we need to dig deeper, especially using tools such as WISE processes.

Differentiating the Superclass from the Miasm

A common question that comes up is what the difference between Miasm and Superclass is. Here we also have to add the 3rd coordinate namely the kingdom.

The Superclass corresponds to the basic dynamic. The Miasm is a measure of the pace, and coping mechanism. The Kingdom gives the area of sensitivity.

The Superclass is a quality of the sensation not the miasm. We must not confuse the two co-ordinates. For example, in Staphysagria the main dynamic is that he is so sensitive that he withdraws inside. This is the first Superclass. The pace is that he experiences as everything going out of control. He needs to bring everything into control. Control is cancer miasm and withdrawal which is the first superclass. The sensitivity and reactivity pertains to the kingdom-plant.

Let us give some more examples:

Ars alb
Pulsatilla
Arg nit
Lac can

Ars alb is in 4th Superclass and 4th Row of the periodic table. This means its main dynamic is to look for and maintain stability. The area of sensitivity is structure: the lack or loss of resources. The Miasm is cancer. Which means its main experience is one of losing control and consequently the desperate attempt to keep control. When we combine this, we see that Ars alb is desperately trying to maintain stability in the area of material resources. This combines the superclass and miasm and kingdom.

Pulsatilla is in the 1st Superclass and 1st subclass of the Dicotyledons. This means its main dynamic is the desire to be in its own world. Area of sensitivity: Sensation and reaction. The miasm is sycotic, which means its main coping mechanism is to avoid things. When combined, we see that Pulsatilla avoids any situation where its sensitivity will be triggered. She does this by going within. This combines the kingdom, superclass and miasm.

Arg nit is in the 5th superclass and the 5th row, this means its main dynamic is to achieve, to explore the new. Area of sensitivity is structure: the lack or loss of resources, its miasm is cancer. This means its main experience is one of losing control. Therefore, the desperate attempt to keep control. When we combine this, we see that Arg nit is desperately trying to maintain its standards in performance. This combines the superclass, kingdom and miasm.

Lac can is in the 4th Superclass and a part of mammals. Area of sensitivity: comparison, survival. This means its main dynamic is to look for and maintain stability within the hierarchy. The miasm is sycotic, which means its main coping mechanism is to avoid things. When combined, we see that Lac can avoids any situation where hierarchy will be disturbed. This combines the kingdom superclass and miasm.

If a person says I avoid something, we have to examine what he means by 'avoid'. Does he mean withdraw or does he mean that he doesn't face the situation. Going inside is a dynamic and belongs to the first superclass. If a person says. "I want to avoid my image getting damaged." This is a situation of avoidance which indicates the miasm (Sycotic). The idea of maintaining an image belongs to the 3rd row of the periodic table. To stay within expected boundaries would characterize the 3rd Superclass. So the remedy Silica would stay within boundaries (3rd Superclass), to maintain his or her image (3rd row of periodic table) and avoid any damage to it (Sycotic miasm)

Words can be misleading. We need to go behind the words. We need to see if the specific words are representing a pace which is the miasm or a dynamic which is the Superclass.

Remedies with more than one Superclass

What happens in remedies like salts, such as Calcarea silicata. Is it in 3rd or 4th superclass? In my understanding, Calc sil will have features of both the Superclasses. The Superclass and sensations are interrelated. If it is a salt and has elements which belong to two Superclasses, the patient will have the qualities of both Superclasses. There are also other remedies such as the Carnivorous plants which will show features of more than one Superclass.

The story of Calcarea-silicata:

Calcarea silicata is a remedy that I have studied extensively, and used a lot in my practice. In my experience, the situation of Calcarea silicate is like that of teenagers belonging to the middle class of Indian society. Especially boys who feel that a lot of expectations rests on them. They feel the need to come up to a certain standard to get the approval of their parents (whose security they seek). You can also extend this idea to the feeling that one needs to come up to a certain standard so that one may find a job or maintain the job.

This feeling has two aspects. The first is that one needs to meet certain expectations and the second is that one needs to maintain the job. When we look at these two aspects, we see that the idea of having to meet expectations is also at a deeper level the idea to stay within a certain boundary, to stay within a certain image. This dynamic corresponds to the 3rd Superclass (Silica). And the idea to maintain one's job corresponds to the need for stability as found in the 4th Superclass (Calcarea).

Thus, the remedy Calc-sil has features of both the Superclasses since it has elements Calcarea and Silica from both of them.

The curious case of Drosera:

Drosera is a very interesting remedy to study in terms of Superclasses. First of all, it is a plant remedy but one which has animal like features namely it is a carnivorous plant. We see in it definitely features of the 5th Superclass, namely the feeling of being trapped, the restlessness, the suspiciousness, the feeling of being threatened. The plant itself deceives and traps its prey which gets stuck on it and finds it very difficult to get out. All this points to the 5th Superclass. It evokes comparison with spiders, with Tuberculinum and with the Anacardiaceae.

There is another side to this where the plant is carnivorous because it lacks certain vital nutrients which are not found in its soil. This need for nourishment also gives us indications of the 3rd Superclass. A study of the rubrics of Drosera indicates both these sides of Drosera.

Symptoms indicating 5th Superclass —

CR19 - Mind; Deceitful, sly(61)
CR19 - Mind; Delusions, imaginations; deceived, is(13)
CR19 - Mind; Delusions, imaginations; enemy; surrounded by(21)
CR19 - Mind; Delusions, imaginations; pursued, of being; enemies, by(36)
CR19 - Mind; Delusions, imaginations; trapped, he is(47)
CR19 - Mind; Restlessness, nervousness; move; must, drives one from place to place(205)
CR19 - Mind; Suspiciousness, mistrustfulness; restlessness, with(1)

Symptoms indicating 3rd Superclass —

CR19 - Mind; Fear; alone, being; solitude, of(35)
CR19 - Mind; Fear; children, in(67)
CR19 - Mind; Homesickness, nostalgia(141)
CR19 - Mind; Holding or being held, desire for; amel.(106)

The study of these remedies shows the possibility that there are remedies which may display the features of more than one Superclass.

The basic nature of the patient

When the patient says: Sometimes I am like this, sometimes I am like that. What does this mean? Let us take an example: A patient says, "Sometimes I am yielding and sometimes I am stubborn". How can we understand this?

There are three possibilities —

1. That one is stubborn within a certain framework where one feels secure and is yielding in places where one feels insecure. For example, a child is stubborn within one's home and with one's parents but is yielding in the outside world. This can happen in Superclass 2, 3 and 4.
2. That by essential nature she is yielding but has learnt to compensate for this due to circumstances, job requirements, relationship issues, etc. For example, they are yielding by nature, but is now put in charge of a big business by the parent. They cannot afford to be yielding. They must become stubborn because they cannot afford to be docile. However, the fundamental essence will manifest in a variety of circumstances as well as during inquiries into the nature of childhood.
3. That the person requires a remedy that has both the sides in it. For example, the person may need a salt that has elements from different Superclasses. One from an earlier superclass and one from a later one.

Repertory and the Superclasses

The use of the repertory is an art. If we use it in a mechanical unartistic manner, we will be lost. Usually, we will end up prescribing the same few polychrest remedies. It is very important that the Repertorial analysis reflects the core pattern of the patient. When applying our understanding of the Superclasses to the patient in the analysis it should also go hand in hand with the repertory. The Superclass features should emerge through the Repertorial analysis. The rubrics selected should always be seen in context to each other and to the pattern of the patient. Let us take an example to show how the repertory can highlight the Superclass features of the remedy.

Let us look at the rubric 'Theorising' and at some of the remedies in it:

Reliable Repertory - Mind

Reliable Repertory > Mind

+Theorizing : *CANN-I., Sulph., ang., aur., *chin., cocc., coff., hep., lach., sanic., sel., sep., verat., apis, arg-n., ars., *aur-s., cimic., ephe., flag-l., *hydrog., *kali-c., lac-eq., lac-lox-a., lat-h., lava-ariz., lim-b-c., limus-tory., lsd, lyc., mobil-ph., op., posit., puls., sil.

In a repertory, it looks flat, and every remedy is put there which has 'Theorizing'. The repertory does not differentiate. It does not tell you the quality of each one. We can use this as a small example of how I look at the repertory and rubrics using the idea of the Superclasses.

Let us understand some of the remedies in this rubric in context of the Superclasses. For this we will see what other rubrics are in this remedy and construct a remedy idea based on the combination of rubrics. Let us take the remedy Cocculus.

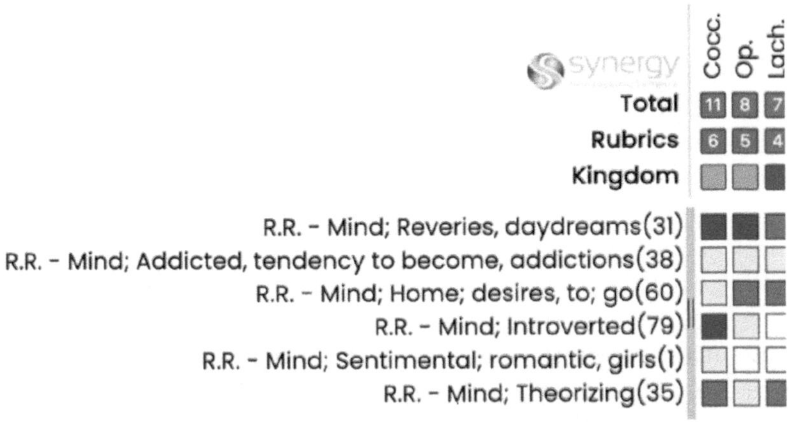

In Cocculus you can see that 'Theorizing' is associated with other rubrics such as sentimental, romantic girls, introverted, tendencies to addictions, reveries and daydreams and the desire to go home. We need to understand this pattern. We can gather from these rubrics that Cocculus sits at home; is introverted which means withdrawn. She is thinking of romantic things and reveries without acting upon it, living in a world of fantasy. Not facing the world, wanting to go home, introverted. Sitting inside the cosiness of the home she is occupying the mind with romantic and other fancies. It is little bit like an addiction. We know that Cocculus belongs to the 1st Superclass. This is the withdrawal, theorising with withdrawal. This is Cocculus. When we associate the Superclass quality with the rubric you get the whole picture.

We can take another example, of Cannabis indica —

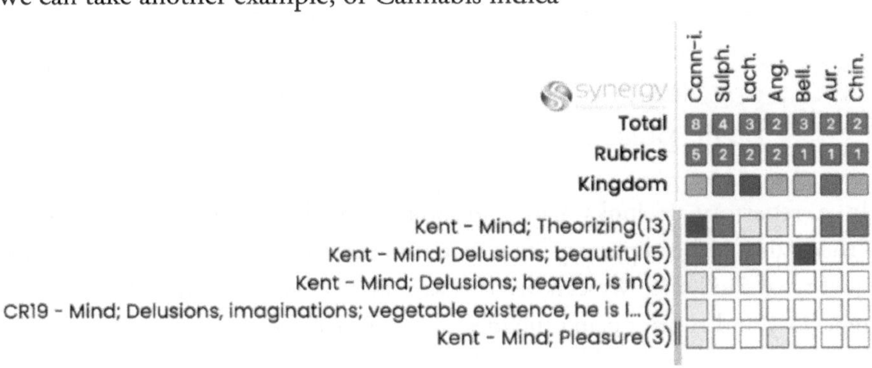

What is the Theorizing of Cannabis indica associated with? The delusion beautiful, delusion he is in heaven, delusion he is leading a vegetable existence and Pleasure. Here, you can see there is a contrast between living a vegetable existence. A feeling as if I have no life, I am like a vegetable there is no excitement, no joy, no pleasure, no sensory stimulation. And on the other hand, beautiful, heaven and pleasure. There are two sides to it. This is the open and shut of the second Superclass.

Let us examine Sulphur —

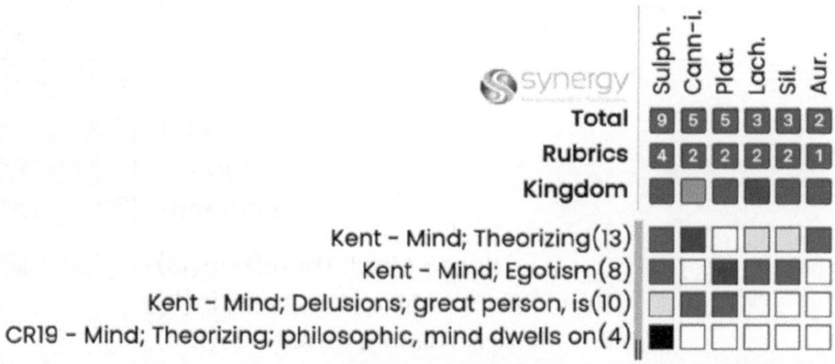

We can see in Sulphur the Theorizing is associated with egotism, Delusion he is a great person and dwells on philosophic things. The main theme of Sulphur is ego. Ego in Sulphur is expressed as "I know better than you". It is like a child telling the parents, "Who are you to limit me to your ideas and opinions, I have my own theories about things." In Phatak's Materia Medica it is written "Contemptuous to men of knowledge" and "he thinks he is a great person." So, he will say, "What do you know." The Theorising of Sulphur is associated with Egotism and the desire to break the limits. This is the 3rd Superclass.

Then we can look at Lycopodium —

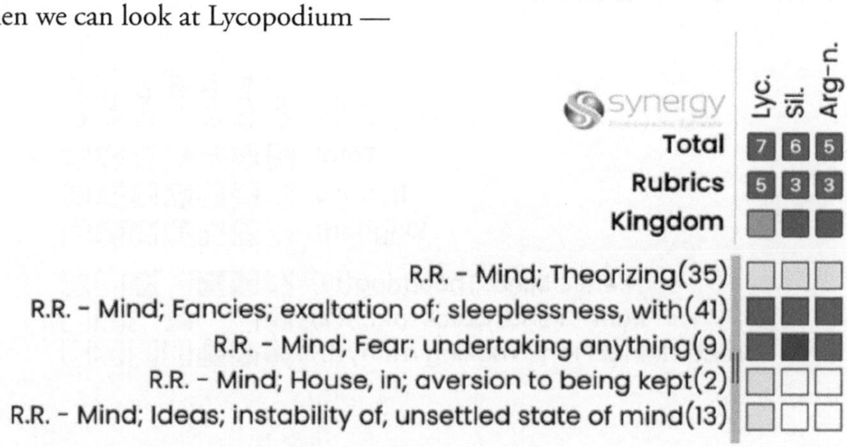

Theorising in Lycopodium is associated with exaltation of fancies, sleeplessness, fear of undertaking anything new, instability, an unsettled mind. The word instability is a big word for the 4th Superclass. He likes stability and therefore the fear of undertaking anything new, of anything taking him away from the routine. In the evening, Lycopodium is sitting and thinking what he could possibly do. This is his 'theorizing'.

Then in the 5th Superclass we have the remedy Angustura —

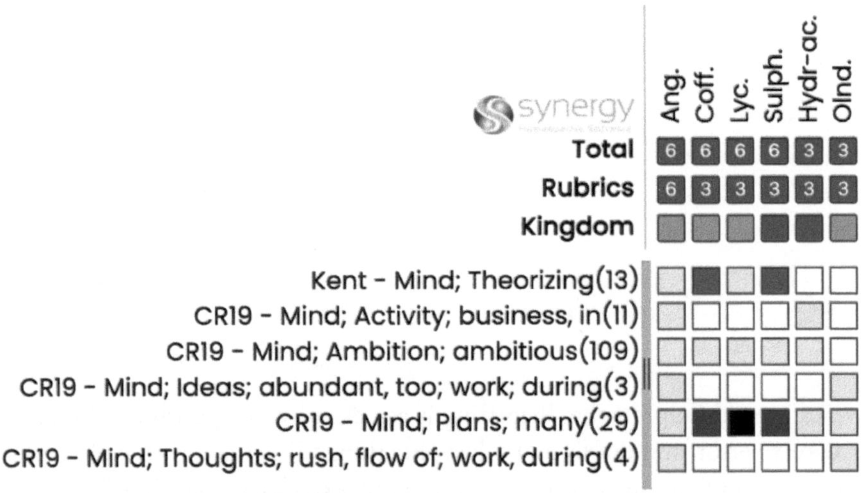

Angustura comes from the same family as Ruta. Theorizing is associated with a lot of ambitiousness, ambitious ideas. Making many plans, rush, and flow of thoughts, too much activity. This is the 5th Superclass, too much activity, wants to do something out of the box.

Finally let us look at Coffea —

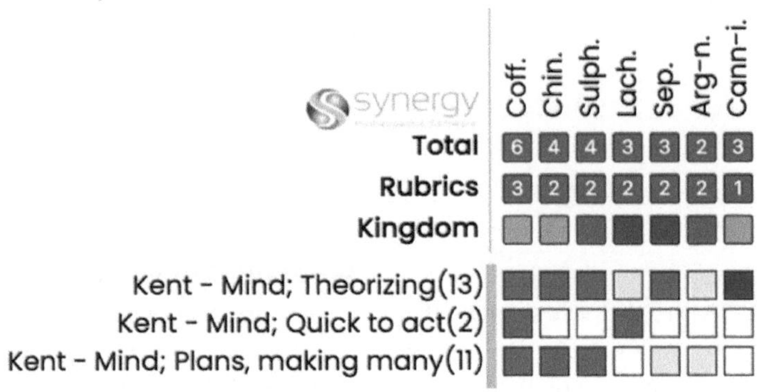

Here theorizing is associated with 'quick to act' and 'making many plans'. They have to be on the go, they either have to fight or flee, they have to think quickly on their feet. The Theorizing here is associated with activity, quick responses such as in the dynamic response of the sixth Superclass.

In the Animal Kingdom, you can see Lachesis —

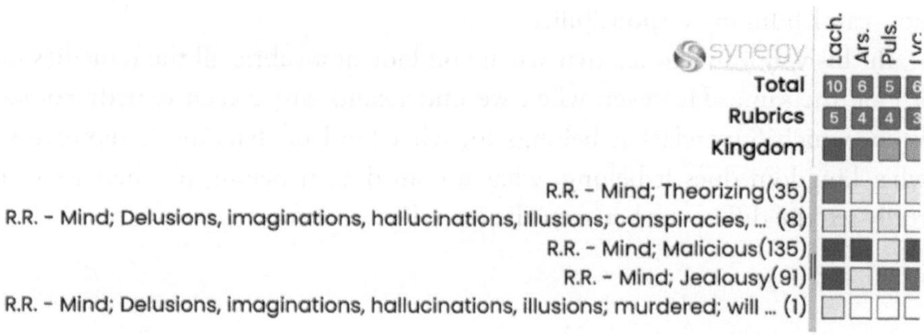

The theorizing is associated with conspiracies. Theorizing that this one and that one is conspiring against me. They will kill me. Therefore, I have to be malicious, suspicious, and jealous because I have the feeling that I can be murdered. This is the animal quality in the 6th superclass with the idea of theorizing.

Also, from the 6th Superclass but from the Mineral kingdom we have Aurum —

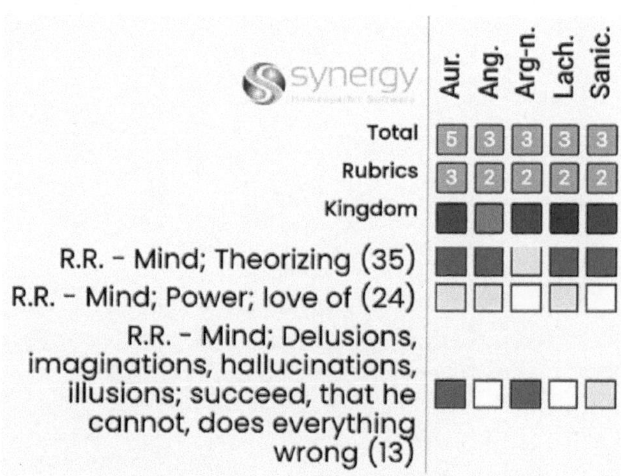

Aurum has 'Theorizing' with the love of power. Aurum is the king. The delusion is that he does everything wrong, he has failed, he could not do his duty. People have lost confidence in him. What do Prime Ministers have to face? What is the worst moment for them. The vote of no confidence. People say we have no faith or confidence in you. That is when they lose their power. So, 'Theorizing ' here is associated with the thought of what more can I do, how can I fulfil my responsibility.

In this way you can see that when you look at a rubric all the remedies in it look the same. However, when we understand where each remedy comes from, which Superclass it belongs to, what kind of dynamic it represents, what kingdom does it belong, what miasm does it belong to, then we can really see the difference between the remedies.

Validity of the previous system

When I look back on my cases from the past, I can see the dimension of Superclass quite clearly in hindsight.

I remember an early case of a gentleman in his late 50s who had come for a non-healing ulcer on his foot. He was a diabetic, hypertensive with a history of ischemic heart disease and cardiac failure. The ulcer was deep and had produced osteolysis of his metatarsals. On enquiry I found out that he was an income tax officer who had the reputation of being very honest, straightforward highly principled. Even his bosses were afraid of him because he could confront anybody. He had a very strong sense of duty and also had a deep interest in music. Especially religious music which would give him great relief.

The remedy Aurum metallicum did wonders on him and in fact even restored his bones. At that time, it was based on the prominent mental symptoms, namely a strong sense of duty, much relief from music and a religious nature.

In hindsight I am able to see that his nature which was very strong, courageous, and confrontational fits in very well with the idea of the 6th super class.

Another case that I remember was of a man in his mid 70s. He had come with acute retention of urine due to cancer of the prostate with multiple metastasis. His chief complaint however was of pain in the rectum. He described it as a cutting pain when he passed stools. There was a sensation as if the rectum was delicate and could be easily torn. One thing peculiar about him was that he never laughed or smiled. On inquiry, he said he was very careful not to laugh lest it be misunderstood by his daughter-in-laws. Such a misunderstanding might cause a rift in the family. Thus, leading to a separation or breaking apart of the family unit. He was greatly helped by the remedy Thuja. This not only relieved his retention but also had a long-term effect on his cancer. At that time, I had based the prescription on the sensation and the miasm. The sensation being fragility and the miasm being sycotic. Now I am able to see that the idea behind his fear was the possibility of a change in the status quo of the family. This is the main dynamic of the 4th superclass.

The above examples illustrate that successful cases were those which the Superclass also matched even if we were not aware of it at that time. It also shows that the right remedy also matches the Superclass even though we understand it only now. The addition of this dimension to the case understanding and to the remedy understanding is of great value in being even more sure of the remedy selected.

Superclasses and life

If we understand the idea of Superclasses, we will know what to expect and what not to expect from others (and ourselves) and respond accordingly.

Let us say you are dealing with your employees. You will have employees from different Superclasses. If a certain employee is from the 5th Superclass, s/he may not remain in your employ for very long. This person is likely to be individually minded. He is inventive and creative, but may not be steady. Creativity is one quality, the other side of which could be being rebellious.

If you want a very creative person in your team, it would be important not to tie the person to a routine. The person will want to get out. You will need to give them a free rein. If you want the benefits of their talent, you may consider an arrangement where they are not tied to you.

If we want people for doing routine work efficiently, we should look in the fourth Superclass, and probably in the Mineral kingdom. We should look for people in the middle columns of the periodic table. On the left-hand side, they are somewhat dependent and on the right side, they are slightly hopeless.

When we expect from someone (or ourselves) the qualities of a Superclass other than what is theirs (or ours) then we are disappointed. We cannot be selective. Each one of us is a package of the qualities of a specific Superclass (and also a specific kingdom and miasm). For example, we like the caring quality of someone but don't like their slow pace or lack of focus. One comes with the other, all these being qualities of a specific Superclass. It is likely that if you had a very focused and fast-paced individual, that individual may not have the qualities of caring or giving. Such a person is likely to be more self-centred and ambitious.

If someone who has leadership qualities is also very egotistical, we must understand that both these qualities go together in the same Superclass (6th).

The same idea applies to kingdoms and miasms. We need to see this and modify our expectations as well as know how to respond to or how to position people so that they are best suited to the position.

Superclass case analysis

Looking at our cases from Section 1 we will be giving the rationale and discussion of the analysis of the Superclass in each case. It is our strong suggestion that before going through the answers here you familiarize yourselves with the cases. Do your best to come up with your own analysis beforehand. Try to focus on the basic nature of the patient and see what the fundamental response in each case is and which Superclass this would correlate with. Once you have analyzed then check your answers here with our solutions. If there is any discrepancy between your answer and ours then try to see where we have placed the emphasis in our analysis. We feel this is the best way to learn from our mistakes and also to grow confidence in the easy use of the Superclass system.

Answer to Case 1

The patient's fundamental essence is immediately apparent at the outset of the case. He is forceful and combative, as is evident. The Superclasses 4-6 quickly come to mind when we hear this. The first three are significantly more subdued and non-confrontational. Further investigation reveals that he also has a high speed. We can tell that he is highly decisive and he completes things swiftly. This also illustrates the notion of performance. He puts forth excellent work and demands that others do the same. Everything here points to the last three Superclasses. It draws even more attention to the patient's aggression. He talks about how he would not just confront but also turn violent. We can see that his initial response was to act violently before speaking. The extreme irritation and aggression are evident. The emphasis is on his internal tempo, anger, irritation, and performance. We are dealing with the sixth Superclass, as is evident. The themes of brutality and a severe circumstance are once more apparent. Aggression and a sense of going all the way to the end are present. We can observe that the fundamental emotion in this situation is significantly more male. The first three Superclasses are far more reserved. They stay away from confrontation and controversy. The feminine aspects would be more apparent. The emphasis would be on love and caring. The sensitivity and emotion would be more than they are with this patient. He is far more forceful, combative, and outgoing in his underlying personality and responses. Everything here points to the sixth Superclass. We are able to distinguish between his efforts and those of the Fifth Superclass. In this instance, the patient's anger and irritation are more prominent. He anticipates that others will do as he says. He is not a follower; he is a leader. In the fifth Superclass there is a bigger emphasis on original and creative thinking in performance and achievement. Instead of using force to solve problems, they would utilise their minds. The remedy for the patient was Nux vomica.

He responded exceptionally well, demonstrating the need for a 6th Superclass remedy.

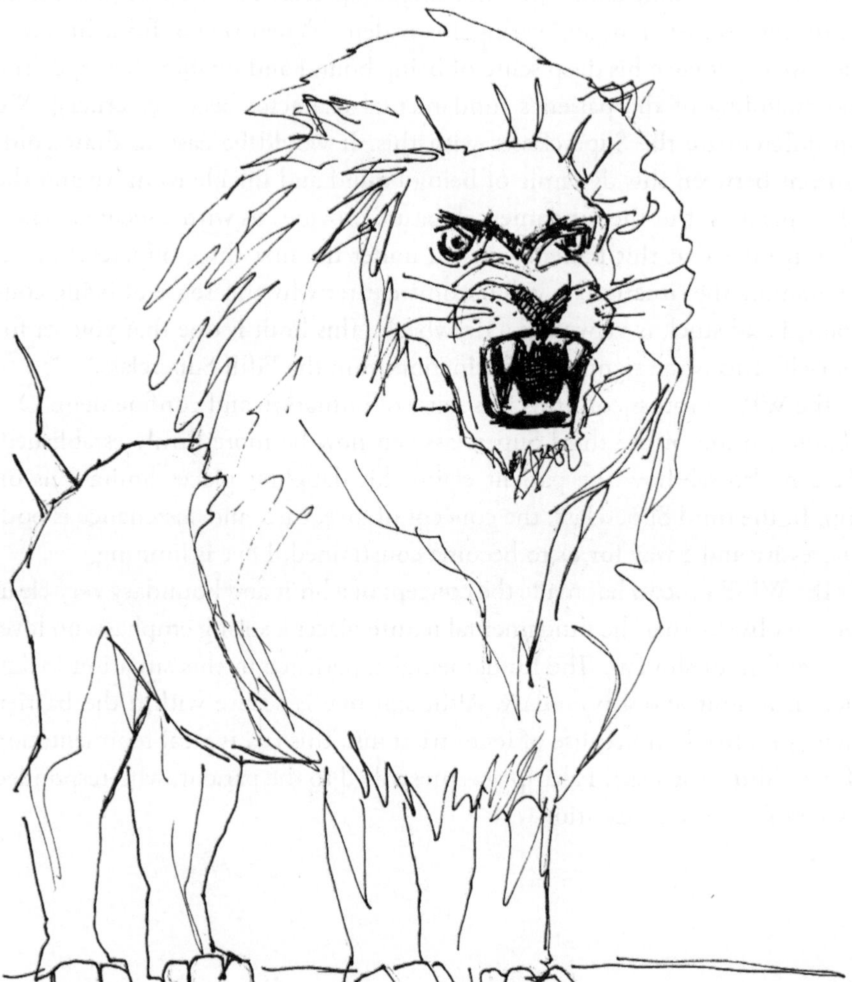

Stoyanov

SC 6⊕ MONICA & MOMCHIL STOYANOV / AGO 2021

Answer to Case 2

We can infer the fundamental characteristics of this patient from his early self-descriptions. In some ways, he is gentler and more sentimental. This provides a little hint about the first three Superclasses. The components of nurturing, compassion, and caring are evident. When we confront his anxieties, we experience his deep sense of being bound and unable to escape. The understanding of the patient's fundamental character becomes crucial. We can differentiate the Superclasses with this. It would be easy to draw comparisons between this dynamic of being bound and unable to move and the 5th Superclass. But the fundamental nature provides us with a secure anchor. We can infer that this patient will fall under the first three Superclasses. As we examine the situation, it will become clearer why this sense of being constrained and stuck is viewed as a drawback. This limit is one that you set for yourself. This is the significant distinction from the Fifth Superclass.

The WISE process confirms this sense of limitation and confinement. Our comprehension of the third Superclass can now be more firmly established. We can also see how the patient claims his daughter places limitations on him. In the third Superclass, the concept of love, care, and sustenance is both a necessity and a way for us to become constrained. Love is limiting.

The WISE process has made the concept of a limit and boundary very clear. We can observe that the fundamental nature places a strong emphasis on love, care, and nourishment. The fundamental experience in this situation is that there is a limit and a boundary. Although one is secure within the barrier, there is no freedom because of its restrictions. This is a typical representation of the Third Superclass. Falco-p was prescribed to the patient, who responded favourably to the medication.

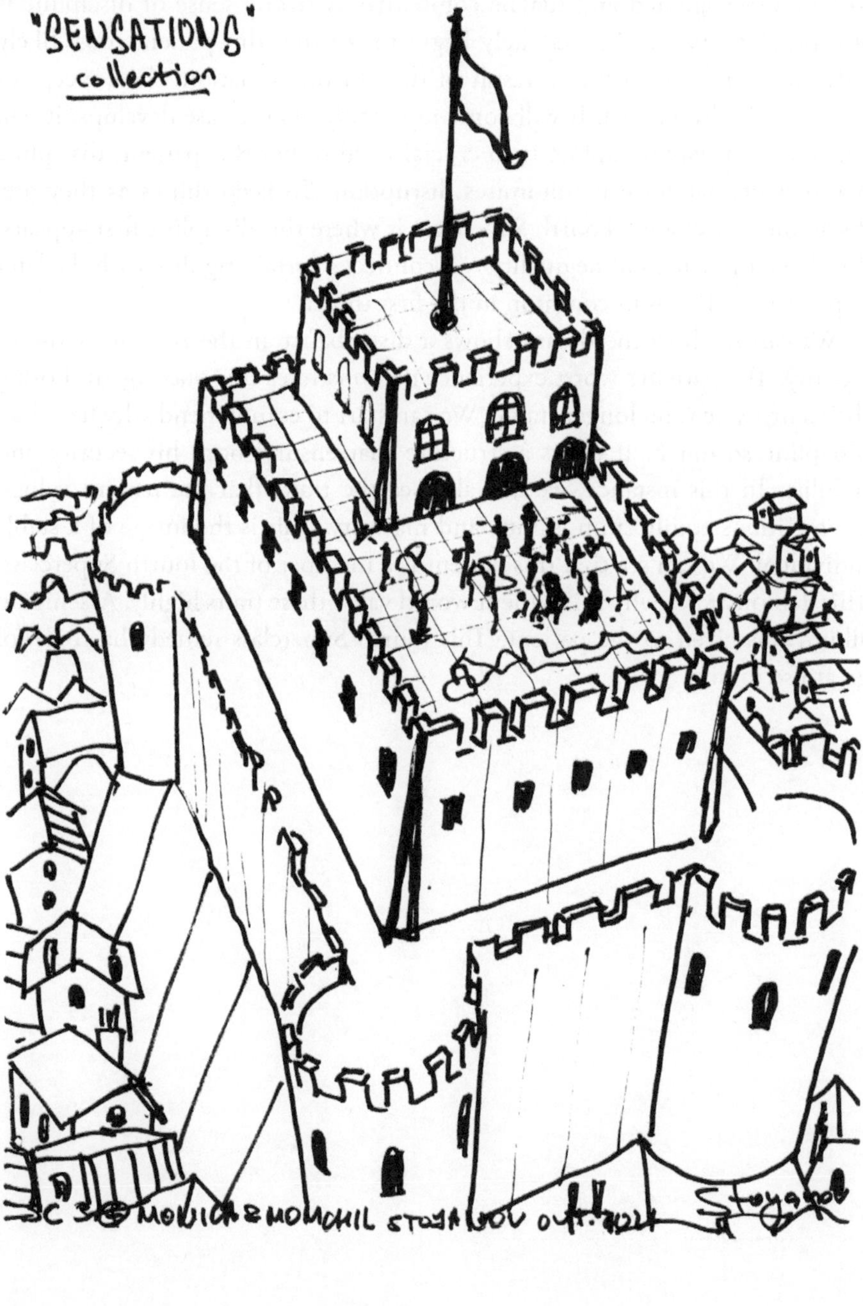
"SENSATIONS"
collection
MONICA & MOMCHIL STOYANOV
Stoyanov

Answer to Case 3

At first, we can see a lot about the patient's fundamental character. He appears to be a little agitated and maybe combative. A strong sense of discipline is also present. We can immediately begin to see that this patient most likely falls into Superclass 4-6 as a result of this. In this situation, the concept of discipline is also crucial. It will come repeatedly. As the case develops, it will become clear why discipline is so crucial to him. For this patient, discipline becomes crucial since it minimises disruption. To keep things as they are, discipline is necessary. Fourth Superclass is where this discipline first appears. This has a more masculine quality. We connect a certain rigidity with the later Superclasses. This is uncommon in the first three.

We can see how the dream shows a disturbance in the patient's sense of security. The patient's worst experience demonstrates this once again. Losing the security, he is no longer stable. We can start to comprehend why he values discipline so much. It offers a structure that ensures both his security and stability. In this instance, we can also see the traits that the patient values. He mentions equilibrium, sanity, and maturity. This is the image of a stable individual. We can see that this patient is a member of the fourth Superclass. This demonstrates why this patient would value these traits highly. Arsenicum album was given to the patient. This fourth Superclass remedy has been of great use to him.

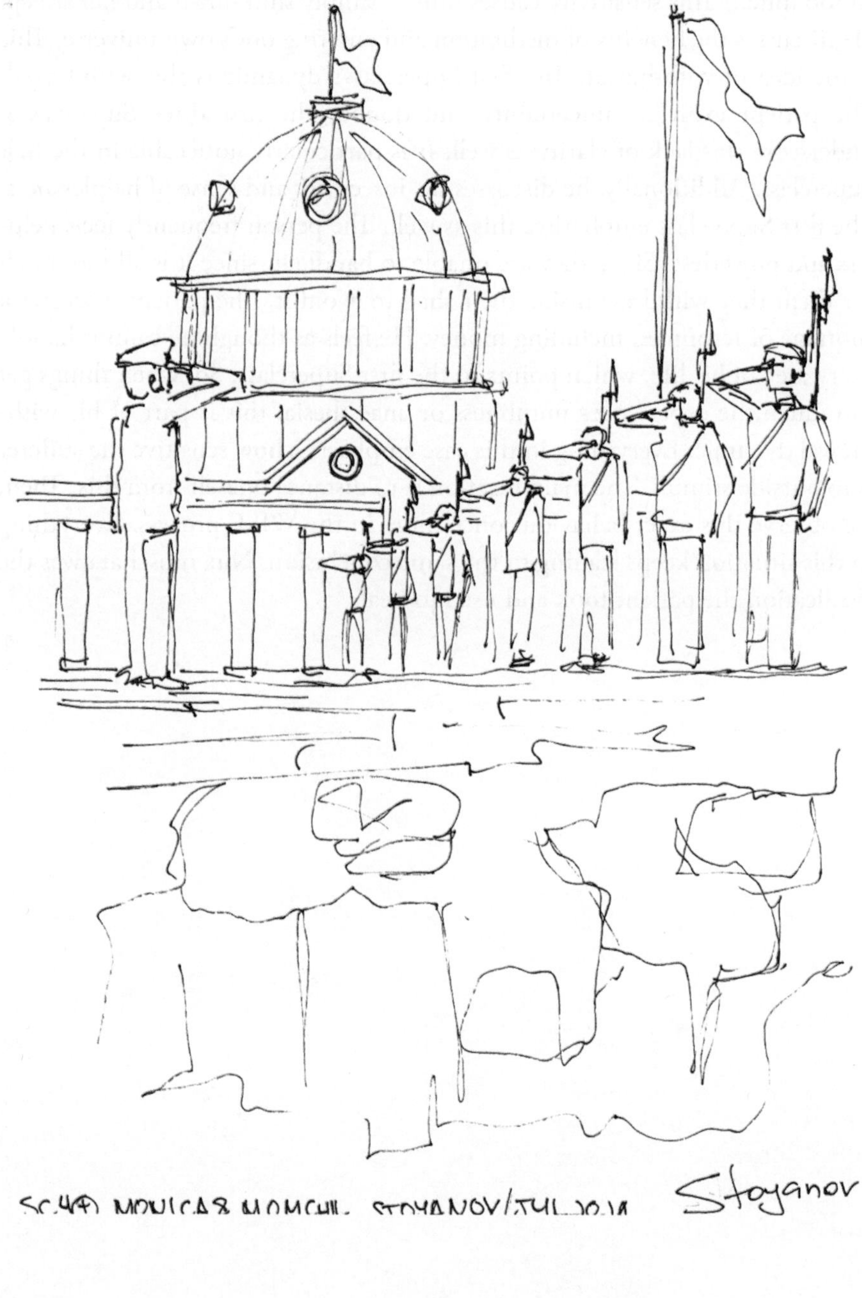
SC.49 MONICA & MOMCHIL STOYANOV/JUL 2014
Stoyanov

Answer to Case 4

We can see the patient's sensitivity in this situation. He can not take it; it is all too much. This sensitivity causes him to simply shut down and fall asleep. He discusses the benefits of meditation and entering one's own universe. This is the idea of withdrawal. The first Superclass's dynamic is this withdrawal. The patient expresses uncertainty and doubt. The first three Superclasses underscore this lack of clarity as well. It is particularly noticeable in the first Superclass. Additionally, he discusses his insecurity and sense of helplessness. The first Superclass emphasises this as well. The person frequently feels helpless and powerless. Since they are unable to handle it, since it is all too much for them they withdraw inside their shell to avoid it. The patient discusses a shortage of resources, including money. He feels as though he cannot handle every area of his life, which points to the first Superclass. So, when things get too much, he experiences numbness or anaesthesia; this is part of his withdrawal dynamic. Everything in this case emphasises how sensitive the sufferer is to outside stimuli. The main reaction is to distance oneself from this. Then, we observe this exact behaviour once more in the WISE process. Everything in this situation keeps leading to the same conclusion. Nux moschata was the medication the patient took and used to heal.

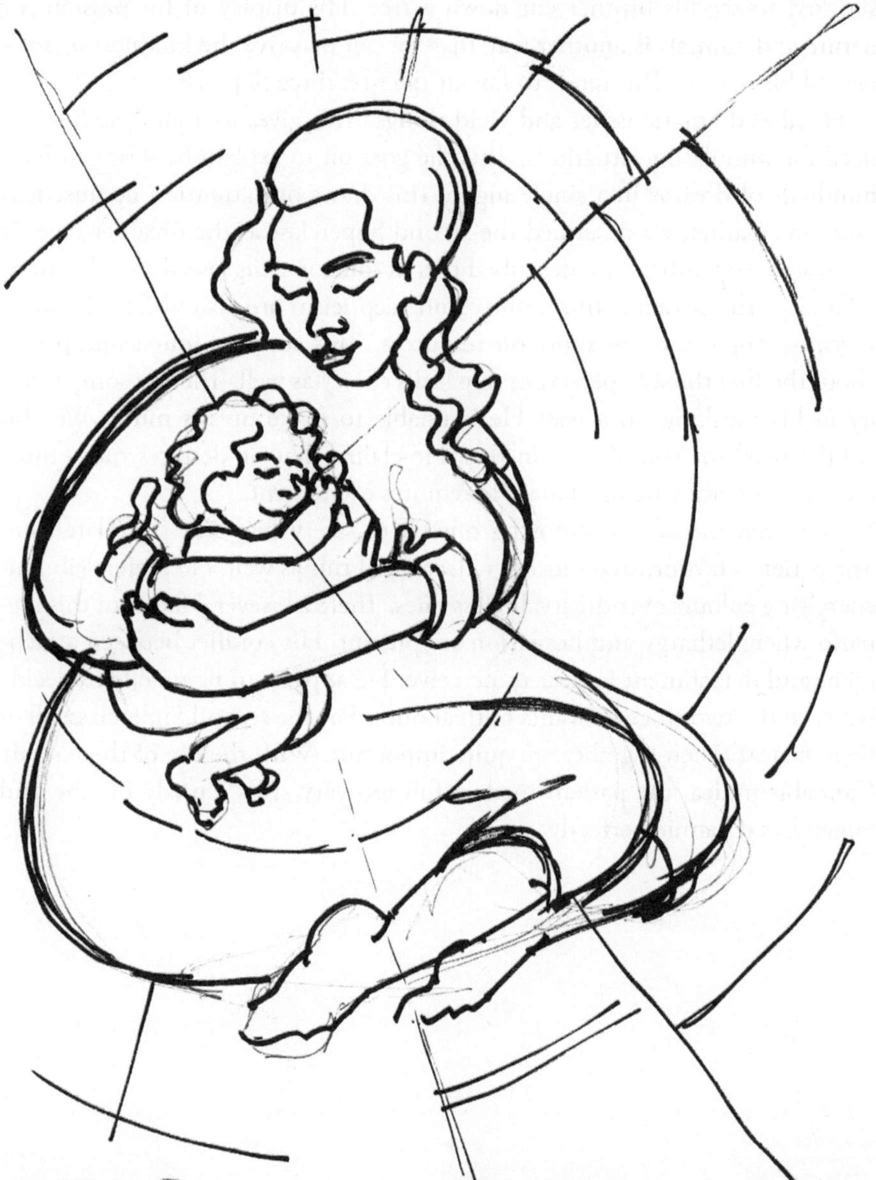
SC 1.6.1 (+)
MONICA & MOMCHIL STOYANOV/0721

Answer to Case 5

In this instance, it seems that the patient is also quite sensitive. He was greatly shocked to see his brother cut down a tree. His display of his passion for nature and animals is another way that we can perceive the kindness or softness of his nature. This tends to favour the first three Superclasses.

He likes dramatic issues and vivid things. This gives us a glimpse into his need for stimulating situations. Then he goes on to explain how he can have hundreds of dreams in a single night. This draws our attention because it is excessive. Earlier, we described the second Superclass as the dreamer type. If the reader remembers, we described this as someone engrossed in a dream or a fantasy. The patients' uncertainty and scepticism are also visible. In some ways, he appears to be short on resources. This supports our assumptions about the first three Superclasses. He lacks clarity as well. There is some rigidity in his thinking, in a way. He is unable to make up his mind. We also see the need for stimulation in this. He claims that he despises quiet time. He does not enjoy being alone. He requires excitement.

However, the act of removing oneself to safety may not stimulate him. The patient's favourite colour is a reflection of this as well. He prefers vibrant, energising colours over dreary, lifeless ones. There are several facets of this scenario where lethargy and hesitation are present. His conflict between attachment and detachment is clear to perceive. He appears to be unable to decide between the two since he wants both at once. For the second Superclass, all of these factors taken together are quite important. With the use of the remedy Cannabis indica, the patient made a full recovery. This remedy fits the 2nd Superclass dynamic perfectly.

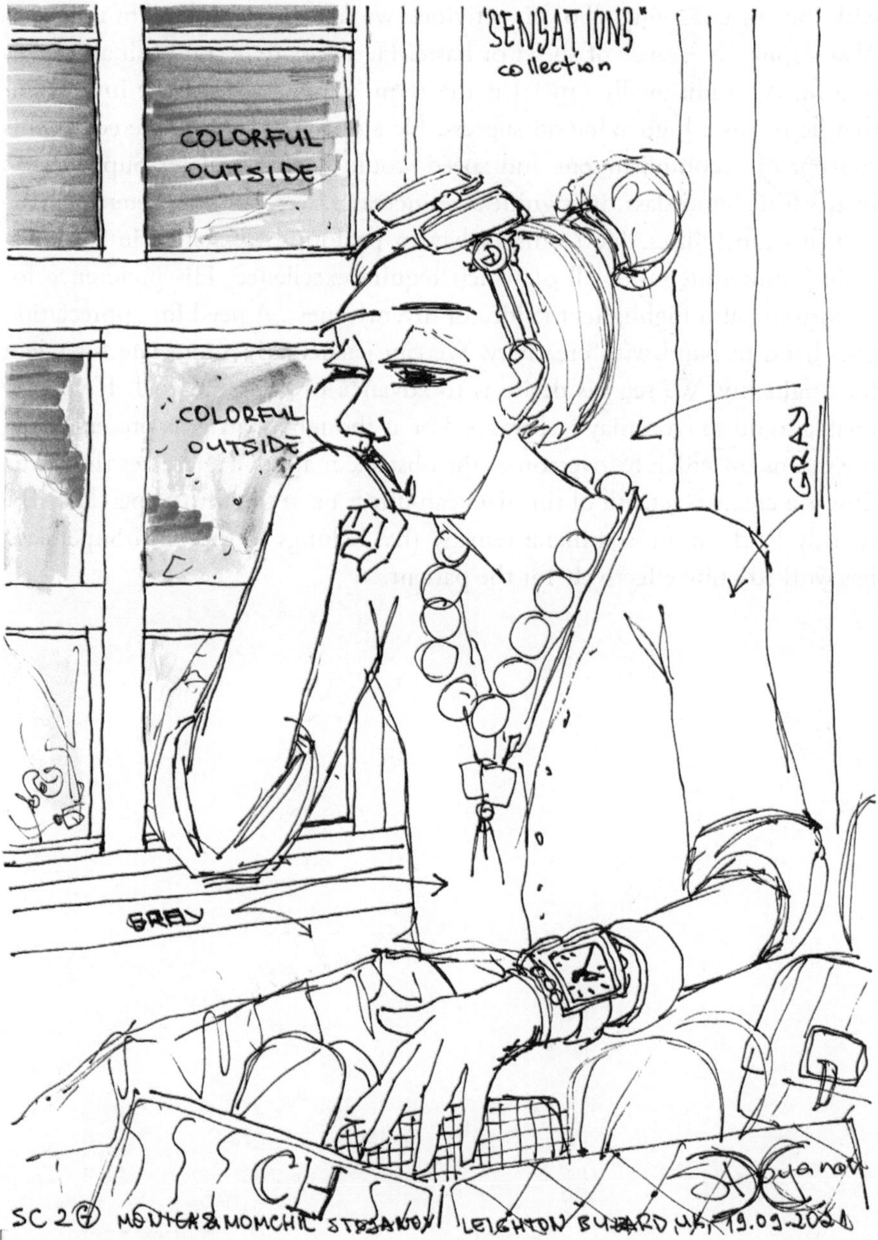
"SENSATIONS"
collection
COLORFUL
OUTSIDE
COLORFUL
OUTSIDE
GRAY
GREY

Answer to Case 6

The patient is explaining how much exercise he needs. He must move. Along with this, by observing all of his activities, we can gauge his level of intensity. Also implied is a sense of speed or haste. He needs to accomplish all of this in a hurry. Additionally crucial is the term 'attain'. We get the impression that he places a high value on success. He also has a competitive edge. This concept of accomplishment and speed would appear in later Superclasses. In the fifth Superclass, its significance increases. We can also determine the patient's capabilities. He seems to have a profound capacity. He is undertaking numerous tasks, all of which require excellence. His preference for performing also highlights the idea of inventiveness. A need for appreciation goes hand in hand with creativity. We can particularly appreciate his talent for originality. We see his desire is to advance towards the goal. If you are unable to do so, you may feel trapped or as though a barrier is present. Even the means by which he overcomes the obstacle matters. He creates the route. This is a creative act. All of this data can direct us to the fifth Superclass. The remedy Ruthenium, a mineral remedy that belongs to the Fifth Superclass, has worked quite effectively for the patient.

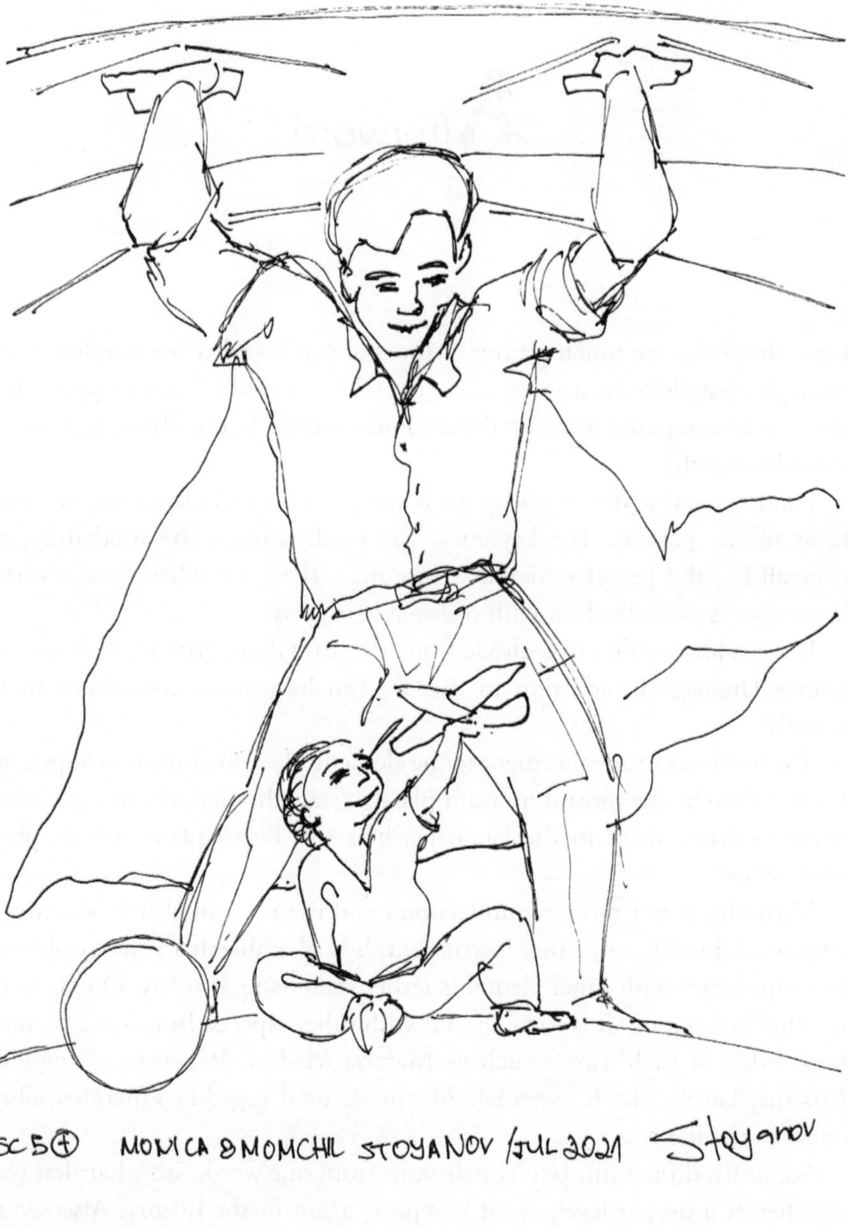
SC5 MONICA & MOMCHIL STOYANOV /JUL 2021 Stoyanov

Afterword

I saw that there are much greater chances of success when we employ several strategies parallelly in a given case. By taking a multi-faceted approach to the case as compared to a one-dimensional approach, our chances of success considerably rise.

Fundamental to the homeopath is the peculiar and characteristic symptoms of the patient. The keynotes, the small rubrics, the modalities, the generalities, the peculiar mental symptoms. These are what generations of homeopaths prescribed on with reasonable success.

If we additionally cross-check from the Kingdom, Miasm, Genius, and Source language in addition to this we can have more confidence in the remedy.

The most recent advancement to the elements described above is Superclass. It appears to be the most important place to start the analysis. As soon as one becomes accustomed to the language, it is also rather plain and simple to understand.

Naturally, if not properly understood and used, it can also be a source of confusion, just like any other instrument. It is advisable that you to utilise this in conjunction with other elements rather than using it solely. One is to not use this in isolation, it is to be used it with other aspects. In this, a systematic knowledge of each aspect such as Materia Medica, Repertory, Kingdoms, Miasms, Levels, etc. is essential. All this is used together synergistically to come to the remedy.

Secondly, do not jump to conclusions from one word. See what that word signifies at a deeper level, see if it repeats again in the history. Also see the entire constellation of qualities to come to a kingdom, miasm or superclass.

Thirdly, the case taking is the most important step. It is an art of being exact, complete, and deep. Several techniques including the WISE process need to be used in very skilful ways. Without a good case taking the rest of it has little use.

Hopefully this book will help to give the whole picture of each Superclass as well as illustrate its applicability in cases, so that it becomes one more effective tool in our technique.

At the same time, this idea gives a paradigm through which we can understand both others and ourselves.

Remedy and Superclass index

Please note all plant groups are according to Cronquist system of botanical classifications

Abbreviation	Remedy Name	Sub-group	Superclass
abel.	Abelmoschus	Malvaceae	Superclass 4; Subclass 4 (Dilleniidae)
abrom-aug.	Abroma augusta	Sterculiaceae	Superclass 4; Subclass 4 (Dilleniidae)
abrot.	Abrotanum	Asteraceae	Superclass 6; Subclass 6 (Asteridae)
absin.	Absinthium	Asteraceae	Superclass 6; Subclass 6 (Asteridae)
acal.	Acalypha indica	Euphorbiaceae	Superclass 5; Subclass 5 (Rosidae)
acon.	Aconitum napellus	Ranunculaceae	Superclass 1; Subclass 1 (Magnolidae)
act-sp.	Actaea spicata	Ranunculaceae	Superclass 1; Subclass 1 (Magnolidae)
adam.	Adamas (Diamond)	Carbon	Superclass 2
adon.	Adonis vernalis	Ranunculaceae	Superclass 1; Subclass 1 (Magnolidae)
aegle-f.	Aegle folia	Rutaceae	Superclass 5; Subclass 5 (Rosidae)
aegle.	Aegle marmelos	Rutaceae	Superclass 5; Subclass 5 (Rosidae)
aesc-g.	Aesculus glabra	Hippocastanaceae	Superclass 5; Subclass 5 (Rosidae)

aesc.	Aesculus hippocastanum	Hippocastanaceae	Superclass 5; Subclass 5 (Rosidae)
aeth.	Aethusa cynapium	Apiaceae	Superclass 5; Subclass 5 (Rosidae)
agar.	Agaricus muscarius	Fungi	Superclass 6
agn.	Agnus castus	Verbenaceae	Superclass 6; Subclass 6 (Asteridae)
agri.	Agrimonia eupatoria	Rosaceae	Superclass 5; Subclass 5 (Rosidae)
ail.	Ailanthus glandulosa	Simaroubaceae	Superclass 5; Subclass 5 (Rosidae)
alum.	Alumina	Row 3	Superclass 3
anac.	Anacardium orientale	Anacardiaceae	Superclass 5; Subclass 5 (Rosidae)
ang.	Angustura vera	Rutaceae	Superclass 5; Subclass 5 (Rosidae)
anh.	Anhalonium lewinii	Cactaceae	Superclass 3; Subclass 3 (Caryophyllidae)
anis.	Anisum stellatum	Illiciaceae	Superclass 1; Subclass 1 (Magnolidae)
ant-t.	Antimonium tartaricum	Row 5	Superclass 5
apis	Apis mellifica	Insects	Superclass 5
ap-g.	Apium graveolens	Apiaceae	Superclass 5; Subclass 5 (Rosidae)
apoc.	Apocynum cannabinum	Apocynaceae	Superclass 6; Subclass 6 (Asteridae)
aral.	Aralia racemosa	Araliaceae	Superclass 5; Subclass 5 (Rosidae)
aran.	Aranea diadema	Spiders	Superclass 5
aran-ix.	Aranea ixobola	Spiders	Superclass 5
arg-n.	Argentum nitricum	Row 5	Superclass 5
arist-cl.	Aristolochia clematitis	Aristolochiaceae	Superclass 1; Subclass 1 (Magnolidae)
arn.	Arnica montana	Asteraceae	Superclass 6; Subclass 6 (Asteridae)
ars.	Arsenicum album	Row 4	Superclass 4
art-v.	Artemisia vulgaris	Asteraceae	Superclass 6; Subclass 6 (Asteridae)
asaf.	Asafoetida	Apiaceae	Superclass 5; Subclass 5 (Rosidae)

asar.	Asarum europapeum	Aristolochiaceae	Superclass 1; Subclass 1 (Magnolidae)
aspin.	Aspidosperminum	Asclepiadaceae	Superclass 6; Subclass 6 (Asteridae)
atista	Atista indica	Rutaceae	Superclass 5; Subclass 5 (Rosidae)
atro.	Atropinum purum	Solanaceae	Superclass 6; Subclass 6 (Asteridae)
aur.	Aurum metallicum	Row 6	Superclass 6
bapt.	Baptisia tinctoria	Fabaceae	Superclass 5; Subclass 5 (Rosidae)
bar-c.	Baryta carbonica	Row 6	Superclass 6
bell.	Belladonna	Solanaceae	Superclass 6; Subclass 6 (Asteridae)
bell-p.	Bellis perennis	Asteraceae	Superclass 6; Subclass 6 (Asteridae)
berb.	Berberis vulgaris	Berberidaceae	Superclass 1; Subclass 1 (Magnolidae)
berul-e.	Berula erecta	Apiaceae	Superclass 5; Subclass 5 (Rosidae)
beryl.	Beryllium metallicum	Row 2 - Left side	Superclass 1
bism-met.	Bismuthum metallicum	Row 6	Superclass 6
biti-at	Bitis atropos	Snakes	Superclass 6
bor.	Borax veneta	Row 2 - Left side	Superclass 1
bor-met.	Boron metallicum	Row 2 - Left side	Superclass 1
bos-s.	Boswelia serrata	Burseraceae	Superclass 5; Subclass 5 (Rosidae)
both-l.	Bothrops lanceolatus	Snakes	Superclass 6
brom.	Bromium	Row 4	Superclass 4
bry.	Bryonia alba	Cucurbitaceae	Superclass 4; Subclass 4 (Dilleniidae)
bufo	Bufo rana	Amphibians	Superclass 6
bung-f.	Bungaris fasciatus	Snakes	Superclass 6
cac.	Cacao	Sterculiaceae	Superclass 4; Subclass 4 (Dilleniidae)
cact.	Cactus grandiflorus	Cactaceae	Superclass 3; Subclass 3 (Caryophyllidae)
cadm.	Cadmium metallicum	Row 5	Superclass 5
calc.	Calcarea carbonica	Row 4	Superclass 4

calen.	Calendula officinalis	Asteraceae	Superclass 6; Subclass 6 (Asteridae)
camp g	Campanula glomerata	Campanulaceae	Superclass 6; Subclass 6 (Asteridae)
camph.	Camphora	Lauraceae	Superclass 1; Subclass 1 (Magnolidae)
cann-i.	Cannabis indica	Cannabaceae	Superclass 2; Subclass 2 (Hamamelidae)
cann-s.	Cannabis sativa	Cannabaceae	Superclass 2; Subclass 2 (Hamamelidae)
canth.	Cantharis	Insects	Superclass 5
caps.	Capsicum annuum	Solanaceae	Superclass 6; Subclass 6 (Asteridae)
carb-an.	Carbo animalis	Carbon	Superclass 2
carc.	Carcinosinum burnett	Nosode	Superclass 5
card-m.	Carduus marianus	Asteraceae	Superclass 6; Subclass 6 (Asteridae)
caul.	Caulophyllum thalictroides	Berberidaceae	Superclass 1; Subclass 1 (Magnolidae)
caust.	Causticum hahnemanni	Row 4	Superclass 4
cean.	Ceanothus americanus	Rhamnaceae	Superclass 5; Subclass 5 (Rosidae)
cedr.	Cedron	Simaroubaceae	Superclass 5; Subclass 5 (Rosidae)
cench.	Cenchris contortrix	Snakes	Superclass 6
cere-b.	Cereus bonplandii	Cactaceae	Superclass 3; Subclass 3 (Caryophyllidae)
cham.	Chamomilla vulgaris	Asteraceae	Superclass 6; Subclass 6 (Asteridae)
cheir.	Cheiranthus cheiri	Brassicaceae	Superclass 4; Subclass 4 (Dilleniidae)
chel.	Chelidonium majus	Papaveraceae	Superclass 1; Subclass 1 (Magnolidae)
chelo.	Chelone glabra	Scrophulariaceae	Superclass 6; Subclass 6 (Asteridae)
chin.	China officinalis	Rubiaceae	Superclass 6; Subclass 6 (Asteridae)
chion.	Chionanthus virginica	Oleaceae	Superclass 6; Subclass 6 (Asteridae)
choc.	Chocolate	Sterculiaceae	Superclass 4; Subclass 4 (Dilleniidae)

cic-m.	Cicuta maculata	Apiaceae	Superclass 5; Subclass 5 (Rosidae)
cimic.	Cimicifuga racemosa	Ranunculaceae	Superclass 1; Subclass 1 (Magnolidae)
cina	Cina maritima	Asteraceae	Superclass 6; Subclass 6 (Asteridae)
cist.	Cistus canadensis	Cistaceae	Superclass 4; Subclass 4 (Dilleniidae)
cob.	Cobaltum metallicum	Row 4	Superclass 4
coca	Cocaerythroxylon coca	Erythroxylaceae	Superclass 5; Subclass 5 (Rosidae)
cocc.	Cocculus indicus	Menispermaceae	Superclass 1; Subclass 1 (Magnolidae)
cod.	Codeinum purum	Papaveraceae	Superclass 1; Subclass 1 (Magnolidae)
coff.	Coffea cruda	Rubiaceae	Superclass 6; Subclass 6 (Asteridae)
coloc.	Colocynthis	Cucurbitaceae	Superclass 4; Subclass 4 (Dilleniidae)
com.	Comocladia dentata	Anacardiaceae	Superclass 5; Subclass 5 (Rosidae)
conch.	Conchiolinum	Bivalve	Superclass 1
con.	Conium maculatum	Apiaceae	Superclass 5; Subclass 5 (Rosidae)
cop.	Copaiva	Caesalpiniaceae	Superclass 5; Subclass 5 (Rosidae)
crat.	Crataegus oxyacantha	Rosaceae	Superclass 5; Subclass 5 (Rosidae)
crot-c.	Crotalus cascavella	Snakes	Superclass 6
crot-h.	Crotalus horridus	Snakes	Superclass 6
croto-t.	Croton tiglium	Euphorbiaceae	Superclass 5; Subclass 5 (Rosidae)
cub.	Cubeba officinalis	Piperaceae	Superclass 1; Subclass 1 (Magnolidae)
cupr.	Cuprum metallicum	Row 4	Superclass 4
cur.	Curare woorari	Loganiaceae	Superclass 6; Subclass 6 (Asteridae)
cycl.	Cyclamen europaeum	Primulaceae	Superclass 4; Subclass 4 (Dilleniidae)
cypra-e.	Cypraea eglantina	Gastropod	Superclass 2

daph.	Daphne indica	Thymelaeaceae	Superclass 5; Subclass 5 (Rosidae)
stram-se	Datura stramonium	Solanaceae	Superclass 6; Subclass 6 (Asteridae)
delphin.	Delphininum staphysagrium	Ranunculaceae	Superclass 1; Subclass 1 (Magnolidae)
dendro-p.	Dendroaspis polylepis (Black mamba)	Snakes	Superclass 6
dig.	Digitalis purpurea	Scrophulariaceae	Superclass 6; Subclass 6 (Asteridae)
dion-m.	Dionaea muscipula	Droseraceae	Superclass 3; Subclass 3 (Caryophyllidae) & Superclass 5
dol.	Dolichos pruriens	Fabaceae	Superclass 5; Subclass 5 (Rosidae)
dros.	Drosera rotundifolia	Droseraceae	Superclass 3; Subclass 3 (Caryophyllidae) & Superclass 5
dulc.	Dulcamara	Solanaceae	Superclass 6; Subclass 6 (Asteridae)
echi.	Echinacea angustifolia	Asteraceae	Superclass 6; Subclass 6 (Asteridae)
echi-p.	Echinacea purpurea	Asteraceae	Superclass 6; Subclass 6 (Asteridae)
elaps	Elaps corallinus	Snakes	Superclass 6
elat.	Elaterium officinarum	Cucurbitaceae	Superclass 4; Subclass 4 (Dilleniidae)
eug.	Eugenia jambosa	Myrtaceae	Superclass 5; Subclass 5 (Rosidae)
eup-per.	Eupatorium perfoliatum	Asteraceae	Superclass 6; Subclass 6 (Asteridae)
euphr.	Euphrasia officinalis	Scrophulariaceae	Superclass 6; Subclass 6 (Asteridae)
fagu.	Fagus silvatica	Fagaceae	Superclass 2; Subclass 2 (Hamamelidae)
falco-p.	Falcon peregrinus	Birds	Superclass 3
ferr.	Ferrum metallicum	Row 4	Superclass 4
fl-ac.	Fluoricum acidum	Row 2 - Right side	Superclass 5
frax.	Fraxinus americana	Oleaceae	Superclass 6; Subclass 6 (Asteridae)
galph.	Galphimia glauca	Malpighiaceae	Superclass 5; Subclass 5 (Rosidae)

gels.	Gelsemium sempervirens	Loganiaceae	Superclass 6; Subclass 6 (Asteridae)
germ.	Germanium metallicum	Row 4	Superclass 4
goss.	Gossypium herbaceum	Malvaceae	Superclass 4; Subclass 4 (Dilleniidae)
gran.	Granatum	Lythraceae	Superclass 5; Subclass 5 (Rosidae)
gran.	Granatum	Myrtaceae	Superclass 5; Subclass 5 (Rosidae)
gran.	Granatum	Punicaceae	Superclass 5; Subclass 5 (Rosidae)
graph.	Graphites naturalis	Carbon	Superclass 2
grat.	Gratiola officinalis	Scrophulariaceae	Superclass 6; Subclass 6 (Asteridae)
grin.	Grindelia robusta	Asteraceae	Superclass 6; Subclass 6 (Asteridae)
gymne.	Gymnema sylvestre	Asclepiadaceae	Superclass 6; Subclass 6 (Asteridae)
haliae-lc.	Halieetus Leucocephalus	Birds	Superclass 3
helia-ol	Helianthus annuus	Asteraceae	Superclass 6; Subclass 6 (Asteridae)
helia.	Helianthus annuus	Asteraceae	Superclass 6; Subclass 6 (Asteridae)
helx.	Helix tosta	Gastropod	Superclass 2
hell.	Helleborus niger	Ranunculaceae	Superclass 1; Subclass 1 (Magnolidae)
herin.	Heroinum	Papaveraceae	Superclass 1; Subclass 1 (Magnolidae)
hist.	Histaminum muriaticum	Sarcode	Superclass 5
hura	Hura brasiliensis	Euphorbiaceae	Superclass 5; Subclass 5 (Rosidae)
hydr.	Hydrastis canadensis	Hydrastidaceae	Superclass 1; Subclass 1 (Magnolidae)
hydrc.	Hydrocotyle asiatica	Apiaceae	Superclass 5; Subclass 5 (Rosidae)
hyos.	Hyoscyamus niger	Solanaceae	Superclass 6; Subclass 6 (Asteridae)
hyper.	Hypericum perforatum	Clusiaceae	Superclass 4; Subclass 4 (Dilleniidae)
iber.	Iberis amara	Brassicaceae	Superclass 4; Subclass 4 (Dilleniidae)

ign.	Ignatia amara	Loganiaceae	Superclass 6; Subclass 6 (Asteridae)
ip.	Ipecacuanha	Rubiaceae	Superclass 6; Subclass 6 (Asteridae)
irid.	Iridium metallicum	Row 6	Superclass 6
jug-r.	Juglans regia	Juglandaceae	Superclass 2; Subclass 2 (Hamamelidae)
kali-c.	Kali carbonicum	Row 4	Superclass 4
kola.	Kola nut	Sterculiaceae	Superclass 4; Subclass 4 (Dilleniidae)
lac-c.	Lac caninum	Mammals	Superclass 4
lac-eq.	Lac equinum	Mammals	Superclass 5
lac-h.	Lac humanum	Mammals	Superclass 3
lac-leo.	Lac leoninum	Mammals	Superclass 6
Lac-d.	Lac vaccinum defloratum	Mammals	Superclass 4
lach.	Lachesis muta	Snakes	Superclass 6
lact.	Lactuca virosa	Asteraceae	Superclass 6; Subclass 6 (Asteridae)
lath.	Lathyrus sativus	Fabaceae	Superclass 5; Subclass 5 (Rosidae)
lat-h.	Latrodectus hasellti	Spiders	Superclass 5
lat-m.	Latrodectus mactans	Spiders	Superclass 5
led.	Ledum palustre	Ericaceae	Superclass 4; Subclass 4 (Dilleniidae)
leon.	Leonurus cardiaca	Lamiaceae	Superclass 6; Subclass 6 (Asteridae)
lept.	Leptandra virginica	Scrophulariaceae	Superclass 6; Subclass 6 (Asteridae)
lith-c.	Lithium carbonicum	Row 2 - Left side	Superclass 1
lob.	Lobelia inflata	Lobeliaceae	Superclass 6; Subclass 6 (Asteridae)
lycpr.	Lycopersicum esculentum	Solanaceae	Superclass 6; Subclass 6 (Asteridae)
mag-c.	Magnesium carbonicum	Row 3	Superclass 3
mand.	Mandragora officinarum	Solanaceae	Superclass 6; Subclass 6 (Asteridae)
mang.	Manganum carbonicum	Row 4	Superclass 4
mangi.	Mangifera indica	Anacardiaceae	Superclass 5; Subclass 5 (Rosidae)

mati.	Matico (Piper angustifolium)	Piperaceae	Superclass 1; Subclass 1 (Magnolidae)
meli.	Melilotus officinalis	Fabaceae	Superclass 5; Subclass 5 (Rosidae)
merc.	Mercurius solubilis hahnemanni	Row 6	Superclass 6
mesc.	Mescalinum	Cactaceae	Superclass 3; Subclass 3 (Caryophyllidae)
mez.	Mezereum	Thymelaeaceae	Superclass 5; Subclass 5 (Rosidae)
mill.	Millefolium	Asteraceae	Superclass 6; Subclass 6 (Asteridae)
morph.	Morphinum	Papaveraceae	Superclass 1; Subclass 1 (Magnolidae)
murx.	Murex purpurea	Gastropod	Superclass 2
mygal.	Mygale lasiodora	Spiders	Superclass 5
myris.	Myristica sebifera	Myristicaceae	Superclass 1; Subclass 1 (Magnolidae)
myt-e.	Mytilus edulis	Bivalve	Superclass 1
naja	Naja tripudians	Snakes	Superclass 6
nat-c.	Natrum carbonicum	Row 3	Superclass 3
nat.	Natrum metallicum	Row 3	Superclass 3
nelum.	Nelumbo nucifera	Nymphaeaceae	Superclass 1; Subclass 1 (Magnolidae)
nicc.	Niccolum metallicum	Row 4	Superclass 4
nuph.	Nuphar luteum	Nymphaeaceae	Superclass 1; Subclass 1 (Magnolidae)
nux-m.	Nux moschata	Myristicaceae	Superclass 1; Subclass 1 (Magnolidae)
nux-v.	Nux vomica	Loganiaceae	Superclass 6; Subclass 6 (Asteridae)
nyct.	Nyctanthes arbor-tristis	Verbenaceae	Superclass 6; Subclass 6 (Asteridae)
oci-s.	Ocimum sanctum	Lamiaceae	Superclass 6; Subclass 6 (Asteridae)
oena.	Oenanthe crocata	Apiaceae	Superclass 5; Subclass 5 (Rosidae)
olnd.	Oleander	Apocynaceae	Superclass 6; Subclass 6 (Asteridae)
opun-v.	Opuntia vulgaris	Cactaceae	Superclass 3; Subclass 3 (Caryophyllidae)

orig-v.	Origanum vulgare	Lamiaceae	Superclass 6; Subclass 6 (Asteridae)
oxyg.	Oxygenium	Row 2 - Right side	Superclass 5
ozone	Ozonum	Row 2 - Right side	Superclass 5
paeon.	Paeonia officinalis	Paeoniaceae	Superclass 4; Subclass 4 (Dilleniidae)
pareir.	Pareira brava	Menispermaceae	Superclass 1; Subclass 1 (Magnolidae)
passi.	Passiflora incarnata	Passifloraceae	Superclass 4; Subclass 4 (Dilleniidae)
Pect.	Pecten Jacobeus	Bivalve	Superclass 1
petr.	Petroleum	Carbon	Superclass 2
petros-c.	Petroselinum crispum	Apiaceae	Superclass 5; Subclass 5 (Rosidae)
phos.	Phosphorus	Row 3	Superclass 3
phyt-fr	Phytolacca decandra	Phytolaccaceae	Superclass 3; Subclass 3 (Caryophyllidae)
phyt.	Phytolacca decandra	Phytolaccaceae	Superclass 3; Subclass 3 (Caryophyllidae)
pip-m.	Piper methysticum	Piperaceae	Superclass 1; Subclass 1 (Magnolidae)
pip-n.	Piper nigrum	Piperaceae	Superclass 1; Subclass 1 (Magnolidae)
plan.	Plantago major	Plantaginaceae	Superclass 6; Subclass 6 (Asteridae)
plat.	Platinum metallicum	Row 6	Superclass 6
plb.	Plumbum metallicum	Row 6	Superclass 6
prun.	Prunus spinosa	Rosaceae	Superclass 5; Subclass 5 (Rosidae)
pulse	Pulsatilla pratensis	Ranunculaceae	Superclass 1; Subclass 1 (Magnolidae)
queb.	Quebracho (Aspidosperma)	Apocynaceae	Superclass 6; Subclass 6 (Asteridae)
oak-b.	Quercus robur	Fagaceae	Superclass 2; Subclass 2 (Hamamelidae)
ran-a.	Ranunculus acris	Ranunculaceae	Superclass 1; Subclass 1 (Magnolidae)
ran-b.	Ranunculus bulbosus	Ranunculaceae	Superclass 1; Subclass 1 (Magnolidae)
raph.	Raphanus sativus	Brassicaceae	Superclass 4; Subclass 4 (Dilleniidae)

rheum	Rheum palmatum	Polygonaceae	Superclass 3; Subclass 3 (Caryophyllidae)
rhus-a.	Rhus aromatica	Anacardiaceae	Superclass 5; Subclass 5 (Rosidae)
rhus-g.	Rhus glabra	Anacardiaceae	Superclass 5; Subclass 5 (Rosidae)
rhus-r.	Rhus radicans	Anacardiaceae	Superclass 5; Subclass 5 (Rosidae)
rhus-t.	Rhus toxicodendron	Anacardiaceae	Superclass 5; Subclass 5 (Rosidae)
rhus-v.	Rhus venenata	Anacardiaceae	Superclass 5; Subclass 5 (Rosidae)
rhus-ver.	Rhus vernix	Anacardiaceae	Superclass 5; Subclass 5 (Rosidae)
rob-po	Robinia pseudacacia	Fabaceae	Superclass 5; Subclass 5 (Rosidae)
rob.	Robinia pseudacacia	Fabaceae	Superclass 5; Subclass 5 (Rosidae)
ros-cal.	Rosa california	Rosaceae	Superclass 5; Subclass 5 (Rosidae)
ros-d.	Rosa damascena	Rosaceae	Superclass 5; Subclass 5 (Rosidae)
rumx.	Rumex crispus	Polygonaceae	Superclass 3; Subclass 3 (Caryophyllidae)
ruta	Ruta graveolens	Rutaceae	Superclass 5; Subclass 5 (Rosidae)
samb.	Sambucus nigra	Sambucaceae	Superclass 6; Subclass 6 (Asteridae)
sang.	Sanguinaria canadensis	Papaveraceae	Superclass 1; Subclass 1 (Magnolidae)
scan.	Scandium metallicum	Row 4	Superclass 4
scroph-n.	Scrophularia nodosa	Scrophulariaceae	Superclass 6; Subclass 6 (Asteridae)
sel.	Selenium	Row 4	Superclass 4
senec.	Senecio aureus	Asteraceae	Superclass 6; Subclass 6 (Asteridae)
seneg.	Senega officinalis	Polygalaceae	Superclass 5; Subclass 5 (Rosidae)
sep.	Sepia	Cephalopods	Superclass 5
sil.	Silica terra	Row 3	Superclass 3
sin-a.	Sinapis alba	Brassicaceae	Superclass 4; Subclass 4 (Dilleniidae)

sin-n.	Sinapis nigra	Brassicaceae	Superclass 4; Subclass 4 (Dilleniidae)
sol-n.	Solanum nigrum	Solanaceae	Superclass 6; Subclass 6 (Asteridae)
sol-t.	Solanum tuberosum	Solanaceae	Superclass 6; Subclass 6 (Asteridae)
solid.	Solidago virga aurea	Asteraceae	Superclass 6; Subclass 6 (Asteridae)
spig.	Spigelia anthelmia	Loganiaceae	Superclass 6; Subclass 6 (Asteridae)
staph.	Staphysagria	Ranunculaceae	Superclass 1; Subclass 1 (Magnolidae)
stenoc-a	Stenocereus aragonii	Cactaceae	Superclass 3; Subclass 3 (Caryophyllidae)
ster.	Sterculia	Sterculiaceae	Superclass 4; Subclass 4 (Dilleniidae)
still.	Stillingia sylvatica	Euphorbiaceae	Superclass 5; Subclass 5 (Rosidae)
stram.	Stramonium	Solanaceae	Superclass 6; Subclass 6 (Asteridae)
stront-c.	Strontium carbonicum	Row 5	Superclass 5
stanza-g	Strophanthus gratus	Apocynaceae	Superclass 6; Subclass 6 (Asteridae)
stroph.	Strophanthus hispidus	Apocynaceae	Superclass 6; Subclass 6 (Asteridae)
sulph.	Sulphur	Row 3	Superclass 3
syph.	Syphilinum	Nosode	Superclass 6
syzyg.	Syzygium jambolanum	Myrtaceae	Superclass 5; Subclass 5 (Rosidae)
tab.	Tabacum	Solanaceae	Superclass 6; Subclass 6 (Asteridae)
tarax-po	Taraxacum officinale	Asteraceae	Superclass 6; Subclass 6 (Asteridae)
tarax.	Taraxacum officinale	Asteraceae	Superclass 6; Subclass 6 (Asteridae)
tarent-c.	Tarentula cubensis	Spiders	Superclass 5
tarent.	Tarentula hispanica	Spiders	Superclass 5
teucr.	Teucrium marum verum	Lamiaceae	Superclass 6; Subclass 6 (Asteridae)
thea.	Thea sinensis	Theaceae	Superclass 4; Subclass 4 (Dilleniidae)

ther.	Theridion curassavicum	Spiders	Superclass 5
thiosin.	Thiosinaminum	Brassicaceae	Superclass 4; Subclass 4 (Dilleniidae)
thlaspi	Thlaspi bursa pastoris	Brassicaceae	Superclass 4; Subclass 4 (Dilleniidae)
thul.	Thulium	Row 6	Superclass 6
thymu-v.	Thymus vulgaris	Lamiaceae	Superclass 6; Subclass 6 (Asteridae)
til.	Tilia europea	Tiliaceae	Superclass 4; Subclass 4 (Dilleniidae)
tinos.	Tinospora cordifolia	Menispermaceae	Superclass 1; Subclass 1 (Magnolidae)
titan.	Titanium metallicum	Row 4	Superclass 4
trib.	Tribulus terrestris	Zygophyllaceae	Superclass 5; Subclass 5 (Rosidae)
trif-p.	Trifolium pratense	Fabaceae	Superclass 5; Subclass 5 (Rosidae)
tung.	Tungstenium metallicum	Row 6	Superclass 6
tus-fa.	Tussilago farfara	Asteraceae	Superclass 6; Subclass 6 (Asteridae)
tus-f.	Tussilago fragrans	Asteraceae	Superclass 6; Subclass 6 (Asteridae)
ulm-p.	Ulmus procera	Ulmaceae	Superclass 2; Subclass 2 (Hamamelidae)
urt-u.	Urtica urens	Urticaceae	Superclass 2; Subclass 2 (Hamamelidae)
valer.	Valeriana officinalis	Valerianaceae	Superclass 6; Subclass 6 (Asteridae)
vanad.	Vanadium metallicum	Row 4	Superclass 4
ven-m.	Venus mercenaria	Bivalve	Superclass 1
verbe-o.	Verbena officinalis	Verbenaceae	Superclass 6; Subclass 6 (Asteridae)
vero-o.	Veronica officinalis	Scrophulariaceae	Superclass 6; Subclass 6 (Asteridae)
vib.	Viburnum opulus	Viburnaceae	Superclass 6; Subclass 6 (Asteridae)
viol-o.	Viola odorata	Violaceae	Superclass 4; Subclass 4 (Dilleniidae)
vip.	Vipera berus	Snakes	Superclass 6
visc.	Viscum album	Viscaceae	Superclass 5; Subclass 5 (Rosidae)

with-s.	Withania somnifera	Solanaceae	Superclass 6; Subclass 6 (Asteridae)
wye.	Wyethia helenoides	Asteraceae	Superclass 6; Subclass 6 (Asteridae)
zinc.	Zincum metallicum	Row 4	Superclass 4

Resources

Homoeopathic Medical Publishers (HMP)

(www.rajansankaran.com)

HMP publishes most of the books of Dr Rajan Sankaran. These books are a very important resource to systematically understand the theory and application of Dr Sankaran's ideas. They provide the foundation on which this current development of the Superclasses rests. The reader is strongly recommended to study these books carefully. Please find below a list of books with a short description of each.

The Elements of Homoeopathy Dr. P. Sankaran

This book illustrates practically every aspect of homoeopathic medicine, whether it is the study of Materia medica, Hints on Case-Taking, Value of Repertory, Cross References to the Repertory, Difficulties in Practice and The Scope of Homoeopathy.

The Spirit of Homoeopathy Dr. Rajan Sankaran

This book is divided into four sections: Philosophy, The Mind, Case-Taking and Finding the Remedy, and Materia medica. The first section looks at what disease is - the origin and the dynamics of disease. The second investigates the understanding of delusions, mental state as a whole and body-mind connection. The third section covers the artistic aspect of homeopathy, understanding the patient. The final section furthers the understanding of remedies, and includes remedies as examples.

The Substance of Homoeopathy Dr. Rajan Sankaran

This book illustrates how delusions can be classified using Hahnemann's theory of miasms. A detailed study of homoeopathic drugs with reference to their source reveals the purpose of the traditional classification into plant, animal and mineral kingdom.

The Soul of Remedies Dr. Rajan Sankaran

Clear, concise, confirmed descriptions of the inner view of a hundred different remedies and how they express this in clinicalsituations.

An Insight into Plants (Volumes 1, 2 and 3) Dr. Rajan Sankaran

This book provides a framework of how the plant kingdom can be classified and understood. Tracing the common sensation of each family, this book shows how this sensation can be seen in the remedies in that family. The remedies are differentiated by the miasm to which they belong.

Sankaran's Schema Dr. RajanSankaran

This book aims to bring in a nut shell, in a tabulated form,the different concepts and information spread over Dr. Sankaran's books The Spirit of Homoeopathy, The Substance of Homoeopathy, The System of Homoeopathy, The Sensation in Homoeopathy, and An Insight into Plants (Volume I, II, III), and Sensation Refined.

Structure - Experiences with the Mineral Kingdom (Volumes 1 and 2)
Dr. Rajan Sankaran

The periodic table readily lends itself to the task of classification. Its seven rows and 18 columns can be understood, seen and experienced as stages of human development. Recent explorations into the rows, backed by several clinical-cases, provings and research, have thrown new light on the Mineral Kingdom that makes it significantly easier to recognize the remedies in practice.

Sankaran's Plant Sensation in Picture Dr. Rajan Sankaran Sandra Petri

As they say 'One picture is worth a thousand words'. In this books Sandra Petri's visual representations is aligned to Dr Sankaran'sexperience of the Plant families. The idea of the whole book is to be informal or more at an artistic level rather than something very structured or formal. It is offered to students and practitioners of homeopathy with the trust that it will further help in getting not only the words of each family but an actual live experience by a look at the illustrations.

Survival - The Mollusc Dr. Rajan Sankaran Dr. SudhirBaldota

Within are described the qualities of Mollusca in nature, its subdivisions, and expressions in the human being. Each of these is described with source words, proving information and clinical cases, to make it easy to recognize in clinical practice.

Survival - The Reptile (Volume 1 and 2) Dr. Rajan Sankaran Dr. MeghnaShah

Within are described the qualities of Reptilia in nature, its subdivisions, and expressions in the human being. Each of these is described with source words, proving information and clinical cases, to make it easy to recognize in clinical practice.

The Synergy in Homoeopathy Dr. Rajan Sankaran

An integrated approach to case-takingand analysis. Never before has the connection between the patient and the remedy been so clear - symptoms and system are two sides of the same coin and this results from an integrated approach. Both the factual and conceptual aspects of the patient and the remedy must be seen together. The knowledge of old masters, such as C.M. Boger, is explained in detail. Through illustrative cases, the secret of success is depicted through this integrated approach. Through a seamless blending of the old and new, conventional and contemporary, the results are proof of a quantum leap in homoeopathic practice.

Synergy Synopsis Dr. Rajan Sankaran

This book is a small handbook, updated with the latest developments in advanced homoeopathic practice. It is intended to be a ready reference guide for participants who attend seminars, and for others who wish to have an overview of this system of practice.

From Similia to Synergy Dr. Rajan Sankaran

From Similia to Synergy guides the reader through the full spectrum of homoeopathic knowledge. Sankaran demonstrates integration with actual case sudies. Case- taking discourses have been transcribed and parsed to allow the reader to understand the Sankaran's thought processes. Thoughout, the reader is encouraged to refer to supporting bodies of work for further research and comprehension.

The Art of Follow-Up Dr. Rajan Sankaran

It is often said that it is easier to come to a remedy selection than managing the follow up. Most of the difficulties that arise in follow up management include how and when to repeat a remedy, when to escalate the potency, when to change the remedy and soon.When mastered, the art of follow up is the key to developing a successful and satisfying homoeopathic practice.

Dr. Rajan Sankaran explains the intricacies and importance of the follow up along side illustrative cases with long-term follow ups from his 30 years of practice. He sees a patient beyond their disease, connects to them at a deeper level, manages critical situations faced by the patient (in health or personal lives) as a homeopath, friend, guide and philosopher, and therefore demonstrates how to effectively encourage the patient to adopt essential changes in their lifestyle including diet, exercise, yoga and meditation.

From Shadow to Light Dr. Rajan Sankaran

In this book, Dr. Sankaran introduces his latest approach to case-taking called the WISE (Witnessing the Inner Song Experience) processes.

One of the main benefits of using the unique WISE processes is that it serves as a really good bypass from the patient's life story and situation and takes us directly into his imagination and core experience. What emerges from the process makes the homoeopathic remedy very clear for the physician. The processes also can prove therapeutic for the patient. Through detailed cases Dr. Sankaran takes us step by step into this journey. The WISE processes take Homeopathic case taking to a level far deeper than ever before.

Exact, Complete, Depth The Eight Box Method of Case Analysis
Dr. Rajan Sankaran

The Eight Box method is Dr. Rajan Sankaran's most recent evolution in homeopathic practice. It involves classifying the patient's information into 8 differentaspects.

It compels the physician to look at the different aspects and find the thread that connects all the different aspects. It allows use of several methodologies synergistically in differentcases.

The Sensation in Homoeopathy

This much awaited book describes, using numerous case examples, the concept and use of Rajan Sankaran's latest and perhaps most significant contribution, ‹The Seven Levels of Experience› which enables a homoeopath to know at all times, in any given case, where to begin and where to aim. In this way of working, a definitive pathway for case taking is provided, a means by which to observe and utilize the active energy patterns of the patient (hand gestures and body movements), plus a way of matching the patient›s level to the remedy potency that is required.

Plant Chart - The Sensation in the Subclasses

This is a laminated Plant Chart *(Size A4)* used by Dr. Sankaran in Plant Subclass and Superclass Online course.

All the 6 subclasses and typical remedies discussed in this Plant Subclass course is included in this Plant Chart

Sensation Refined

This latest book by Dr. Rajan Sankaran is the most evolved and comprehensive of his work to date. As he notes at the beginning, it is the fullest representation of his ideas, both new as well as incorporated from his earlier works. It approaches completeness, with regard to formulating a system of homeopathic case taking, analysis, prescribing and management (follow-up), knowledge of remedies, and the understanding of how this practise relates to the fundamental principles of nature. In its totality, Sankaran delivers more profound insights regarding all of the above, in a new way, representing a significant advance in the field of homeopathy. The method is now clearer, easier and more refined than ever before.

Dog, Yogi, Banyan Tree Dr. Rajan Sankaran

"If you are open to learn, everyone and everything becomes your teacher."

Told through a series of fascinating vignettes, Dog, Yogi, Banyan Tree brings alive Dr.. Rajan Sankaran's meetings with various people and situations to form a rich tapestry of his experiences. Starting from his formative years with his father, he takes us on an undulating journey where ordinary people, gurus, a tree and even a dog leave an everlasting impression. The anecdotes, steeped in introspection of ethics, love, friendship, passion, coincidences, criticism, challenges and spirituality, strike a chord with us all. The stories, in sightful yet amusing, may seem unconnected initially, like threads of different hues hanging loosely, but soon they are deftly woven into a larger picture.

It is a tale of personal evolution and spiritual discovery that both touches the heart and heals the soul.

Sankaran DeWise

Sankaran DeWise is a very useful book that resembles a desktop calendar. The DeWise tool is synonymously linked with the WISE Processes (WISE: Witnessing the Inner Song Experience). Sankaran DeWise contains important images used in the WISE processes, along with instructions of use for the homeopath. It is a quick, handy reference, also providing information on many of Dr. Sankaran's concepts such as kingdoms, miasms, levels of experience, and plant subclasses. DeWise also highlights his latest ideas on meditation and awareness, and how both can help in healing. The images within, hand-selected by Dr. Rajan Sankaran, are used as a gateway into the patient's unconscious, and help the patient uncover their own inner pattern.

Manjhi, the Boatman Dr. Rajan Sankaran

'When the disciple is ready the guru will appear', is an old saying. A seemingly chance encounter with a tourist guide in Rishikesh, a town in north India, is the beginning of an incredible adventure for someone going through a crisis in life. "Your experience is your truth. You have to do nothing. Just be aware of whatever there is." the guide advises. With his gentle instruction, the guide shows the way to become aware of what deeply underlies one's personal situations across different aspects of life such as fear, relationships, and death; an awareness that leads to transformation. Who is this enigmatic guide? Where did he come from? And why? What is his message? The mystery gradually unravels to reveal something least expected.

For all the above books please see: **www.rajansankaran.com**

Homoeopathic Medical Publishers

H.O.P.E

H.O.P.E. Homoeopathy Online Portal for Education is the latest advancement in homeopathic e-learning that aims to enhance the quality of homeopathic education globally.

H.O.P.E. is an online platform that provides video seminars and various lecture series that can be accessed on demand right from the individual's home, no matter what level of development. Many renowned homeopaths in the world have contributed to this project with the hopes of advancing our science in which they speak about topics including the Organon,Case-taking,Provings, Posology, Materia Medica, Repertory, contemporary approaches in practice, and many more.

H.O.P.E. establishes a cyberspace education center where affordable and good quality homeopathic education is accessible to homeopaths worldwide.

We see this education platform as the H.O.P.E. for homeopathy. Homeopathy needs good practitioners and this is only possible through good training. Modern technology makes it possible to bring inspirational teachers right into the home of the student, thus saving time and energy for both.

The other song: International Academy of Advanced Homeopathy (TOS) is an integrated Homoeopathic clinic, training and research academy led by Dr. Rajan Sankaran, ably aided by a dedicated team of more than 30 homoeopathic practioners, teachers and authors, of national and international acclaim, dedicated to holistic patient care and well-being, high quality student-practitioner education and training.

TEACHING TOOLS AND METHODOLOGY:

The only thing that homeopathy needs today is good quality homoeopathic practitioners. This can only be produced via clinical and practical training.

Homoeopathy is best learned when a student is exposed to an experienced practitioner in practice and observes the art of case-taking, understanding the totality and the process of coming to a remedy. The academy provides this unique platform where sophisticated video technology connects the clinic consulting rooms to the training auditoriums. Students witness live cases and follow-ups on a daily basis, followed by an in-depth discussion and analysis and discussion of the case with experienced homoeopaths. This helps to connect seamlessly to the theoretic principles being applied in daily practice.The academic faculty comprises of several internationally-acclaimed homoeopaths. Students are exposed to different styles of practising the same method of homeopathy.

Bridging the gap between theory and practice is one of the basic tenets of the academic program at the other song academy. This teaching is done through case based learning and is especially highlighted in our flagship courses such as the 6-month Masters programme in advanced homeopathy as well as our Fellowship course. Teaching and training at the academy is geared towards the all-round development of students and practitioners.

For information about our courses, please visit our website:
www.theothersongacademy.com

WISE retreats

Join us for healing and awareness through the WISE (Witnessing Inner Song Experience) processes. We offer different workshops and retreats using the WISE processes as healing tools as well as instruction on how to use them. These are available online, in India and also abroad. For further information regarding the content and upcoming events please visit the website **www.rajansankaran.com**

WISH (World Institute For Sensation Homeopathy): *WISH* is a worldwide, not-for-profit collaboration of homeopaths who practice the Sensation Method. The core group represents homeopaths from all over the world. WISH was formed to provide a forum of communication and education, ensuring that a certain standard is maintained, whilst allowing development to serve the needs of practitioners and patients in a more effective way.

For more information please visit: **https://www.wish4healing.net**

For more information on Rajan Sankaran,
visit: www.rajansankaran.com

For further details, contact:
Homoeopathic Medical Publishers
201, Dinar Building, Opp. City Plaza, 20, Station Road,
Santacruz (W), Mumbai - 400054, India
Visit: www.onlinehmp.com

Telephone: +91 8657974109
Email: sales@onlinehmp.com

Join us on Facebook:
https://www.facebook.com/onlinehmp

Join us on Instagram:
https://www.instagram.com/homoeopathicmedicalpublishers/

Homoeopathic Medical Publishers

Books by Dr. Rajan Sankaran and Dr. P Sankaran

English Books

1. The Spirit of Homeopathy
2. The Substance of Homeopathy
3. The Soul of Remedies
4. The System of Homeopathy
5. An insight into plants (Vol 1 & 2)
6. An insight into plants (Vol 3)
7. Sankarans Schema
8. The Sensation in Homeopathy
9. Sensation Refined
10. Structure (Vol 1&2)
11. Survival – The Mollusc
12. The Elements of Homeopathy (Vol 1 & Vol 2) - Dr. P. Sankaran
13. The Synergy in Homeopathy
14. Synergy Synopsis
15. From Similia to Synergy (With DVD)
16. Dog, Yogi Banyan Tree
17. The Art of Follow up
18. Exact, Complete, Depth
19. From Shadow to Light
20. Sankaran DeWISE
21. Manjhi the Boatman
22. Plant chart
23. Sankaran Plant Sensation in Picture

German Books

1. Die Substanz Der Homeopathie
2. Das Geistige Prinzip Der Homoopathie
3. Die Seele Der Heilmittel
4. Das System Der Homeopathie
5. Einblicke Ins Pflanzenreich Band (Vol 1 & Vol 2)
6. Einblicke Ins Pflanzenreich Band (Vol 3)
7. Sankarans Tabellan
8. Die Empfindung in Der Homeopathie
9. Die Empfindung – Verfeinerung der methode
10. Struktur Vol (Vol 1 & Vol 2)
11. Uberleben Die Mollusken
12. Patienttenfragebogen
13. Sankaran Pflanzenempfindungen in Bildern
14. Syergie Höopathischer Ansatze
15. Synergie Synopsis

French Books

1. L'Esprit De L'Homeopathie
2. Le Schema De Sankaran
3. Comprendre La Sensation Vitale En Homeopathie

Spanish Books

1. El Espiritu De L'Homeopatia
2. La Substancia De La Homeopatia
3. El Esquema De Sankaran 2007
4. Sensacion Vital En Homeopatia

Dutch Book

1. Homeopathie En Materie

Homoeopathic Medical Publishers

www.rajansankaran.com